Wolfgang See

T0091814

Microsurgery of the Cranial Base

Springer-Verlag Wien New York

Prof. Dr. med. WOLFGANG SEEGER
Medical Director of the Department of General Neurosurgery
and Chairman of Neurosurgery of the Neurosurgical Clinic,
University of Freiburg i. Br., Federal Republic of Germany

With 200 Figures

This work is subject to copyright

All rights are reserved, whether the whole or part of the material is concerned, specifically those of translation, reprinting, re-use of illustrations, broadcasting, reproduction by photocopying machine or similar means, and storage in data banks

© 1983 by Springer-Verlag/Wien
Softcover reprint of the hardcover 1st edition 1983

Design: Hans Joachim Böning, Wien

Library of Congress Cataloging in Publication Data. Seeger, Wolfgang, 1929– . Microsurgery of the cranial base. 1. Basicranium-Surgery. 2. Microsurgery. I. Title. RD529.S44. 1983. 617'.514. 83-14652.

ISBN 978-3-7091-3090-2 ISBN 978-3-7091-3088-9 (eBook)
DOI 10.1007/978-3-7091-3088-9

Preface

The preceding volumes having considered microsurgery of the brain as well as microsurgery of the Medulla spine, with its surrounding structures, it then seemed logical to cover microsurgery of the areas near the brain. In addition to daily work at the operation table, the increasing experience of the University of Freiburg Neurosurgical Hospital in the bordering areas of ophthalmology and ENT was stimulating. Of significance was the work with Prof. Dr. Renate Unsöld, Freiburg University Ophthalmological Hospital (Director: Prof. Dr. G. Mackensen) whose experience, published together with C. B. Ostertag, J. DeGroot, and T. H. Newton in "Computer Reformations of the Brain and Skull Base" offered valuable diagnostic ideas. Some of the findings attributed to Prof. Dr. R. Unsöld and Doz. Dr. C. B. Ostertag are again covered here. I thank Prof. Dr. Chl. Beck, Director of University Freiburg ENT-Hospital, for his critical review of the chapter on oro-nasal hypophysis approach. Special appreciations go to my colleagues Doz. Dr. J. M. Gilsbach, Dr. H. R. Eggert, Dr. W. Hassler, and Dr. E. Gröbner for suggestions and assistance in providing literature. Several anatomical preparations were made possible with the help of Prof. Dr. N. Boehm, Deputy Director of Freiburg University Institute of Pathology and Prof. Dr. J. Staubesand, Director of Freiburg University Anatomical Institute I. The translation of the text was undertaken by my colleague, Dr. E. Gröbner, and Mrs. S. Godine, Freiburg. I am grateful to Mrs. E. Hilsenbeck-Hottek for typing the manuscript.
Once again I am especially grateful to Dr. W. Schwabl, and his colleagues, of the Springer-Verlag, Wien and New York, who have published this extensive work with their usual speed, generous presentation and precision.

Freiburg, October 1983 Wolfgang Seeger

Contents

Introduction 1

Chapter 1
Oronasal Hypophysis Operations (Figs. 1 to 49) 2

Chapter 2
Operations at Sinus cavernosus (Figs. 50 to 99)
Anatomy of Sinus cavernosus (Figs. 50 to 54) 100
Ophthalmic Aneurysms (Figs. 55 to 60) 110
Pneumosinus dilatans (Figs. 61 to 68) 122
Tumors (Figs. 69 to 99) 138

Chapter 3
Frontobasal Operations (Figs. 100 to 134)
Tumor (olfactory groove meningioma) (Figs. 100 to 115) 200
Frontobasal Fracture with Liquorrhea (Figs. 116 to 134) 232

Chapter 4
Extra-intracranial Bypass (Figs. 135 to 167)
"STAMCA" (Figs. 135 to 156) 270
Bypass Between A. occipitalis and A. cerebelli inf. post. (Figs. 157 to 167) 314

Chapter 5
Operative Decompressions of N.V and N.VII in the Cerebellopontine Angle (Figs. 168 to 184) 336

Chapter 6
Operations at the Base of Fossa cranii post. (Figs. 185 to 200)
Epidermoid, Pre- and Paramedullary (Figs. 185 to 194) 370
Extradural Tumor with Shift of Sinus sigmoideus (Figs. 195 to 200) 390

References 403

Subject Index 415

Introduction

Operations in the skull base area are performed by neurosurgeons, ear-nose- and throat physicians and ophthalmologists, as well as by facial surgeons, since the skull base is characterized as a transition area of intracranial space, sinuses and orbitae. In this volume the areas of neurosurgical interest to be covered are basically limited to intra- and extradural relations of dura, cranial nerves and brain. Some of these operative procedures may be carried out in cooperation with colleagues in related fields, as when sinuses or orbitae are opened. Other operations, for example those in the area of A. carotis int. path within Os petrosum, are left completely to specialists in other fields, since the neurosurgeon rarely has sufficient experience in the problematic anatomical topographical relations of the skull base.

A few neurosurgical procedures are not dealt with in this volume, since the author has insufficient personal operative experience in these areas; for example, Glomus tumors of Foramen jugulare and aneurysms of A. basilaris or vertebralis are covered neither in the volume "Microsurgery of the Brain" nor in the present volume. Other operations, relating to but not strictly limited to the skull base, were included because of their great clinical importance, such as extra-intracranial bypass operations. It seemed unsuitable to expand this volume to include processes of the skull convexity and/or convexity dura, since a later volume will cover microsurgical operations in the area of cerebral veins, giving special attention to skull and brain convexity. This volume is already in preparation. The present volume is composed along guide-lines similar to previous volumes. Drawings were done by the author this time as well, since it is impossible to find an artist capable of making drawings from the author's extremely detailed operation sketches, even given years' time. The technical quality of the drawings is less important than providing as detailed as possible microsurgical information. In this connection may I mention that, in this volume as well, only the anatomical structures are enlarged to scale; this scale does not apply to the instruments, usually sketched on a smaller scale. In reality (and contrary to the drawings) the instruments cover a large area of the operation site; therefore a realistic presentation such as photography has less didactic value than these sketches. The author's mode of presentation is justified since this book does not seek to document specific operations. Rather, as in previous volumes, it seeks through individual cases to assist the neurosurgeon who is in training and/or especially interested in microsurgery in his understanding of the anatomical structures of the operation site and, together with his already assimilated anatomical knowledge, to improve his operative technique.

Chapter 1

Oronasal Hypophysis Operations (Figs. 1 to 49)

Fig. 1. Special anatomical features and special techniques of hypophysis operations
Vestibulum oris, varying topographical **relations to Apertura piriformis** (broken-lines) in 5 normal individuals of various age groups

a Distance of Apertura piriformis from juncture of Gingiva and Labium sup.

b Distance between first incisor and juncture of Vestibulum oris or between toothless Processus alveolaris sup. and Vestibulum oris (**C**)

Abbreviations:

(api) Apertura piriformis (projection)

FIG. 1

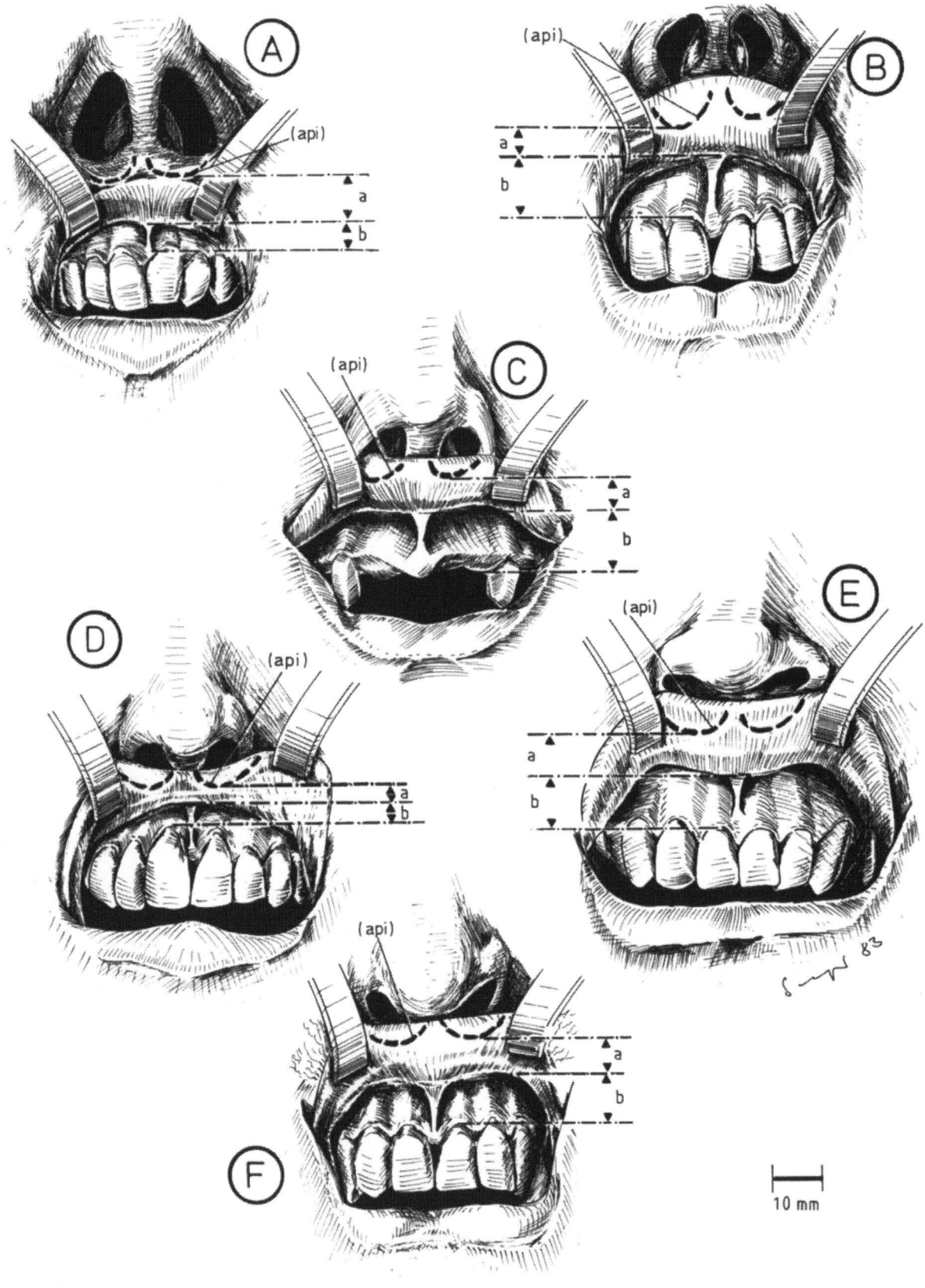

Fig. 2. Special anatomical features and special techniques of hypophysis operations

A – F **Apertura piriformis,** anatomical variants. Section lines **c** and **d** see Fig. 3, note varying width of lower half of Apertura piriformis and its asymmetries

G + G' Upper area of Apertura piriformis with Lamina mediana *–lm–*

G **Lamina mediana** reaches as far as anterior edge of nasal bone and thus to Apertura piriformis (arrow)

G' Lamina mediana *–lm–* does not reach as far as Apertura piriformis (arrow)

Abbreviations:

(cs) Cartilago septi nasi (projection)
lm Lamina mediana

FIG. 2

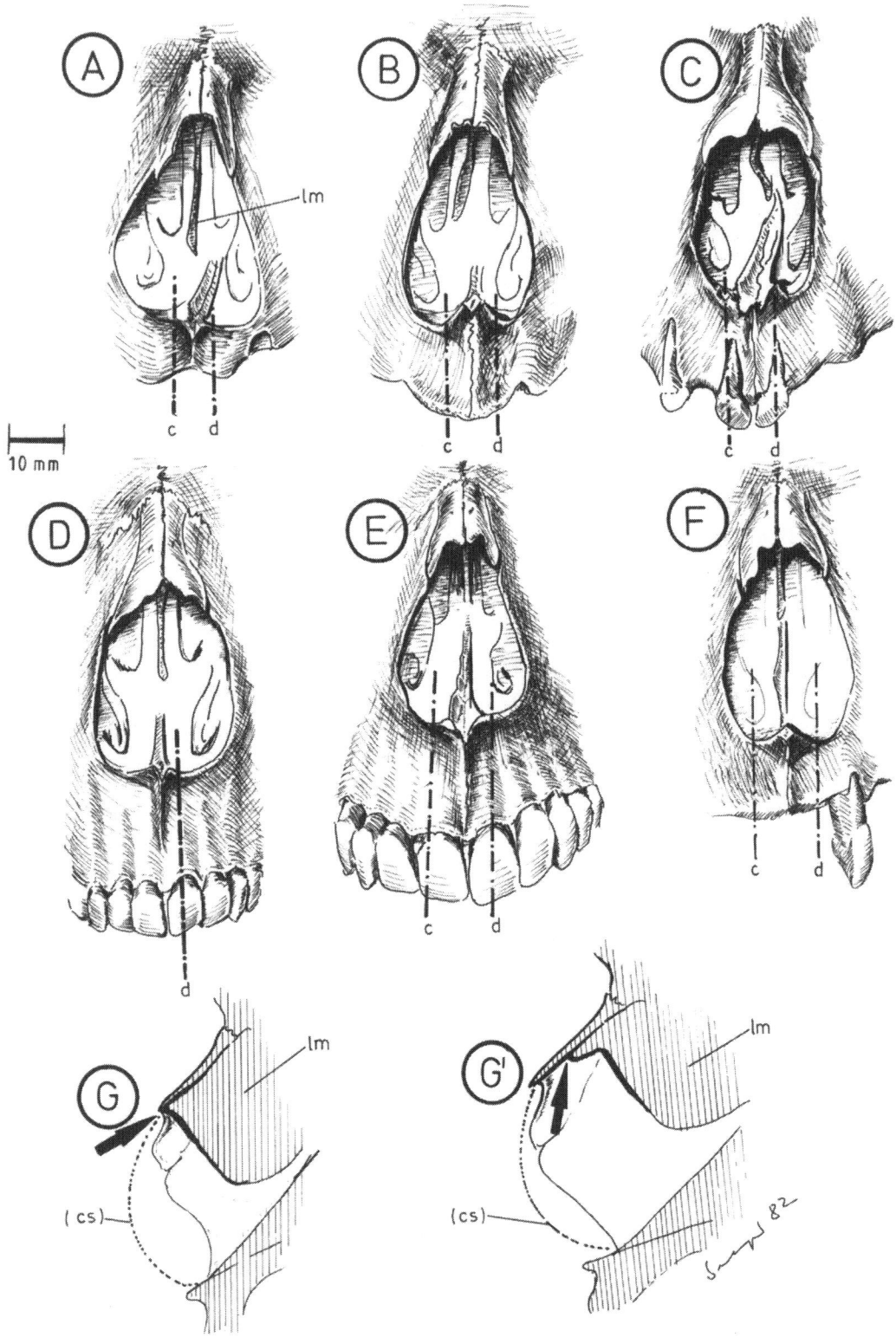

Fig. 3. Special anatomical features and special techniques of hypophysis operations

Floor of nasal cavity. Parasagittal section planes **c** (right side) and **d** (left side) see Fig. 2

A' – F' Showing section sketches of the anatomical samples **A – F** of Fig. 2
Behind Spina nasalis ant. Palatum durum –*p*– is prominent. At this prominence the mucosa of Meatus nasalis inf. may tear if preparation is not carried out carefully

Abbreviations:

c Section right, Fig. 2
d Section left, Fig. 2
p Prominent area of Palatum durum
pd Palatum durum
spa Spina nasalis ant.

FIG. 3

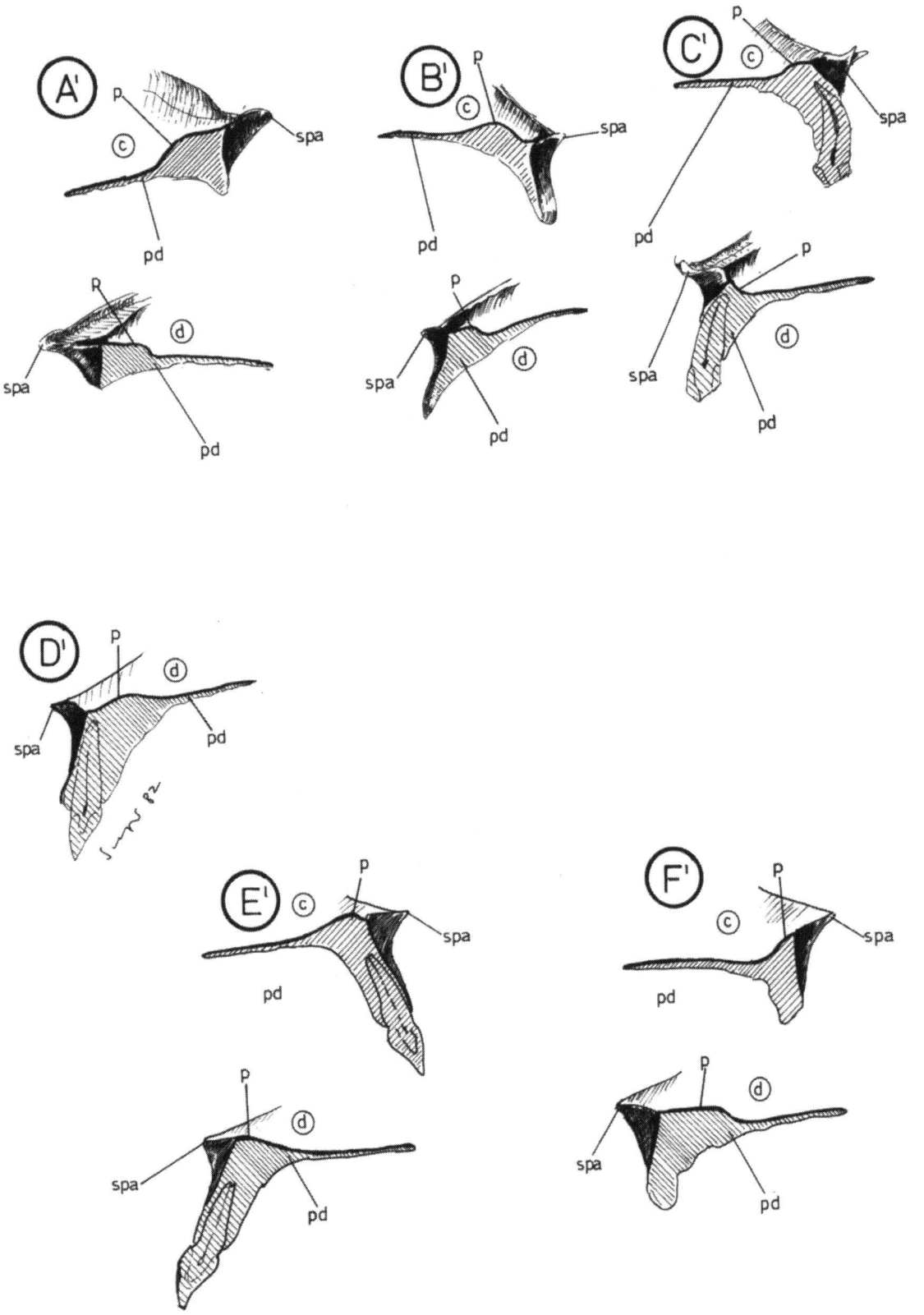
A'
p
c
spa
pd
p
d
spa
pd
B'
p
c
spa
pd
p
d
spa
pd
C'
p
c
spa
pd
p
d
spa
pd
D'
p
d
spa
pd
E'
c
p
spa
pd
p
d
spa
pd
F'
p
c
spa
pd
p
d
spa
pd

Fig. 4. Special anatomical features and special techniques of hypophysis operations
Spina nasalis ant., variants
Five skeletal samples with varying widths and asymmetries of Spina nasalis ant. and adjoining areas of Vomer

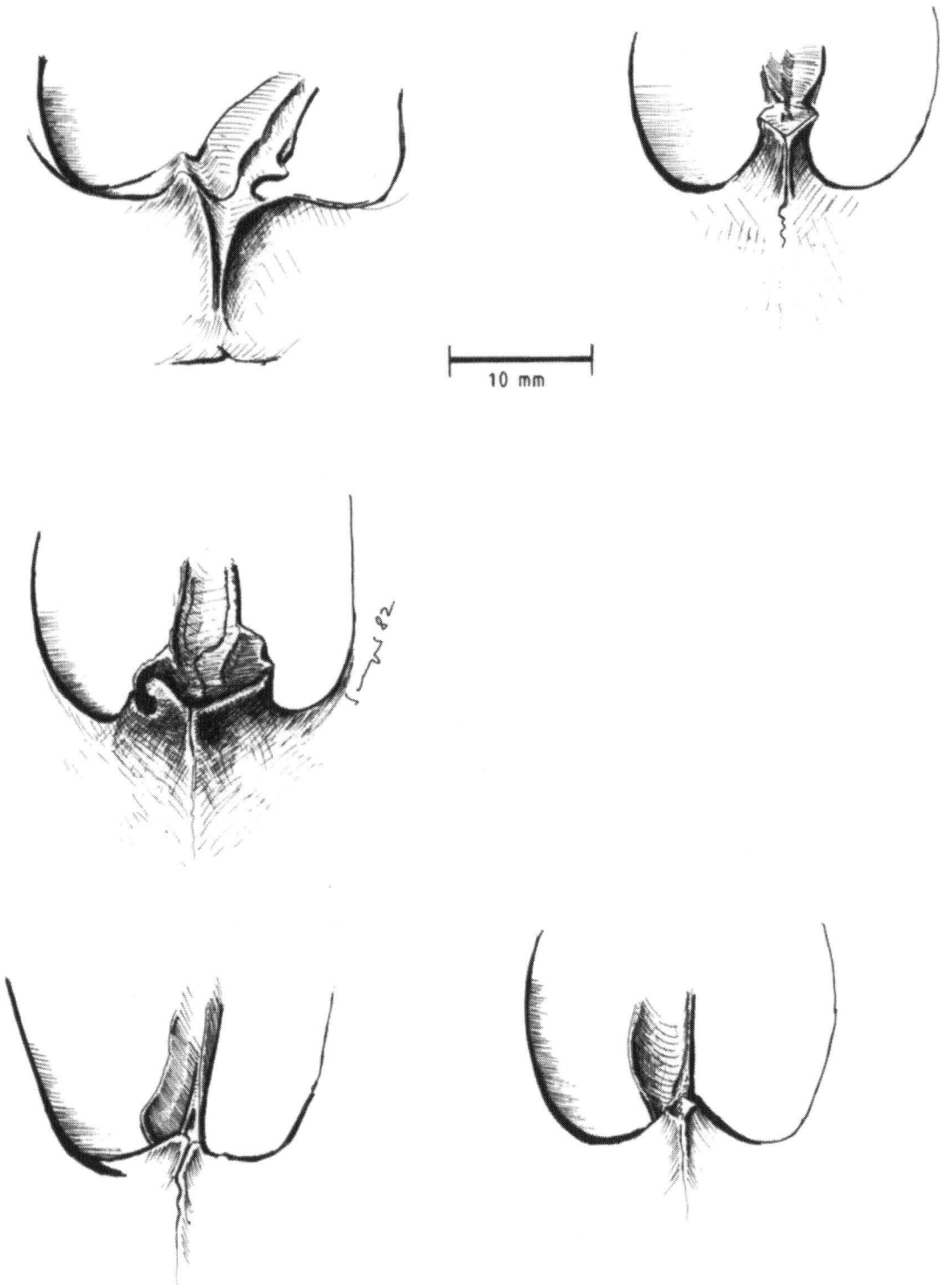
10 mm

Fig. 5. Special anatomical features and special techniques of hypophysis operations

Septum nasi, sample. Slight bony asymmetry, more extensive asymmetry of cartilage *–(cs)–*

A Bone preparation, anterior view

A' Same view, enlarged with Cartilago septi *–(cs)–*. (Transparently sketched)

B Same preparation, anterior-caudal view

B' Same preparation, cartilage not sketched in. This view corresponds to view during operation. Only by slight septum deviation one can see Lamina cribrosa *–lc–* deeper rostrally, still farther rostrally Apertura sphenoidalis *–asp–*, below it Ala vomeris *–av–*. Extensive asymmetry of Spina nasalis ant. *–spa–*

Abbreviations:

asp Apertura sphenoidalis
av Ala vomeris
(cs) Cartilago septi nasi (projection)
lc Lamina cribrosa
lm Lamina mediana
spa Spina nasalis ant.
vo Vomer

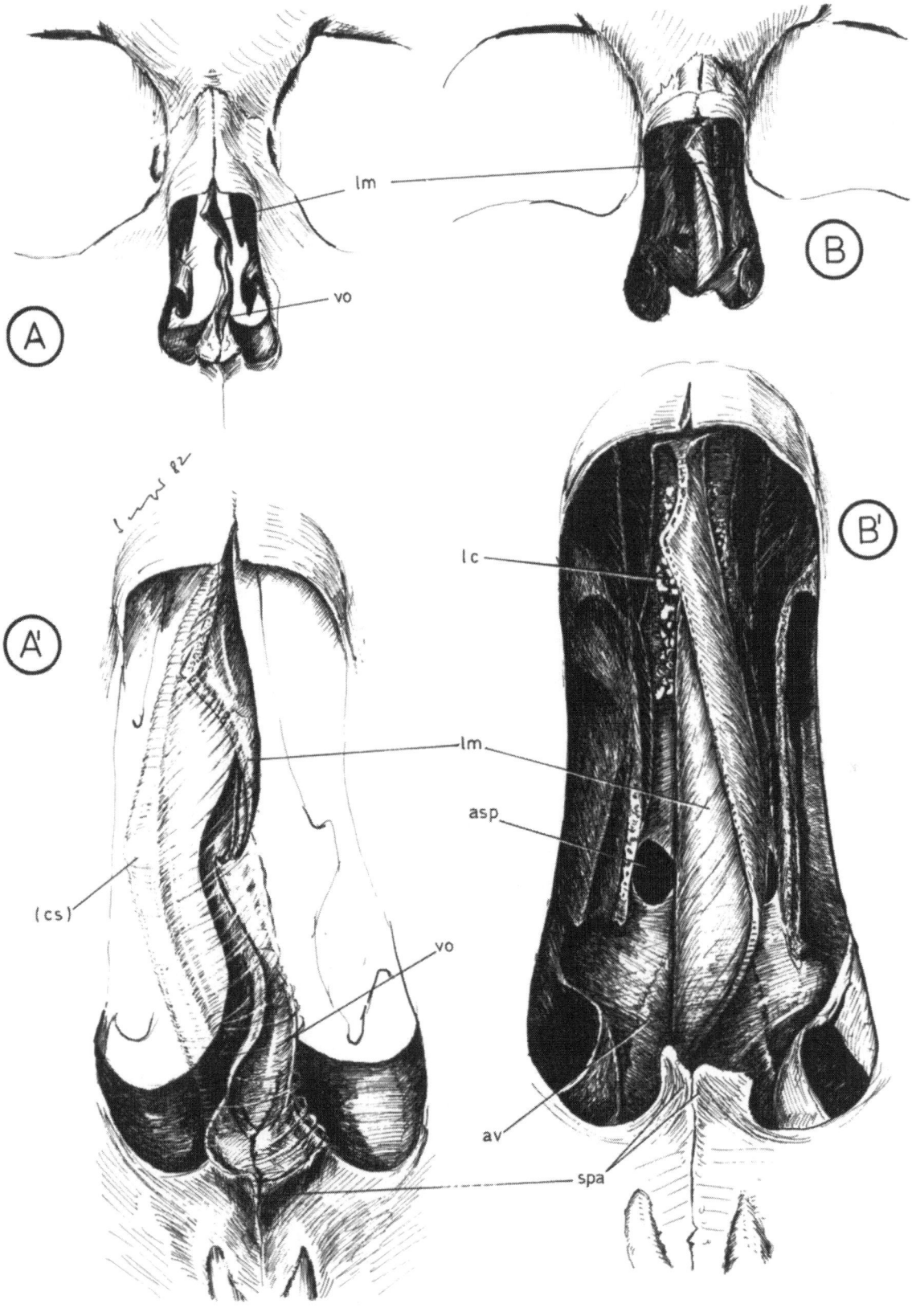
lm
vo
A
B
A'
B'
lc
lm
asp
(cs)
vo
av
spa

Fig. 6. Special anatomical features and special techniques of hypophysis operations

Topography of **Sinus sphenoidalis,** anatomical overview. Sagittal view of preparation is, however, not as low as the view during operation

A Skull preparation, anterior view with removal of parts of Apertura piriformis and Maxilla on the right side, as well as removal of Maxilla, Os zygomaticum and the major portion of Os ethmoideum on the left side. Vomer resected

B Sectional enlargement of **A**

Abbreviations:

apa Ala parva
asp Apertura sphenoidalis
av Ala vomeris
cet Cellulae ethmoidales (residuals)
fos Fissura orbitalis sup.
fosp Facies orbitalis of Os sphenoidale
lc Lamina cribrosa
lm Lamina mediana (resected)
na Os nasale
op Canalis opticus
rt Foramen rotundum
vo Vomer (resected)

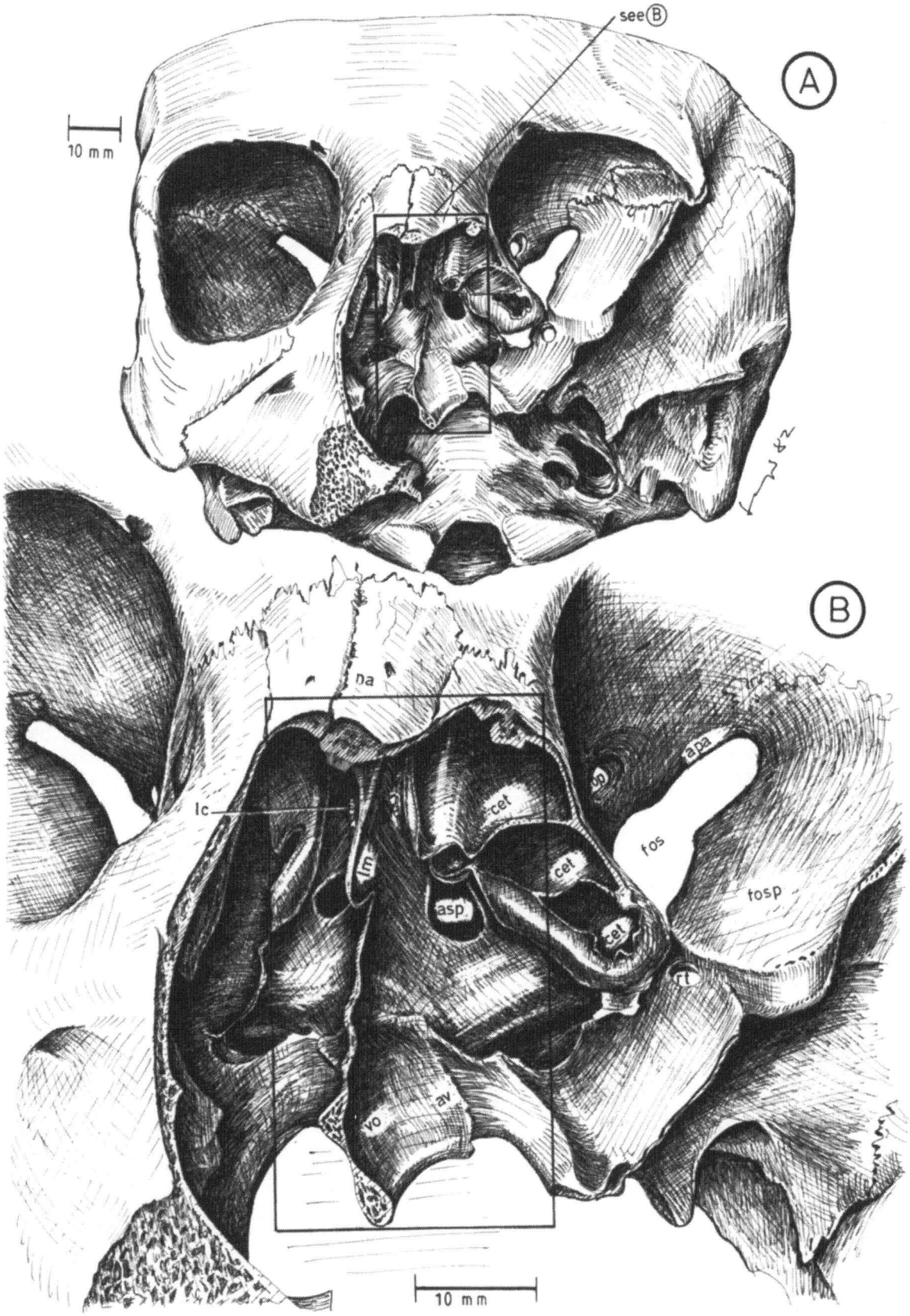
see B
A
10 mm
B
na
lc
lm
cet
cet
cet
asp
vo
av
ug
apa
fos
fosp
rt
10 mm

Fig. 7. Special anatomical features and special techniques of hypophysis operations
Topography of **Sinus sphenoidalis,** anatomical overview. View of Preparation is from an inferior direction as during operation, however obliquely lateral (not sagittal as during operation)

A Skull preparation, oblique view from a left inferior direction

B Detail view of **A**

Abbreviations:

apa Ala parva
asp Apertura sphenoidalis
av Ala vomeris
cet Cellulae ethmoidales (residuals)
fos Fissura orbitalis sup.
fosp Facies orbitalis of Os sphenoidale
lc Lamina cribrosa
lm Lamina mediana (resected)
na Os nasale
op Canalis opticus
rt Foramen rotundum
vo Vomer (resected)

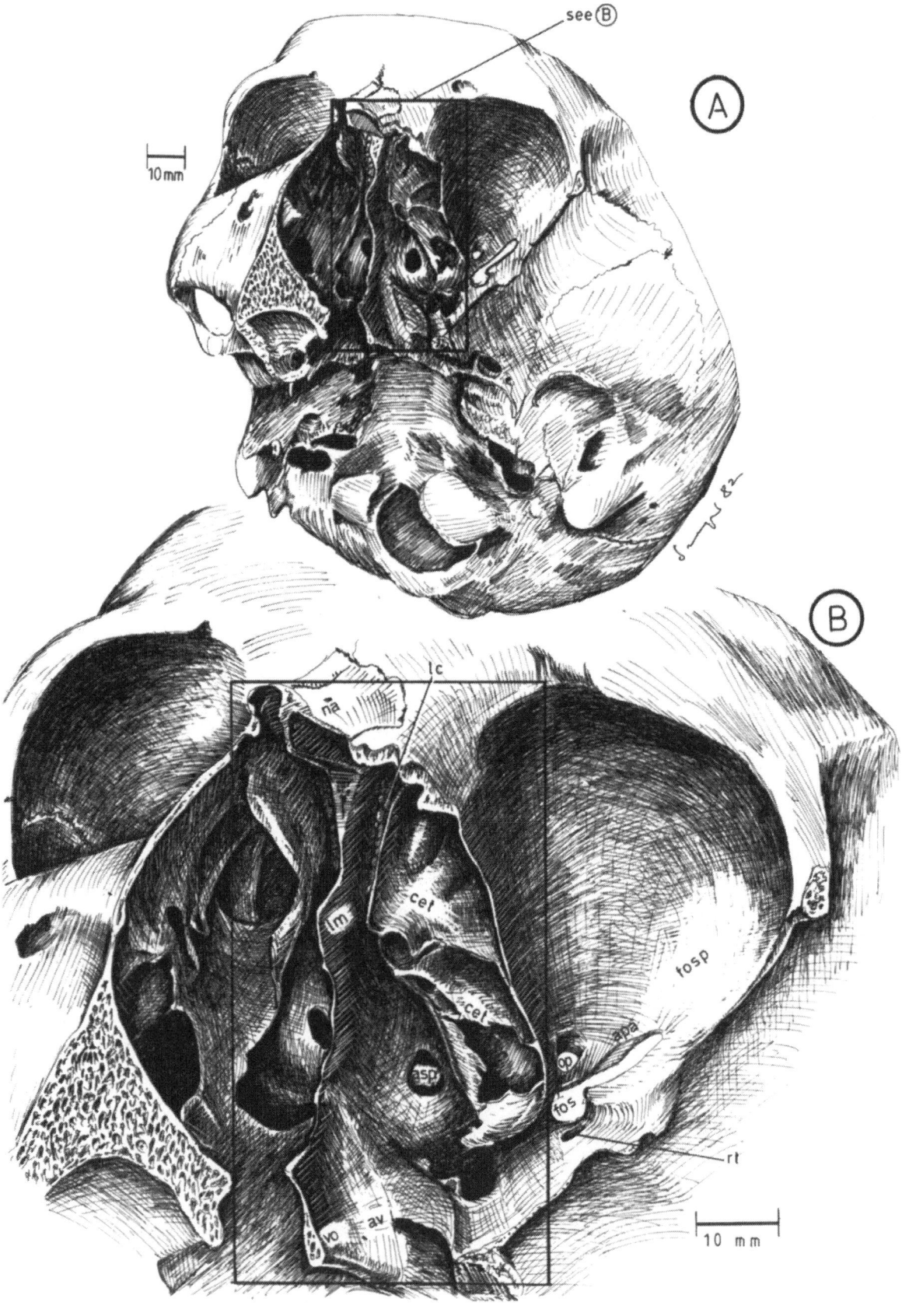
see B
A
10 mm
B
lc
na
cet
lm
tosp
cet
apa
op
asp
fos
rt
vo
av
10 mm

Fig. 8. Special anatomical features and special techniques of hypophysis operations
Topography of **Sinus sphenoidalis,** skull preparation, superior posterior view

A Overview

B Detail, enlarged from **A**. Sella floor, Dorsum sellae, Tuberculum sellae and adjoining posterior portions of Planum sphenoidale are removed, in order to open view into Sinus sphenoidalis. One sees that Sinus sphenoidalis extends so far laterally, that its medial wall can border medial wall of Foramen rotundum *–rt–*. Ridges in the floor of Sinus sphenoidalis *–pe–*; open arrows: Canalis opticus, the medial wall of which is opened up. Beyond Sinus sphenoidalis looking through Apertura sphenoidalis *–asp–* one sees the medial margin of Concha superior *–cs–*

Abbreviations:

asp Apertura sphenoidalis
cs Concha sup.
(csp) Juncture of Concha sup. to the floor of right Sinus sphenoidalis
[csp] Bony cleft at juncture of Concha sup.
op Canalis opticus
pe Bony rigdes in the floor of Sinus sphenoidalis
psp Planum sphenoidale
rt Foramen rotundum
ssp Septum sphenoidale

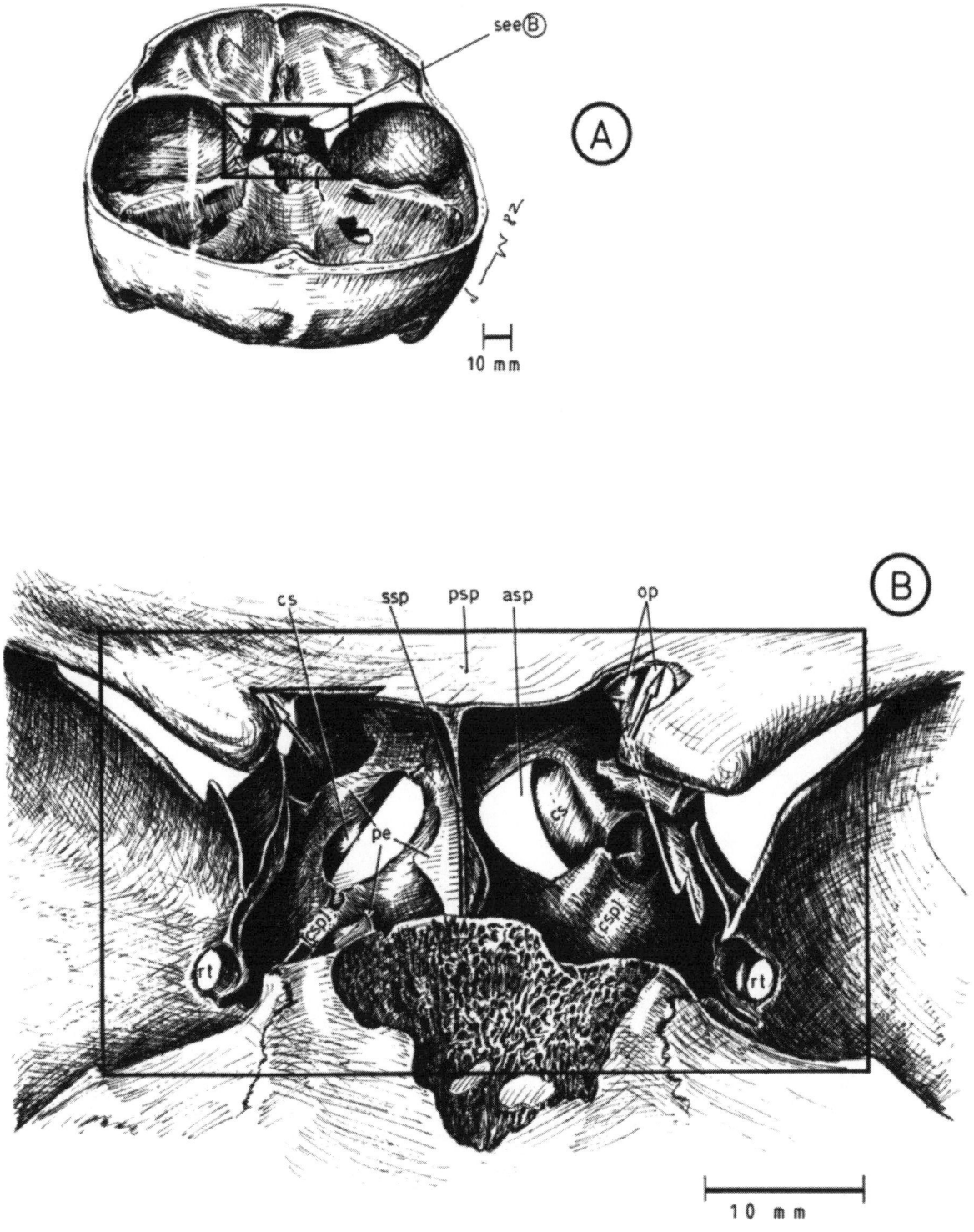
see B
A
10 mm
B
cs
ssp
psp
asp
op
pe
csp
rt
10 mm

Fig. 9. Special anatomical features and special techniques of hypophysis operations

Sinus sphenoidalis, the same skull preparation as in Fig. 8, superior view from above

A – C Progressive enlargements. Irregularily shaped ridges *–pe–* in the floor of Sinus sphenoidalis

Abbreviations:

asp Apertura sphenoidalis
pca Processus clinoideus ant.
pe Ridges in the floor of Sinus sphenoidalis
psp Planum sphenoidale
ssp Septum sphenoidale
rt Foramen rotundum

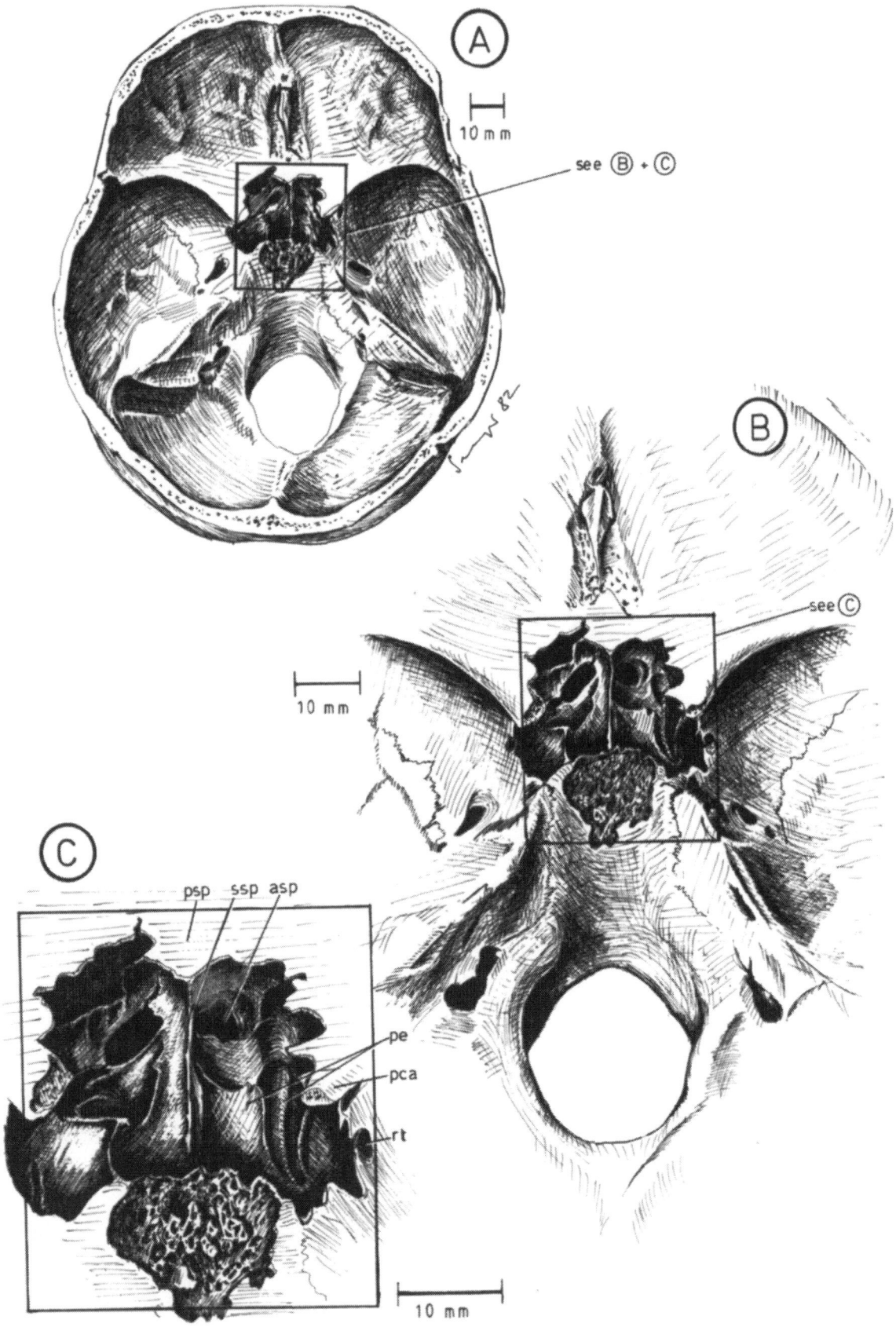
A
10 mm
see B + C
B
see C
10 mm
C
psp
ssp
asp
pe
pca
rt
10 mm

Fig. 10. Special anatomical features and special techniques of hypophysis operations
Anatomy of **Sinus sphenoidalis,** topographical relation to N. opticus, A. carotis int. and N. maxillaris. Asymmetry of Septum sphenoidale

A Position of frontal section planes. View as in Fig. 9 **B**

B Section plane at the level of Apertura sphenoidalis *–asp–*. Medial wall of Canalis opticus *–(wop)–*, which was removed in the preparation, is sketched in. Septum sphenoidale *–ssp–* is nearly at the median (otherwise relation to median is often very asymmetrical). Only the midpoint between Aperturae sphenoidales *–asp–* lies approximately in the median plane of the skull

a Distance between median plane of skull and medial edge of Apertura sphenoidalis

a' The same distance contralaterally

C Farther posterior section plane parallel to **B** through Processus clinoideus ant. and through Foramen rotundum with N. maxillaris -N.V2-. Because roof of Sinus sphenoidalis was removed in preparation, contours were sketched in afterwards. A. carotis int. lies in Sulcus caroticus *–(suc)–*. This portion of the dorso-lateral wall of Sinus sphenoidalis may protrude into Sinus sphenoidalis. A. carotis int. *–cl–* is sectioned in the anterior siphon area

Abbreviations:

asp	Apertura sphenoidalis
cet	Cellula ethmoidalis
cl	A. carotis int.
fos	Fissura orbitalis sup.
fptp	Fossa pterygopalatina
(fse)	Floor of Sella (projection)
lm	Lamina mediana nasi
op	Canalis opticus
pca	Processus clinoideus ant.
pe	Ridges in floor of Sinus sphenoidalis
sip	Sinus sphenoidalis divided (by Septum sphenoidale *–ssp–*) in separate cavities
(suc)	Sulcus caroticus (projection)
(wop)	Wall of Canalis opticus (projection)
(wsuc)	Dorso-lateral wall of Sinus sphenoidalis below Sulcus caroticus (projection)

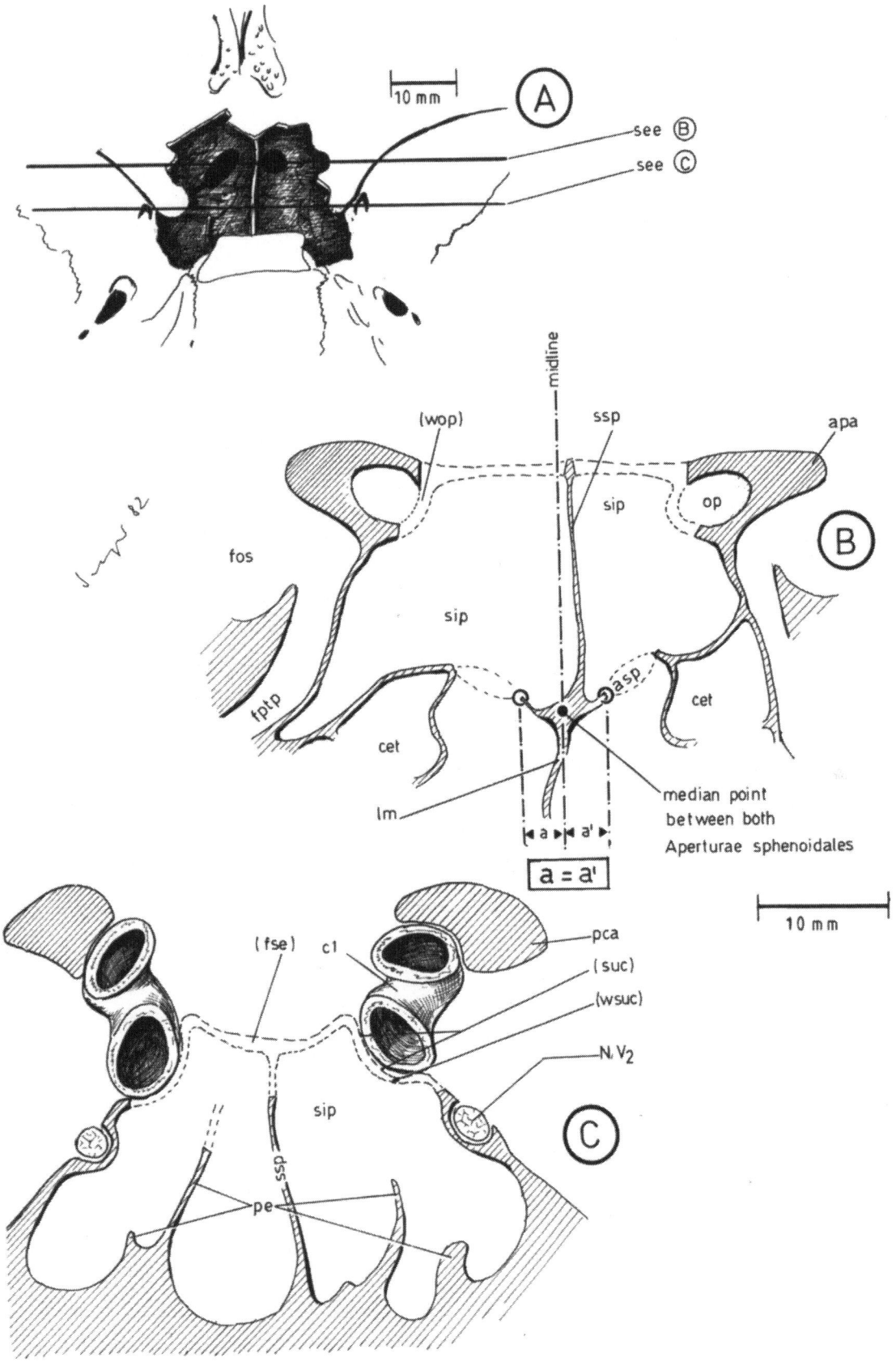
10 mm
A
see B
see C
midline
(wop)
ssp
apa
sip
op
B
fos
sip
fptp
asp
cet
cet
lm
median point
between both
Aperturae sphenoidales
a
a'
a = a'
10 mm
(fse)
c1
pca
(suc)
(wsuc)
N. V2
sip
C
ssp
pe

Fig. 11. Special anatomical features and special techniques of hypophysis operations

Anatomy of **Sinus sphenoidalis** in presence of **intrasellar processus.** Displacement of A. carotis int.

A Schematic frontal section at the level of carotis syphon. Floor of Sella *–fse–* is inferiorly displaced from original position, *–(fse)–*, and A. carotis int. *–cl–* is laterally displaced. Processus clinoideus ant. *–pca–* is thinned out and laterally displaced from original position *–(pca)–*. Note topographical relation of Sinus sphenoidalis *–sip–*, floor of sella *–fse–*, A. carotis int. *–cl–* to N. maxillaris -N.V2-

B The same topographical situation as in **A,** superior view. Here too one sees the lateral displacement of both Aa. carotis intt.

Asymmetries of A. carotis int.:

a short distance between midline and Curvatura ant. of A. carotis int. (variant)

a' short distance of Curvatura post. of A. carotis int. from midline anterior to Dorsum sella *–dos–*

In the presence of intrasellar processus both Aa. carotis intt. are laterally displaced. Displacement of A. carotis int. towards the midline very rarely occurs. Position of A. carotis int. must be ascertained by means of preoperative angiography

Abbreviations:

cl	A. carotis int.
(cl)	A. carotis int. (projection of normal findings)
dos	Dorsum sellae
fse	Floor of Sella
(fse)	Floor of Sella (projection of normal findings)
pca	Processus clinoideus ant.
(pca)	Processus clinoideus ant. (projection of normal findings)
pe	Ridges in the floor of Sinus sphenoidalis
sip	Sinus sphenoidalis
(sip)	Sinus sphenoidalis (projection of normal findings)
(ssp)	Septum sphenoidale (projection of normal findings)
ts	Tuberculum sellae

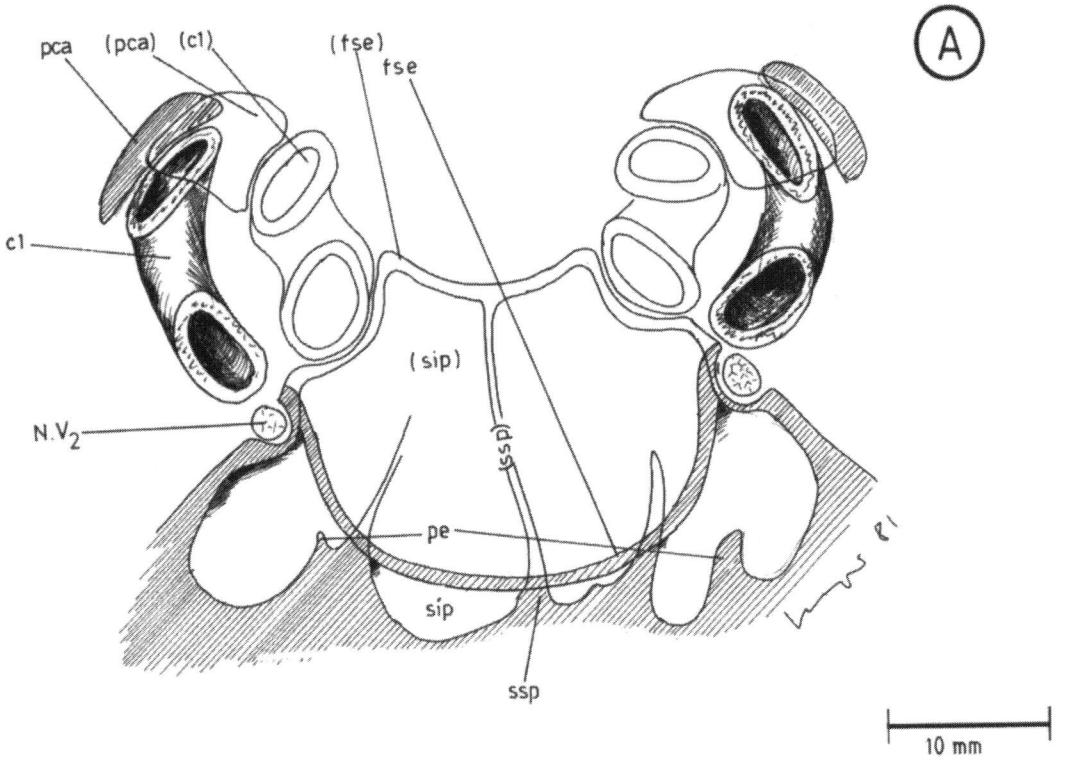
A
pca
(pca)
(cl)
(fse)
fse
cl
(sip)
N.V2
(ssp)
pe
sip
ssp
10 mm

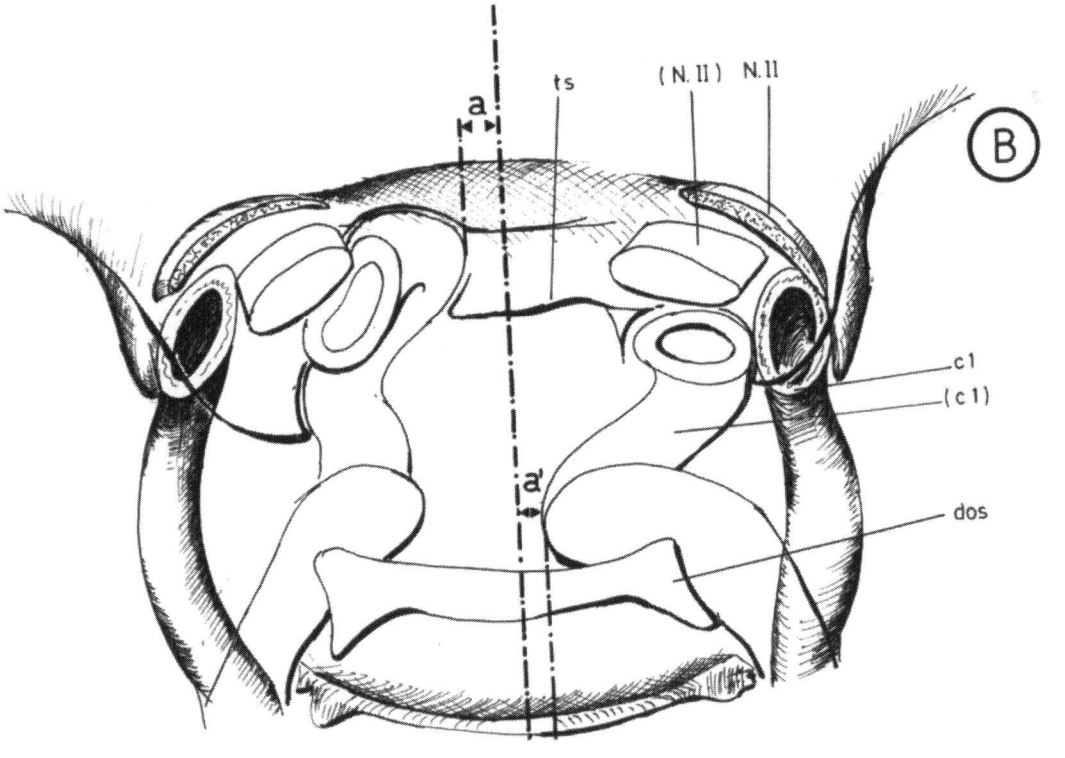
B
a
ts
(N.II)
N.II
cl
(cl)
a'
dos

Fig. 12. Special anatomical features and special techniques of hypophysis operations
Anatomical model of inner sella wall according to observations of hypophysis tumors by transcranial approach. Superior view. Cutting plane *–s–* of Dura corresponds to resection edge of Dura at operation. Dura lining of Sella in the presence of tumors contrary to normal findings is smooth and show numerous round and cleftlike gaps with slight seepage of venous blood (from Sinus cavernosus and Sinus intercavernosi). Both Aa. carotis intt. protrude only slightly into Sella *–p–* in the presence of large intrasellar tumors contrary to the normal findings. This facilitates thorough tumor removal

Abbreviations:

cl A. carotis int.
(cl) A. carotis int. (projection of path within Sinus cavernosus)
p Prominent sella wall along path of A. carotis int.
s Cutting plane of Dura after removal of hypophysis tumor

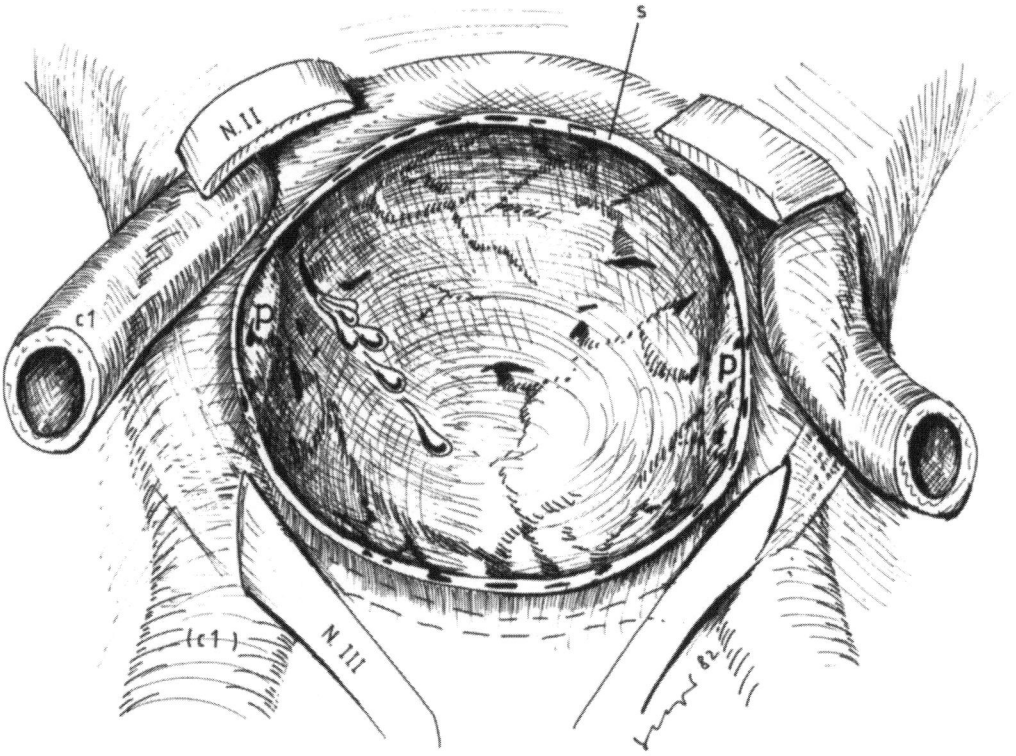
S
N. II
C1
P
P
(C1)
N. III

Fig. 13. Special anatomical features and special techniques of hypophysis operations
Anatomy of **Sinus sphenoidalis,** sagittal section of topographical relationship

A Anatomical preparation, overview

B Sectional enlargement from **A.** Walls of Canalis opticus and Foramen rotundum may stand out prominently against the Sinus sphenoidalis *–wop–* and *–wrt–*. Danger of injury during operations on Sinus sphenoidalis

C Preparation as **B,** with sketch of A. carotis int. *–cl–*. -N.II- and N. maxillaris -N.V2-

Abbreviations:

asp Apertura sphenoidalis
cl A. carotis int.
pca Processus clinoideus ant.
se Sella turcica
wop Wall of Canalis opticus
wrt Wall of Foramen rotundum

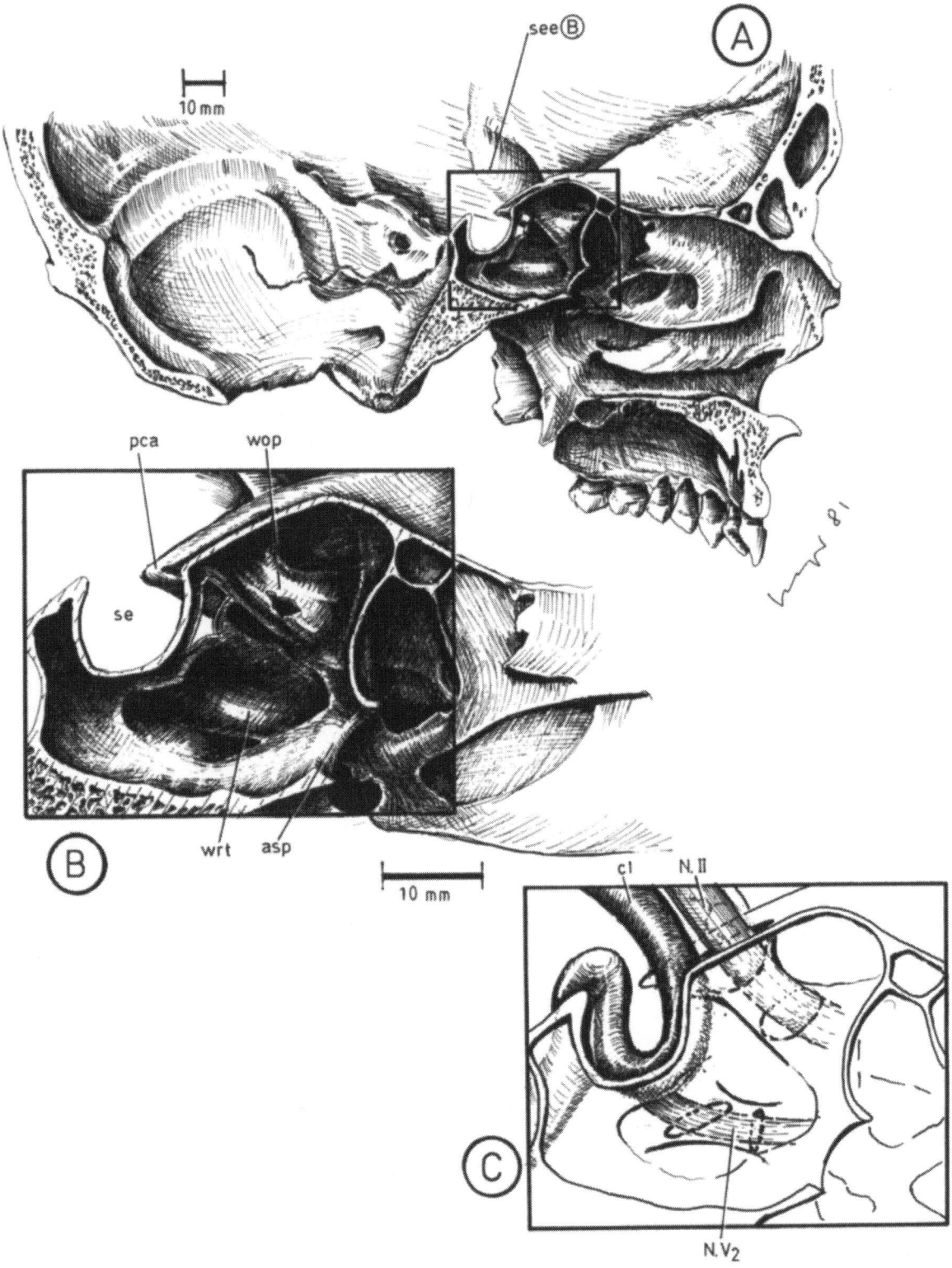
see B
A
10 mm
pca
wop
se
wrt
asp
B
10 mm
cl
N. II
C
N. V2

Fig. 14. Special anatomical features and special techniques of hypophysis operations
Continuation of Fig. 13. Topographical relationship of intrasellar processes

A Path of A. carotis int. *–c1–*, N. opticus -N.II- in the presence of balloon sella

B Path of A. carotis int. *–c1–*, N. opticus -N.II- and N. maxillaris *-(N.V2)-* in the presence of flatly enlarged sella

C Normal findings

Abbreviations:

c1 A. carotis int.
(N.V2) N. maxillaris (projection)

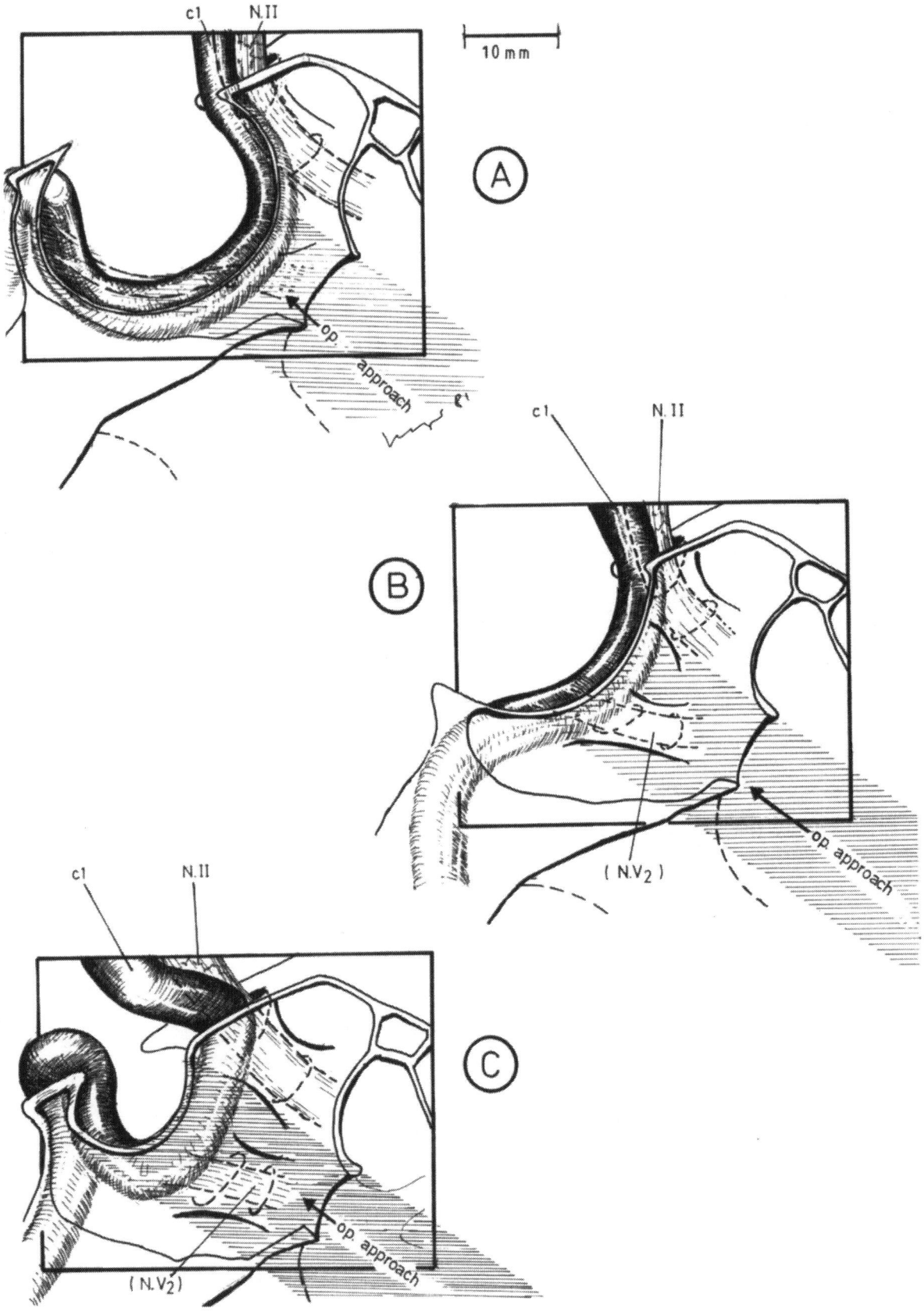
c1
N.II
10 mm
A
op. approach
c1
N.II
B
(N.V2)
op. approach
c1
N.II
C
(N.V2)
op. approach

FIG. 15 30

Figs. 15–24. Special anatomical features and special techniques of hypophysis operations
Principles of operation

Fig. 15. Position of gingiva incision, and operative approach towards sella

A Position of **gingiva incision**

B Fold-back of upper lip after soft tissue incision, **operative approach** sketched (arrow)

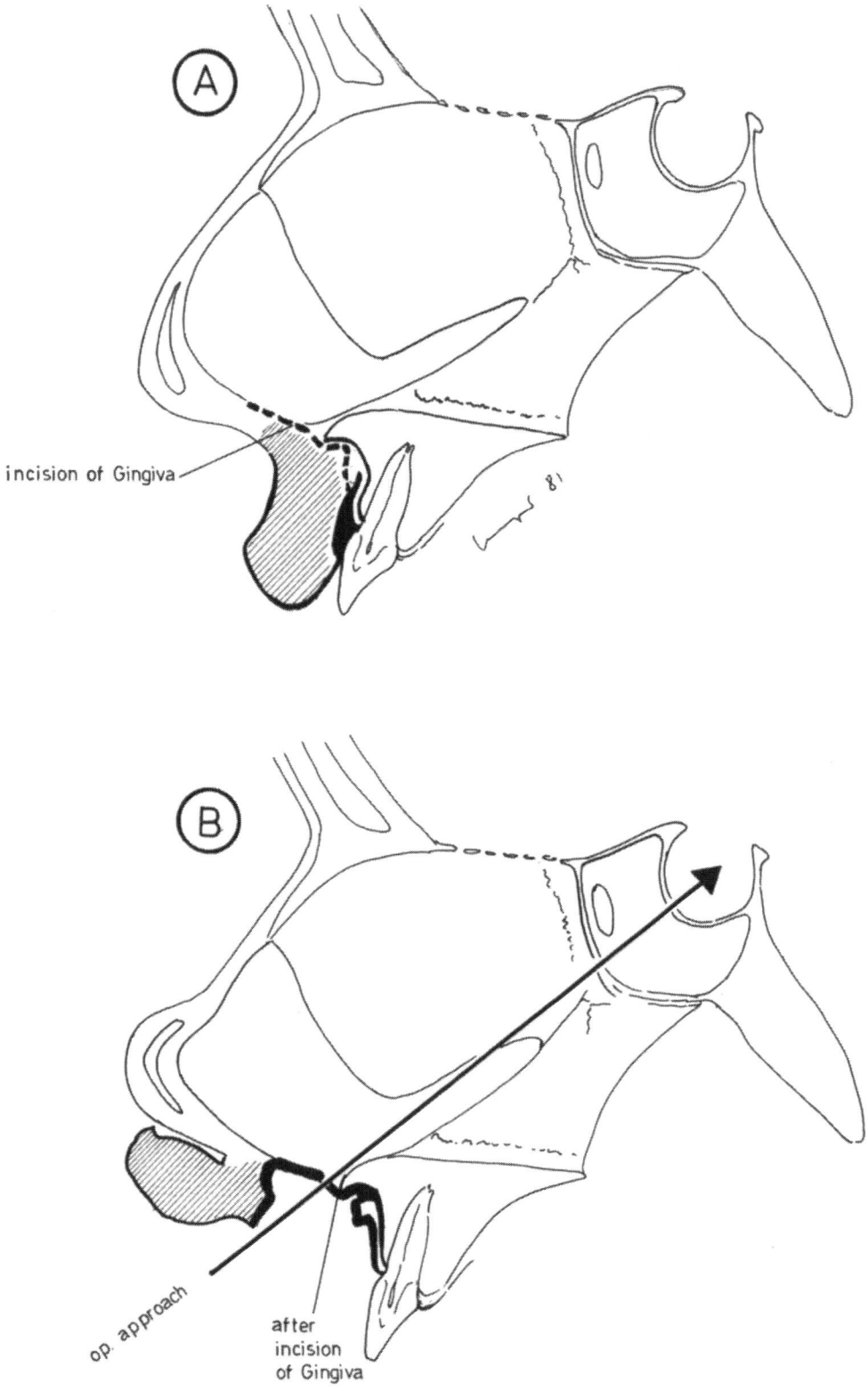
A
incision of Gingiva
B
op. approach
after
incision
of Gingiva

Fig. 16. Special anatomical features and special techniques of hypophysis operations
Principles of operations. **Detachment of nasal mucosa** *–muc–* from the cartilaginious nasal septum *–cs–* and from Spina nasalis ant. *–spa–*, as well as from floor of Meatus nasalis inf. *–fn–*

A Frontal schematic presentation

B Correct detachment of mucosa from floor of nasal cavity with downward-curved instrument

B' Use of upward-curved instrument carries the risk of perforating mucosa

Abbreviations:

cs Cartilaginious Septum nasi
fn Floor of Meatus nasalis inf.
muc Mucosa nasi
pd Palatum durum
spa Spina nasalis ant.

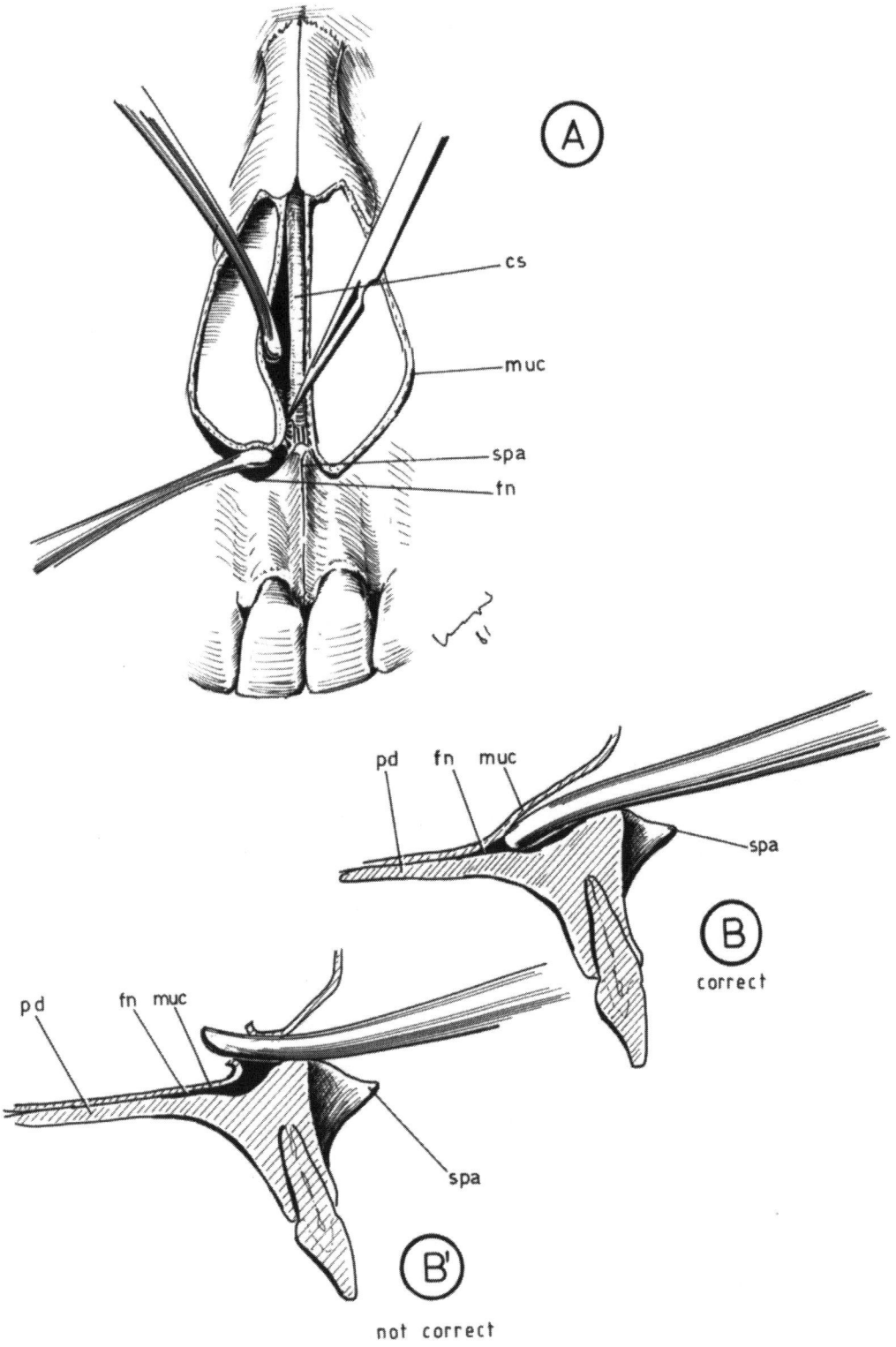
A
cs
muc
spa
fn
pd
fn
muc
spa
B
correct
pd
fn
muc
spa
B'
not correct

Fig. 17. Special anatomical features and special techniques of hypophysis operations

Principles of operation. **Resection of Septum nasi**

A Resection of Septum nasi, measurements. In the area of Spina nasalis ant. *–spa–*, a part of Septum nasi can be saved, if the approach is only from **one** side

B Anatomical preparation, overview. Upper edge of speculum, Apertura sphenoidalis and Canalis opticus lie in **one** plane

C Speculum is at first inserted (see also **A**) only 50 mm deep measured from Spina nasalis ant.

1 Detachment of mucosa from Vomer residual *–vo–*

2 Arrows: Farther insertion of speculum into final position after mucosa preparation. Apertura sphenoidalis (s. also **B**) appears at the upper edges of speculum, on both sides

Abbreviations:

asp Apertura sphenoidalis
cs Cartilaginious Septum nasi
lm Lamina mediana
pd Palatum durum
sip Sinus sphenoidalis
spa Spina nasalis ant.
vo Vomer

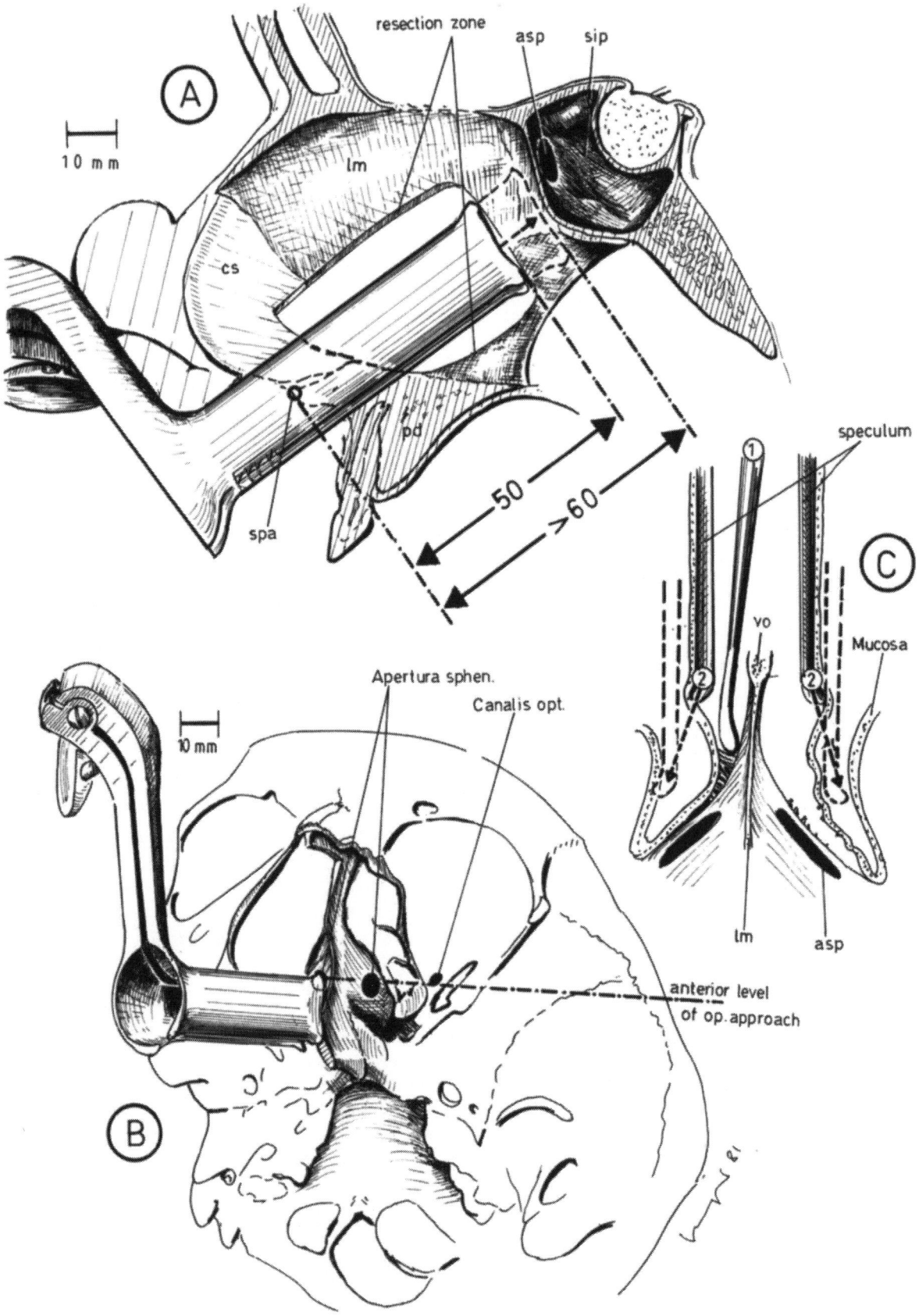
A
10 mm
resection zone
asp
sip
lm
cs
pd
spa
50
>60
B
10 mm
Apertura sphen.
Canalis opt.
anterior level
of op. approach
C
speculum
vo
Mucosa
lm
asp

Fig. 18. Special anatomical features and special techniques of hypophysis operations

Principles of **operation with narrow Apertura piriformis**

A Apertura piriformis too narrow for insertion of speculum

B Alternative procedure 1: resection of bony wall of Apertura piriformis. Disadvantage: Sinus maxillaris and teeth are adjoining (see Fig. 19)

B' Insertion of speculum through operatively enlarged Apertura piriformis

C Alternative procedure 2: Septum nasi is cut anteriorly also in the area of Spina nasalis ant. *–spa–*. Disadvantage: cosmetically unfavourable

C' Speculum can be inserted if cut Septum nasi is pushed aside

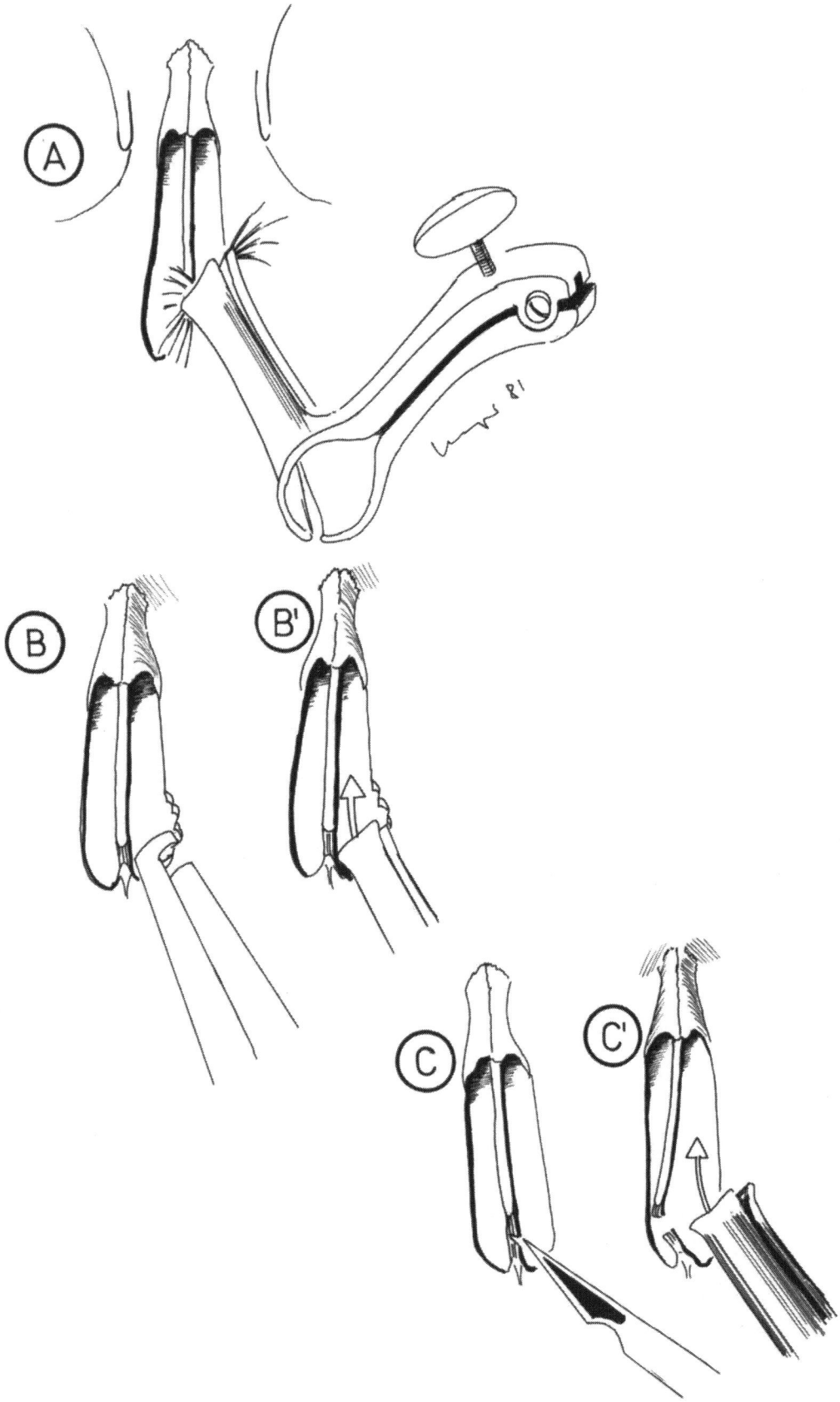
A
B
B'
C
C'

Fig. 19. Special anatomical features and special techniques of hypophysis operations. Dangers in operative widening of **Apertura piriformis**

A Favourable for operation: Sinus maxillaris is located at a considerable distance from Apertura piriformis (thin bony wall of Apertura piriformis)

A' Bone resection of lateral margin of Apertura piriformis

B Unfavourable situation (in younger persons). Sinus maxillaris *–(sma)–* adjoins Apertura piriformis. The bone quickly broadens laterally because it hugs Sinus maxillaris. Dental roots *–(ro)–* approach closely Apertura piriformis

B' If one tries to resect lateral margin of Apertura piriformis, Sinus maxillaris might be opened up and one or several dental roots may be injured. **Preop. X-ray-studies important**

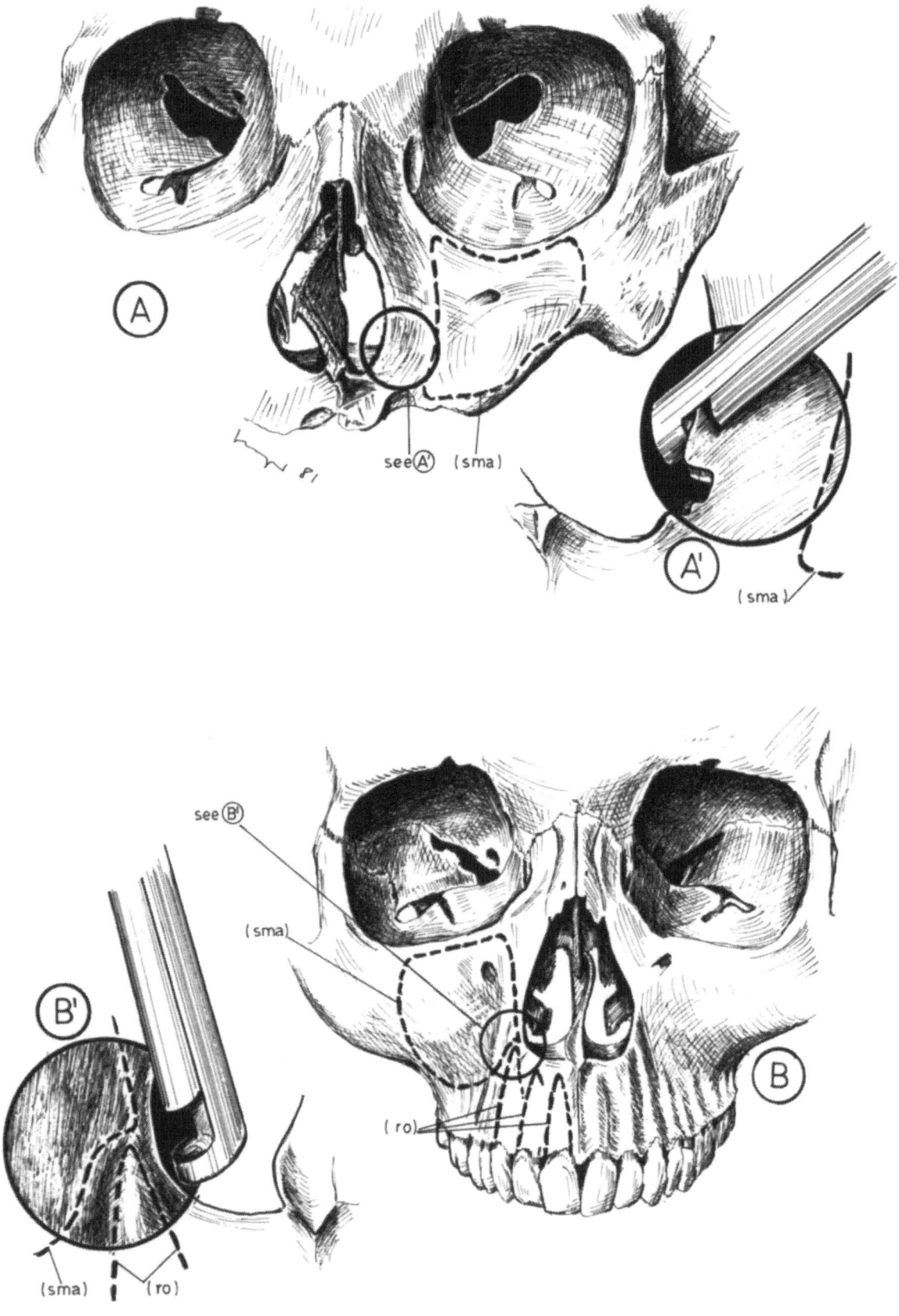
A
see A'
(sma)
A'
(sma)
see B'
(sma)
B'
B
(ro)
(sma)
(ro)

Fig. 20. Special anatomical features and special techniques of hypophysis operations
Principles of operation. Tear of mucosa of Septum nasi with resulting **obstructed approach**
Corrected position of speculum

A – C Anatomical sketch
A' – C' Operation site
A Speculum *–sp–* pushes back mucosa on the right side only. On the left *–L–* mucosa is torn and is not pushed back by speculum *–muc–*
A' The torn mucosa overlaps anterior wall of Os sphenoideum on the left side
B Insertion of two flexible spatulas *–spt–*
B' Operation site corresponding to **B**
- **1a + 1b** Removal of speculum *–sp–* after insertion of the spatula *–spt–*
- **2a + 2b** Bending of spatula tips on both sides of speculum after removal

C Reinsertion of speculum
- **1a + 1b** Branches of speculum are eased forward
- **2a + 2b** Removal of spatulas

C' Operative site, corresponding to **C**

Abbreviations:

muc torn mucosa
sp Speculum
spt Spatula

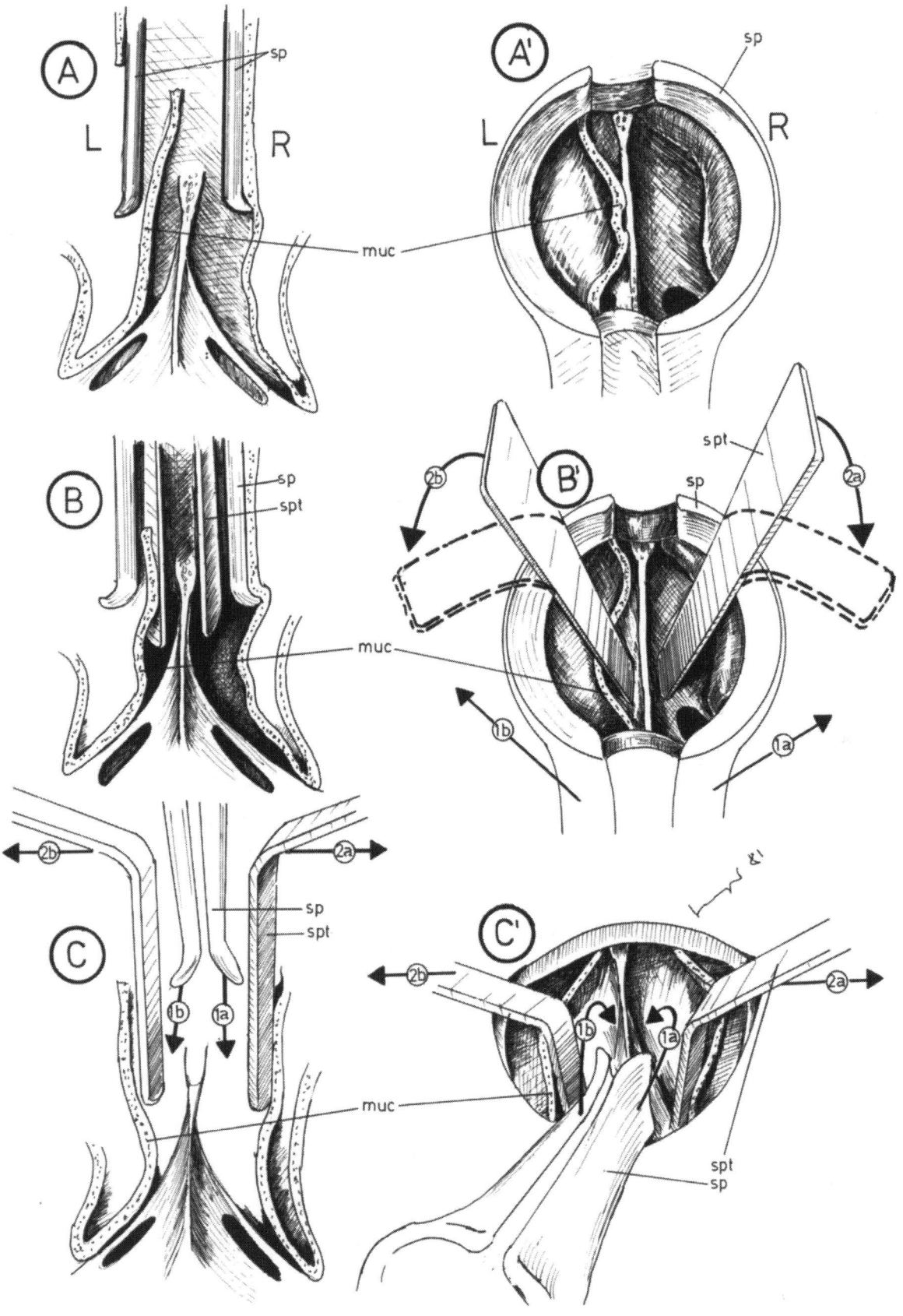
A
sp
L
R
muc
A'
sp
L
R
B
sp
spt
muc
B'
spt
sp
2b
2a
1b
1a
C
2b
2a
sp
spt
1b
1a
muc
C'
2b
2a
1b
1a
spt
sp

Fig. 21. Special anatomical features and special techniques of hypophysis operations
Principles of operation. **Operative approach** into **skull base** sketched in. Basal view after nearly complete resection of facial part of skull, resection planes at Septum nasi (Lamina mediana, Vomer)

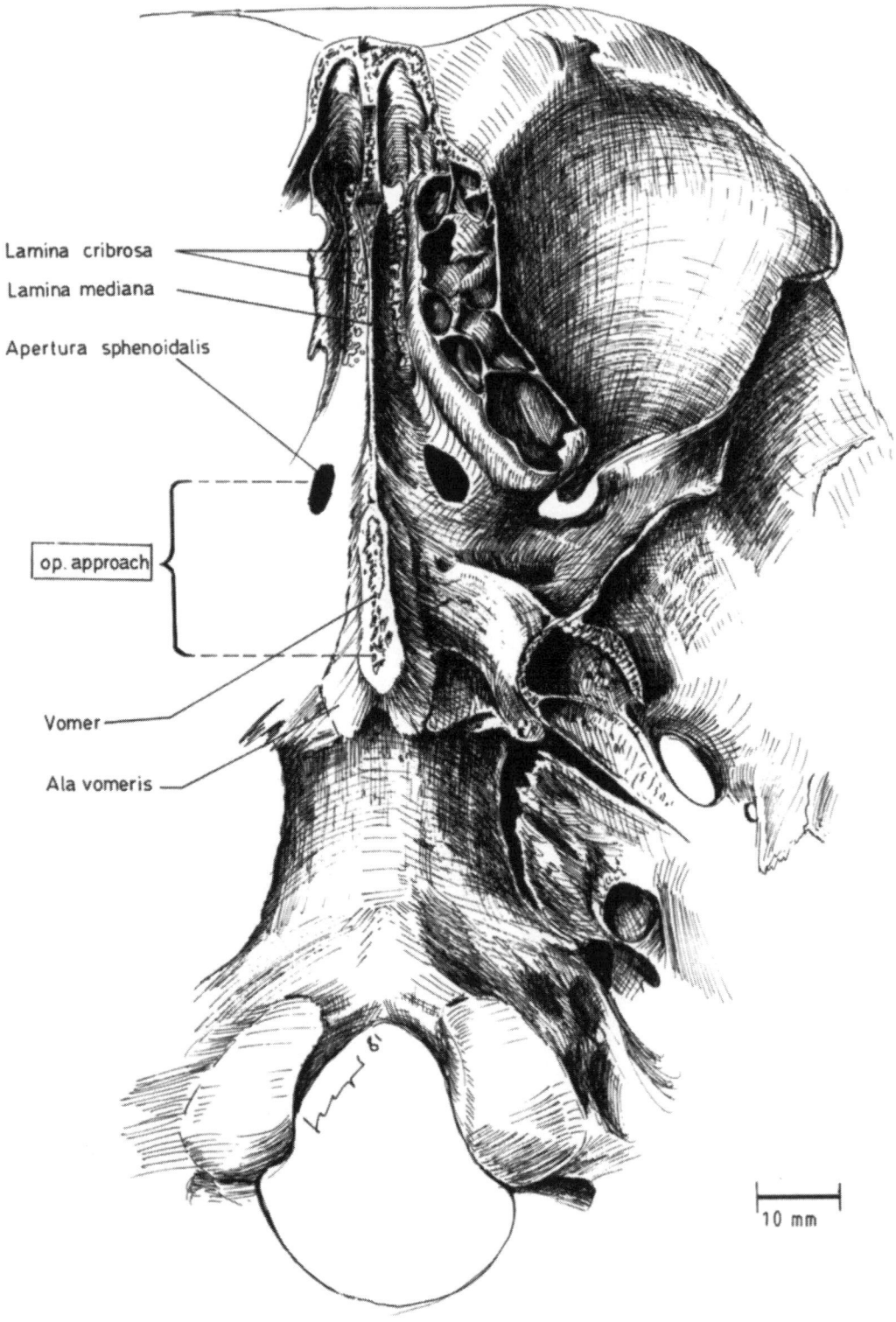
Lamina cribrosa
Lamina mediana
Apertura sphenoidalis
op. approach
Vomer
Ala vomeris
10 mm

Fig. 22. Special anatomical features and special techniques of hypophysis operations
Principles of operation. **Determination of midline and resection of Sinus sphenoidalis floor**

A – C Basal view, detail from Fig. 21

A' – C' Sagittal view, detail

A Detail of preparation, sketched according to Fig. 21. Vomer *–vo–* deviates from midline

A' Situation as **A** during Vomer resection, sagittal section

B After Vomer resection one recognizes that the insertion of Vomer, with juncture to Alae vomerris *–av–*, is in the median position. The midline lies between both Aperturae sphenoidales *–asp–*. Beginning of Sinus sphenoidalis resection

B' Situation as **B,** sagittal section

C Sinus sphenoidalis opened up. Septum sphenoidale nearly always has an oblique path; it seldom lies in the midplane or parasagittaly

C' Situation as **C,** sagittal section

Abbreviations:

asp Apertura sphenoidalis
av Ala vomeris
sip Sinus sphenoidalis
vo Vomer

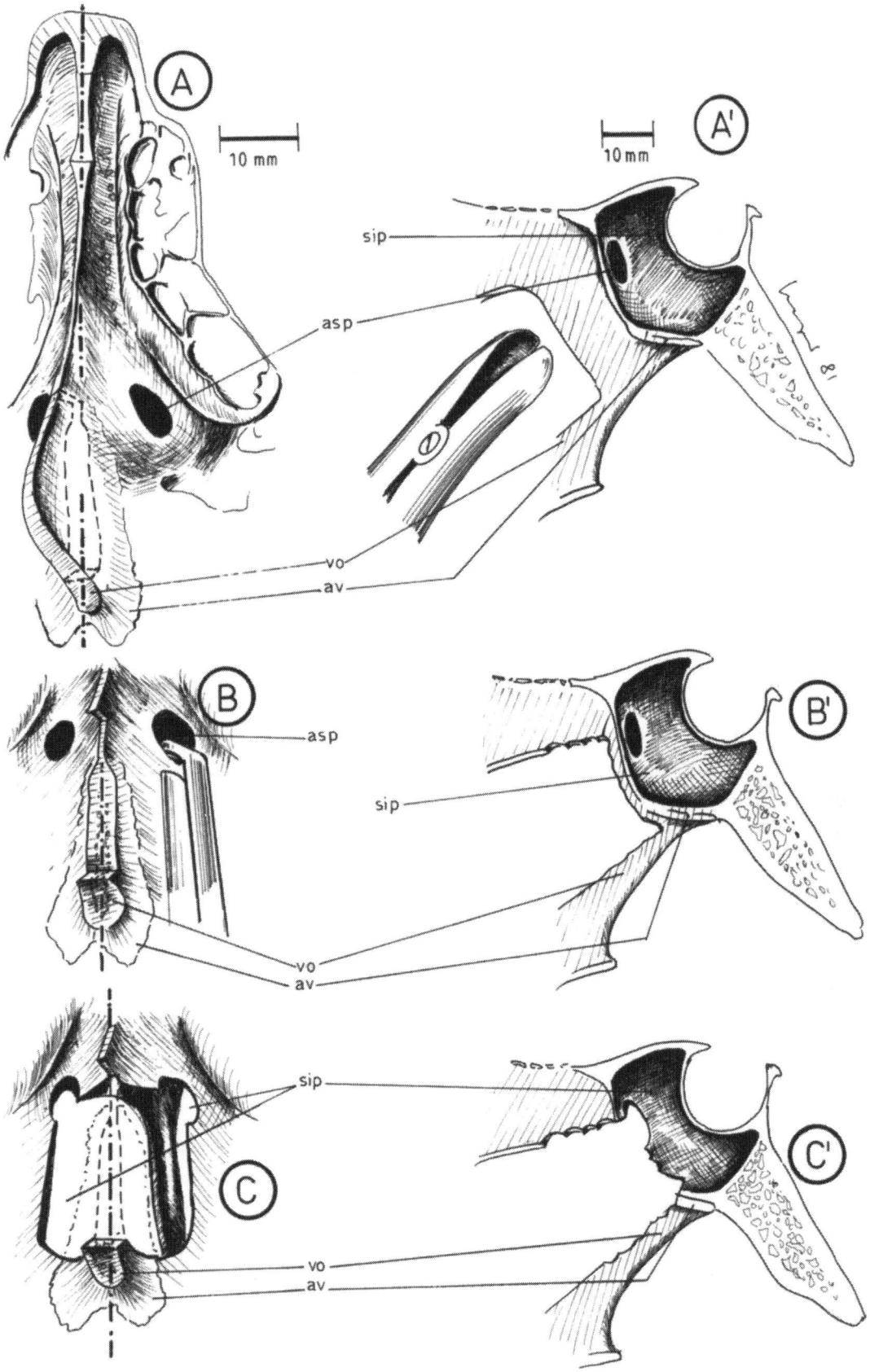
A
10 mm
A'
10 mm
sip
asp
vo
av
B
asp
B'
sip
vo
av
sip
C
C'
vo
av

Fig. 23. Special anatomical features and special techniques of hypophysis operations
Principles of operation. **Os sphenoidale preparation, anterior view, microsurgical operation site** sketched in

A Overview

B Detail enlargement from **A.** Presentation of topographical relation of Vomer and Alae vomeris to Spina sphenoidalis *–spsp–*. Spina sphenoidalis and/or Alae vomeris *–av–*, contrary to Vomer *–vo–*, are of nearly symmetrical configuration. Lamina mediana *–lm–* too is nearly midpositioned at the juncture of Os sphenoidale. In the area of Aperturae sphenoidales *–asp–* slight asymmetries are to be expected.
Portions of Septum nasi are often very asymmetrical; however, the more nearly they approach Os sphenoidale, the more they tend toward midplane-location

Abbreviations:

asp Apertura sphenoidalis
av Ala vomeris
fos Fissura orbitalis sup.
lm Lamina mediana
psp Planum sphenoidale
rt For. rotundum
spsp Spina sphenoidalis

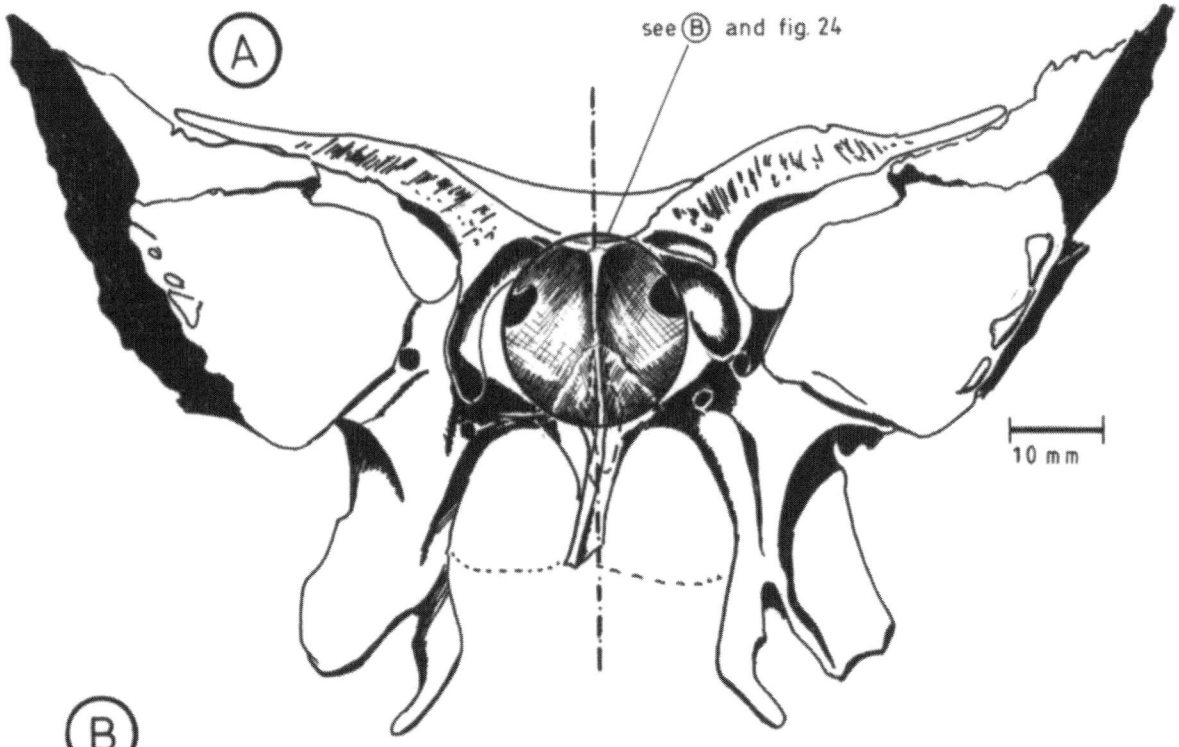
A
see B and fig. 24
10 mm

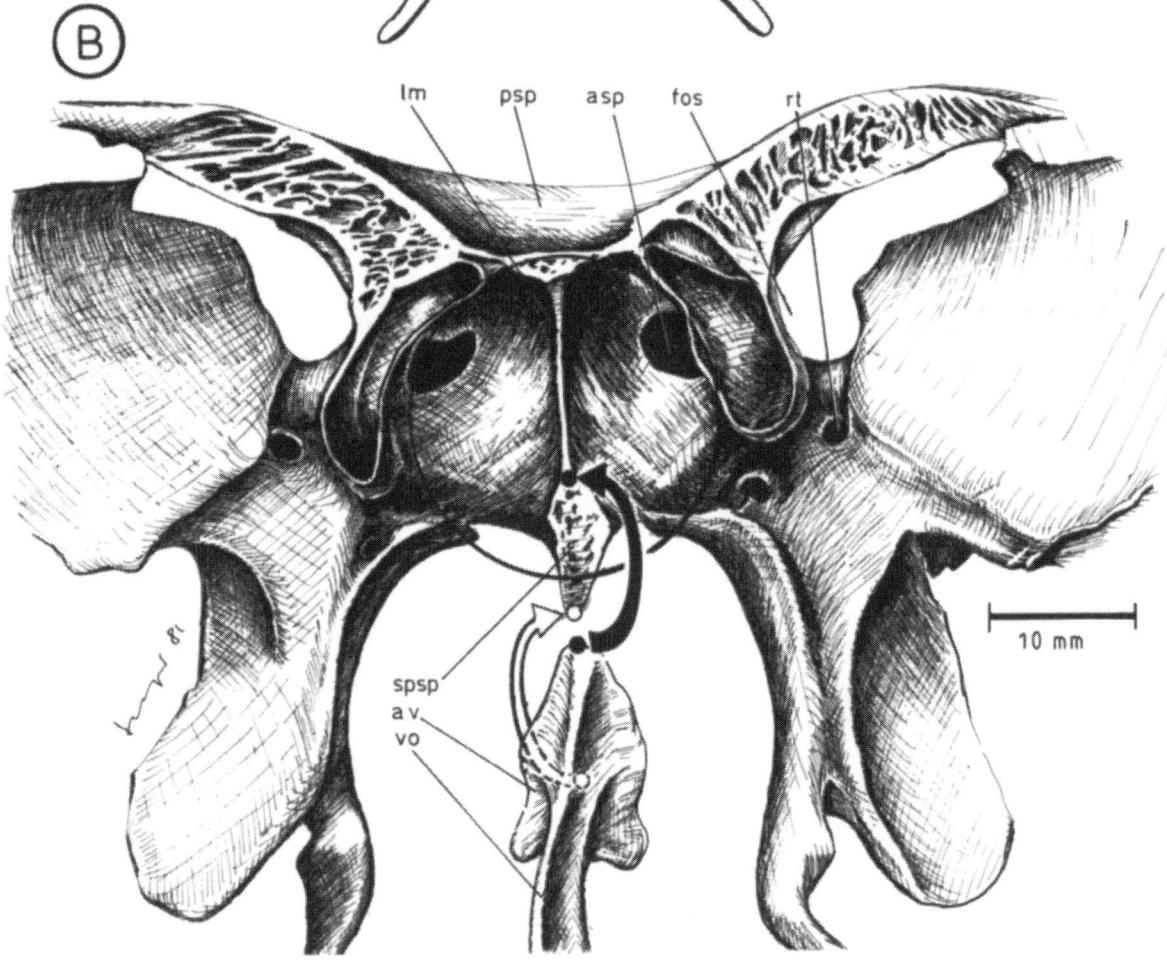
B
lm
psp
asp
fos
rt
spsp
a v
vo
10 mm

Fig. 24. Special anatomical features and special techniques of hypophysis operations
Principles of operation. Continuation of Fig. 23.

Opening up of Sinus sphenoidalis

A – C Microsurgical site

A' – C' Anatomical sketch, sagittal view

A Presentation similar to Fig. 23

A' **1** The exposure of Sinus sphenoidalis starts with the resection at the anterior wall, beginning at Apertura sphenoidalis *–asp–*

B After opening the anterior wall of Sinus sphenoidalis, resection of basal Vomer portions *–vo–*, and resection of Ala vomeris *–av–* one can view grossly asymmetrical Septum sphenoidale *–ssp–*

B' Extirpation of mucosa of Sinus sphenoidalis
- **1** Detachment of mucosa from bone by dissector, if possible throughly, using a **blunt** dissector
- **2** Stretching of mucosa by forceps
- **1** and **2** To be repeated until the mucosa is removed in as few large pieces as possible.

  If small mucosa pieces remain (i.e. in hidden niches), the danger of a later mucocele exists

C Opening up of sella floor
- **1** Opening up of bony sella floor
- **2** Incision of dura lining on sella floor. Watch out for A. carotis int., review angiography!

C' **1** Loosening of tumor by curette

Abbreviations:

asp Apertura sphenoidalis
av Ala vomeris
lm Lamina mediana
ssp Septum sphenoidale
vo Vomer

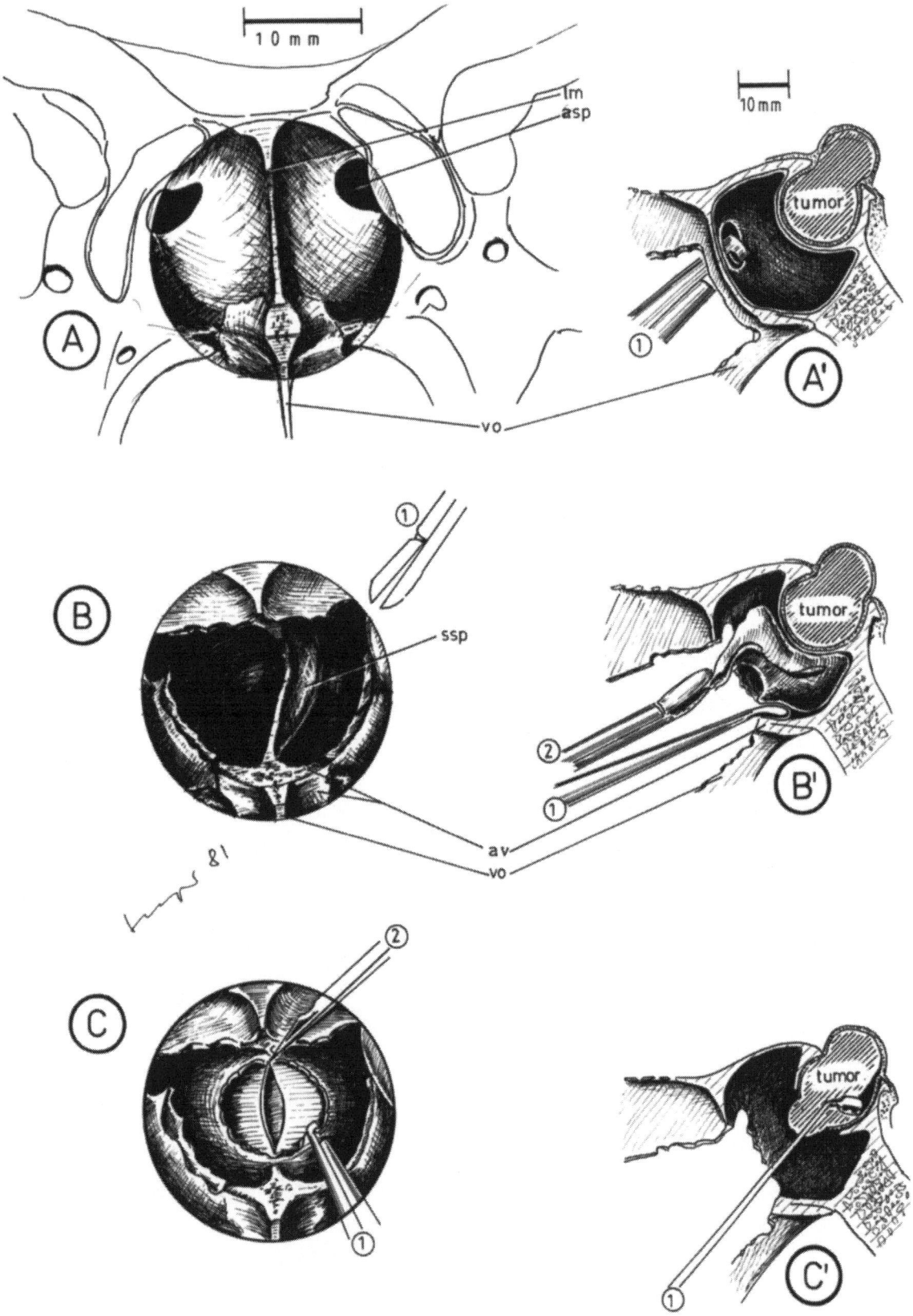
10 mm
lm
asp
10 mm
tumor
A
A'
vo
B
ssp
tumor
B'
av
vo
C
C'
tumor

Fig. 25. Special anatomical features and special techniques of hypophysis operations

Principles of operation. **Problems of tumor removal** in the presence of grossly enlarged sella.

A Typical findings in the presence of hypophysis tumors: sella clearly enlarged; from a narrow approach –*d*– thorough tumor removal is possible

B, C, D Broad sella, approach –*d*– as in **A.** However, a more rostral approach –**C**–, or more posterior approach –**B + D** –, will leave tumor remains

E Broad sella as in **B** and **D.** Atypically wide approach –**d'**–: tumor can be removed throughly, necessitating X-ray control of curette position in relation to sella wall

Abbreviations:

d Sella approach of normal width

d' Enlarged sella approach

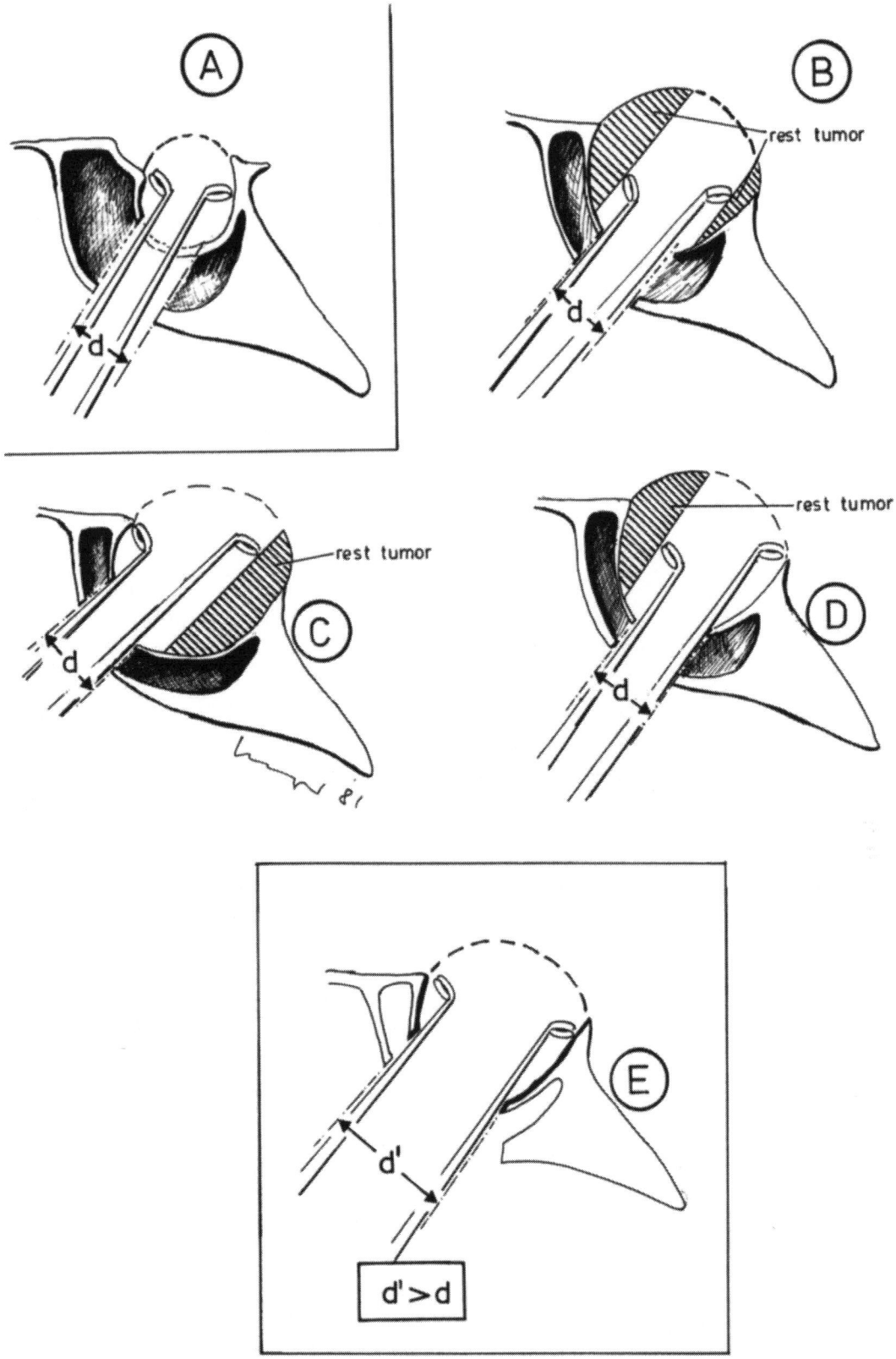
A
d
B
rest tumor
d
C
rest tumor
d
D
rest tumor
d
E
d'
d'>d

Fig. 26. Oro-nasal hypophysis operation according to Hardy (modified*)
Clinical example of a chromophobe hypophysis adenoma; preoperative bitemporal hemianopsia, improved postoperatively. Diagnostic procedures

A – B' Bilateral carotis angiographies. Note the short distance of the Curvatura anterior of A. carotis int. from the midline *–a–* (right side) and *–a'–* (left side). Curvatura post. of A. carotis int. lies farther away *–b–* (right side) and *–b'–* (left side)

C – G Preoperative CT-findings

C Section planes of CT

D Asymmetry of Septum sphenoidale

E Topographical relation of tumor to A. carotis int. *–cl–*. Processus clinoideus ant. *-pca-*, and mesencephalon *–me–*, as well as to A. basilaris *–bl–*

F' reconstruction from **F.** Topographical relation of tumor to third ventricle, basal cisterns *–cis–* and Sinus sphenoidalis *–sis–*, frontal section plane

F Sketch of CT section plane of reconstruction **F'**

G' Position of tumor in sagittal section, reconstruction from **G**

G Sketch of CT section plane of reconstruction **G'**

H Postoperative CT: tumor removed

Abbreviations:

cl A. carotis int.
cis Cisternae basales
bl A. basilaris
me Mesencephalon
pca Processus clinoideus ant.
sis Sinus sphenoidalis
● Curvatura ant. of A. carotis int.
○ Curvatura post. of A. carotis int.

---

* I am greatly obliged to Prof. Dr. R. Fahlbusch, Director of the Neurosurgical Clinic, University of Erlangen, Federal Republic of Germany, for suggestions as to operative technique.

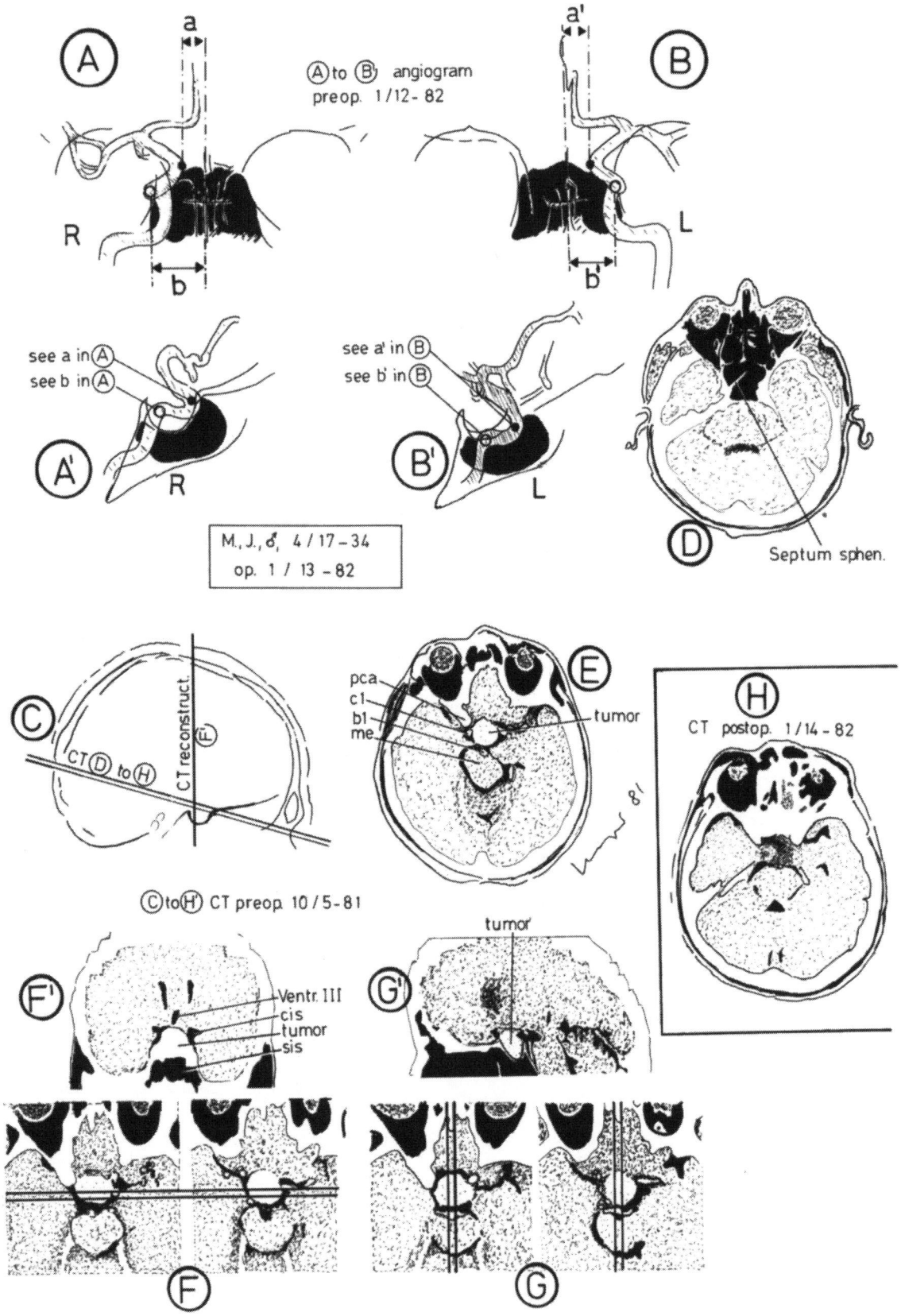
A
a
A to B angiogram
preop. 1/12-82
a'
B
R
L
b
b'
see a in A
see b in A
see a' in B
see b' in B
A'
R
B'
L
M., J., ♂, 4/17-34
op. 1/13-82
D
Septum sphen.
C
CT D to H
CT reconstruct.
E
pca
c1
b1
me
tumor
H
CT postop. 1/14-82
C to H' CT preop. 10/5-81
tumor
F'
Ventr. III
cis
tumor
sis
G'
F
G

Fig. 27. **Instruments** for oronasal hypophysis operation (HARDY)

A	Retractor for holding back the upper lip
B – D	Instruments for gingiva incision
E + F	Dissector for detachment of mucosa from Septum nasi and floor of Meatus nasalis inf.
G	Spatula for holding back mucosa from Septum nasi
I + H	Shapeable spatulas for holding back torn mucosa s. Fig. 20
J	Hardy speculum

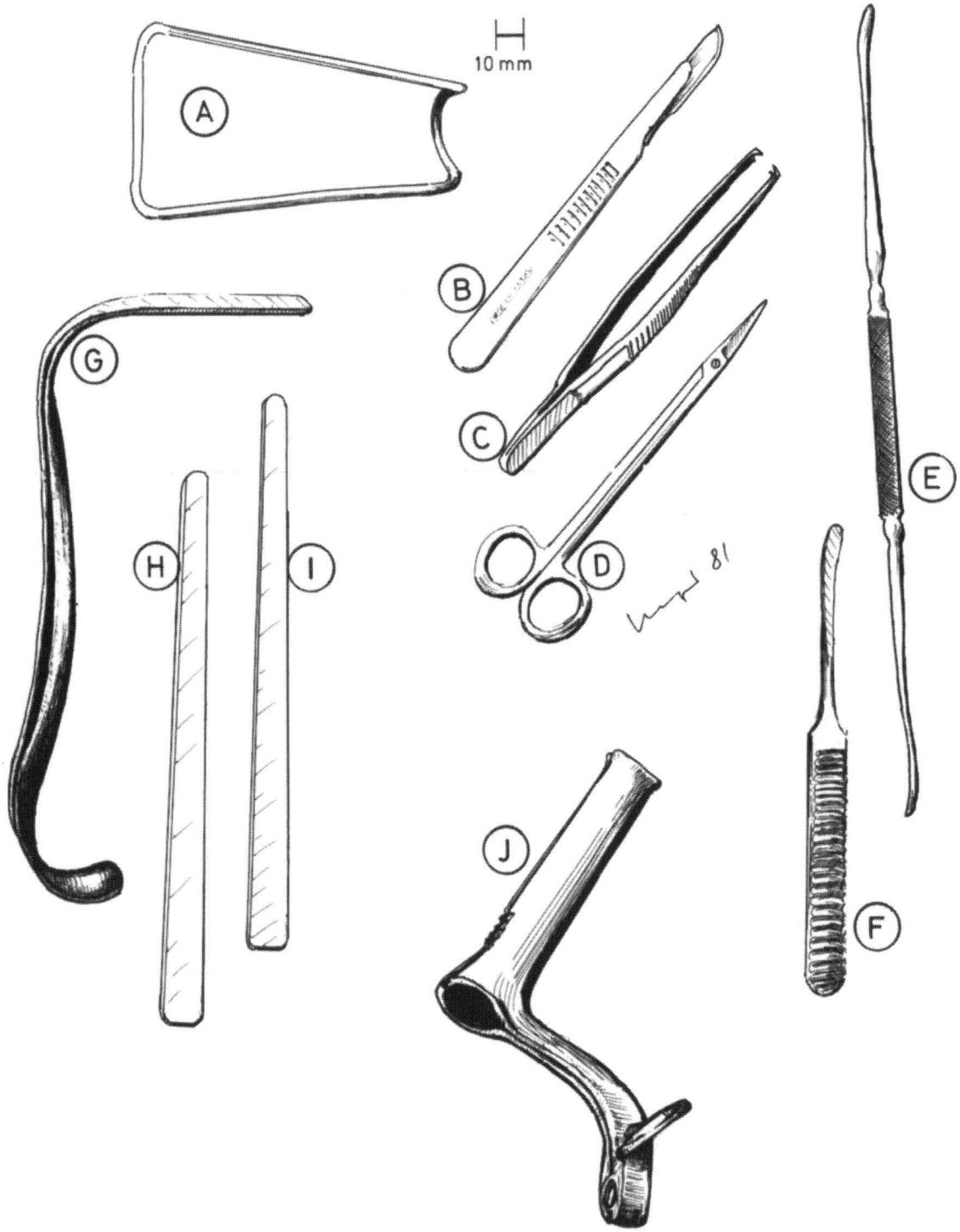
10 mm
A
B
C
D
E
F
G
H
I
J

Fig. 28.

A + B	Instruments for resection of Septum nasi
C	Microdissector for detachment of mucosa from anterior wall of Sinus sphenoidalis (which forms the floor of Sinus sphenoidalis)
D	Enlarged detail from **C**
E – H	Instruments for opening up sella floor (**G + H**), and for resection of Sinus sphenoidalis floor (**E + F**)

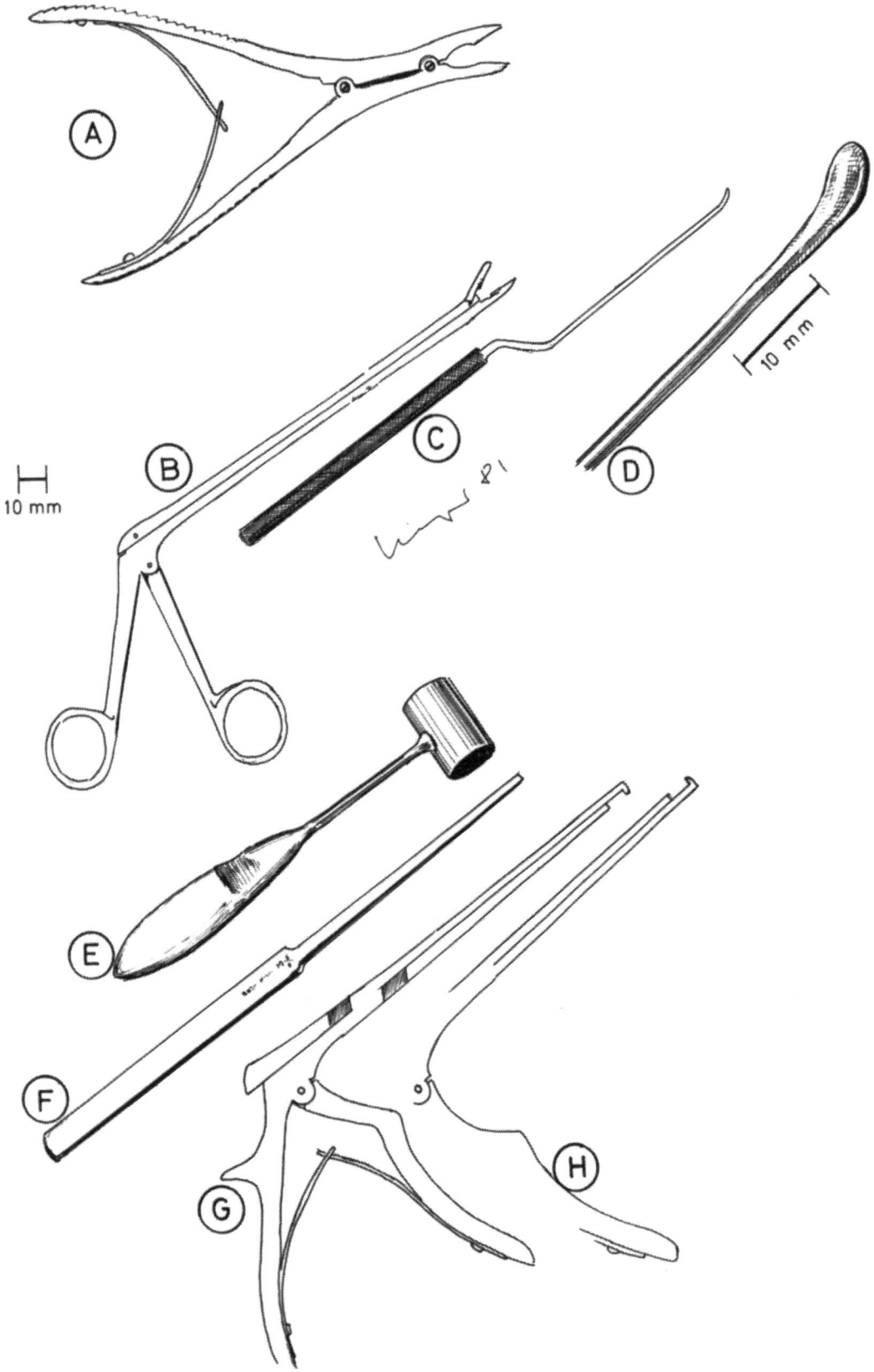
A
B
C
D
E
F
G
H
10 mm
10 mm

Fig. 29. **Instruments** for hypophysis operation

A	Bipolar coagulation forceps: to be used in the mucosa area, but, if possible, **not** in the sella area
B	Sucker (maximum size shown, types with smaller lumen also necessary)
C	Tumor forceps
D	Enlarged detail from **C**
E – L	Hypophysis curettes – Hardy
M	Speculum for spreading nasal opening for tamponage at operation's end

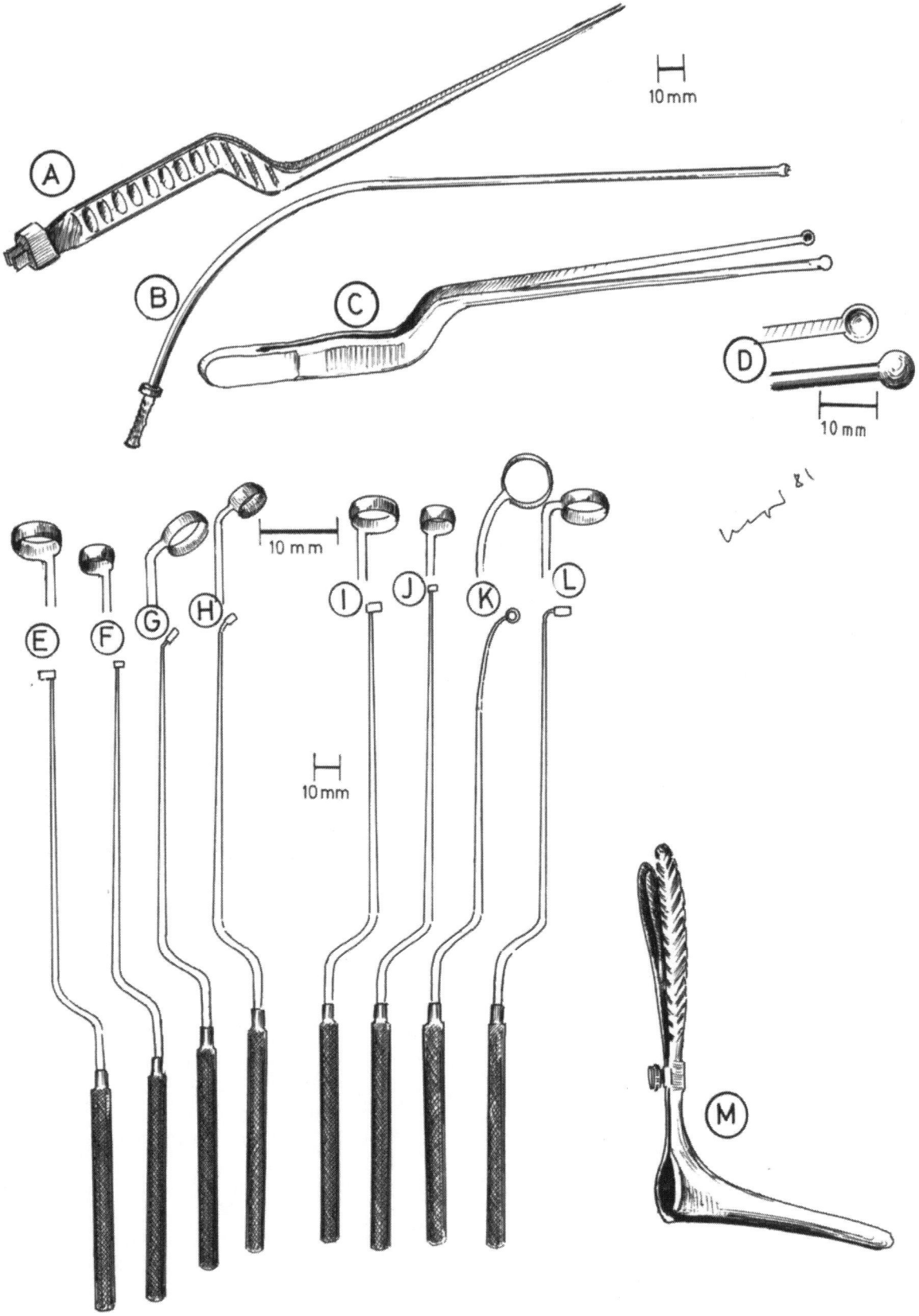
10 mm
A
B
C
D
10 mm
10 mm
E
F
G
H
I
J
K
L
10 mm
M

Figs. 30 to 48. Hypophysis operation

Fig. 30. **Positioning of patient**

A Position of patient on operating table and X-ray position

B Anatomical sketch from **A.** The neurosurgeon does not sit, as is customary, at the side of the patient, but above patient's head as for trepanations. Thus only a slight reclination of patient's head is required

FIG. 30

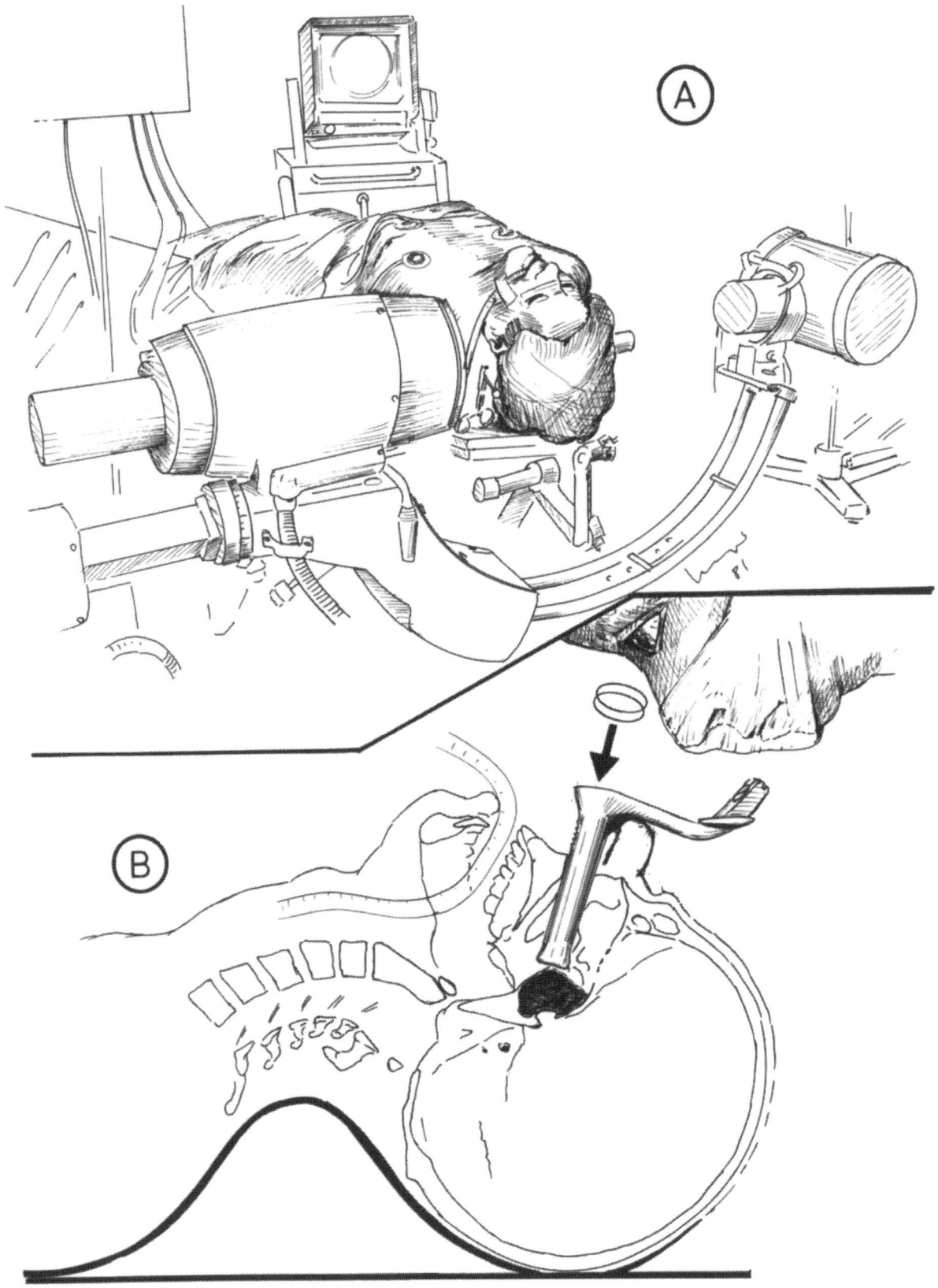

Fig. 31. Hypophysis operation
Local anesthesia

A Injection technique in the presence of gross asymmetry of the anterior Septum nasi area
1a – 2b Positions of injection needle
Broken lines: Position change of needle

A' The same as in **A** shown on anatomical model. Cartilaginous and bony structures can be palpated digitally

B Injection technique in Vestibulum oris. Points of puncture are located at juncture of gingiva and mucosa labii

B' The same as in **B** on the anatomical model. Here an example of a median position of the anterior Septum nasi portions. Cartilaginous and bony structures are palpable

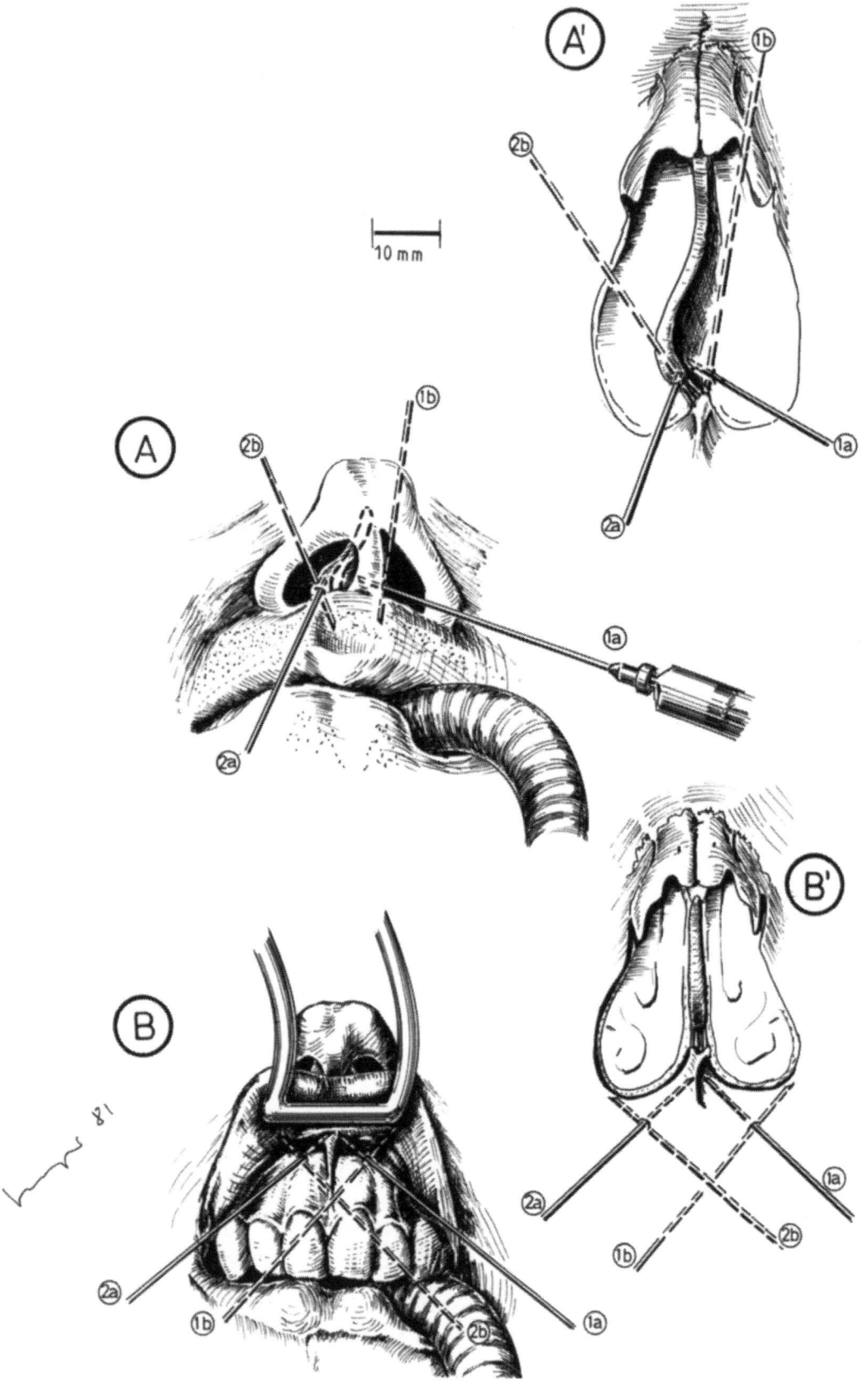
A'
1b
2b
10 mm
1a
2a
A
1b
2b
1a
2a
B'
2a
1a
1b
2b
B
2a
1b
2b
1a

Fig. 32. Hypophysis operation. **Incision and preparation of mucosa** in Vestibulum oris

A Mucosa incision just above juncture of gingiva and mucosa labii. Measurements in mm

B + C Detachment of mucosa from Os maxillare

C Exposure of Spina nasalis ant. and of the inferior medial portion of Apertura piriformis

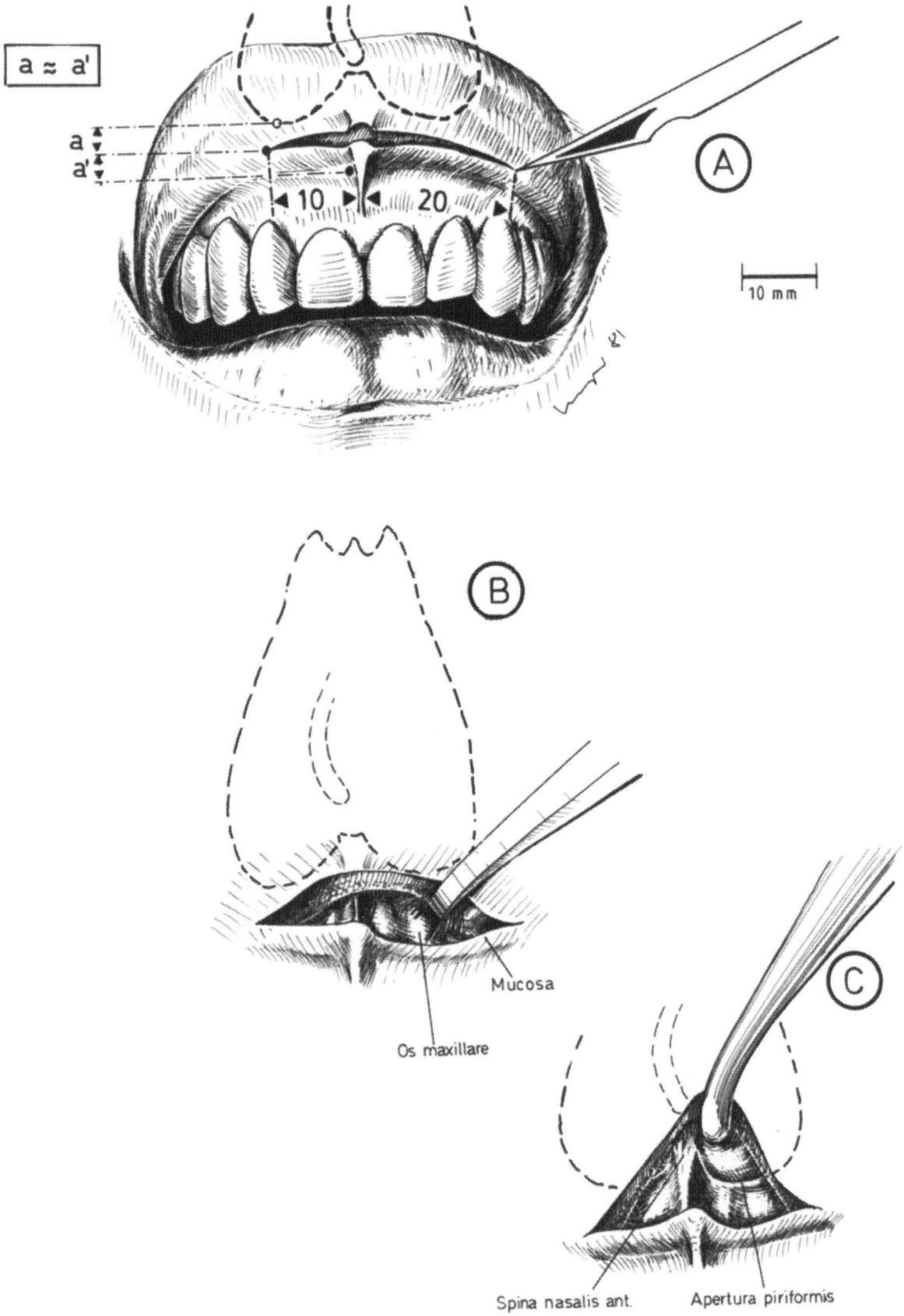
a ≈ a'
a
a'
10
20
A
10 mm
B
Mucosa
Os maxillare
C
Spina nasalis ant.
Apertura piriformis

Fig. 33. Hypophysis operation

D **1a + 1b Detachment of mucosa** upwards

2a Incision over Septum cartilagineum, which is palpable

E **3** **Detachment of perichondrium** *–per–* from Septum cartilagineum *–cart–*

After detachment of perichondrium the incision *–inc–* is extended to Spina nasalis ant. *–spa–*

F **1** Detachment of perichondrium from Septum cartilagineum *–cart–* with spatula

2 Detachment of incised connective tissue between Septum cartilagineum *–cart–* and Spina nasalis ant. *–spa–* with dissector

3 Cutting of fibrous connections between Septum nasi and medial mucosa

G **1 + 3** As in **F**

4 Alternating with **3. At this point there is great danger of perforating the mucosa and opening up Cavum nasi**

Abbreviations:

cart Septum cartilagineum
per Perichondrium
spa Spina nasalis ant.

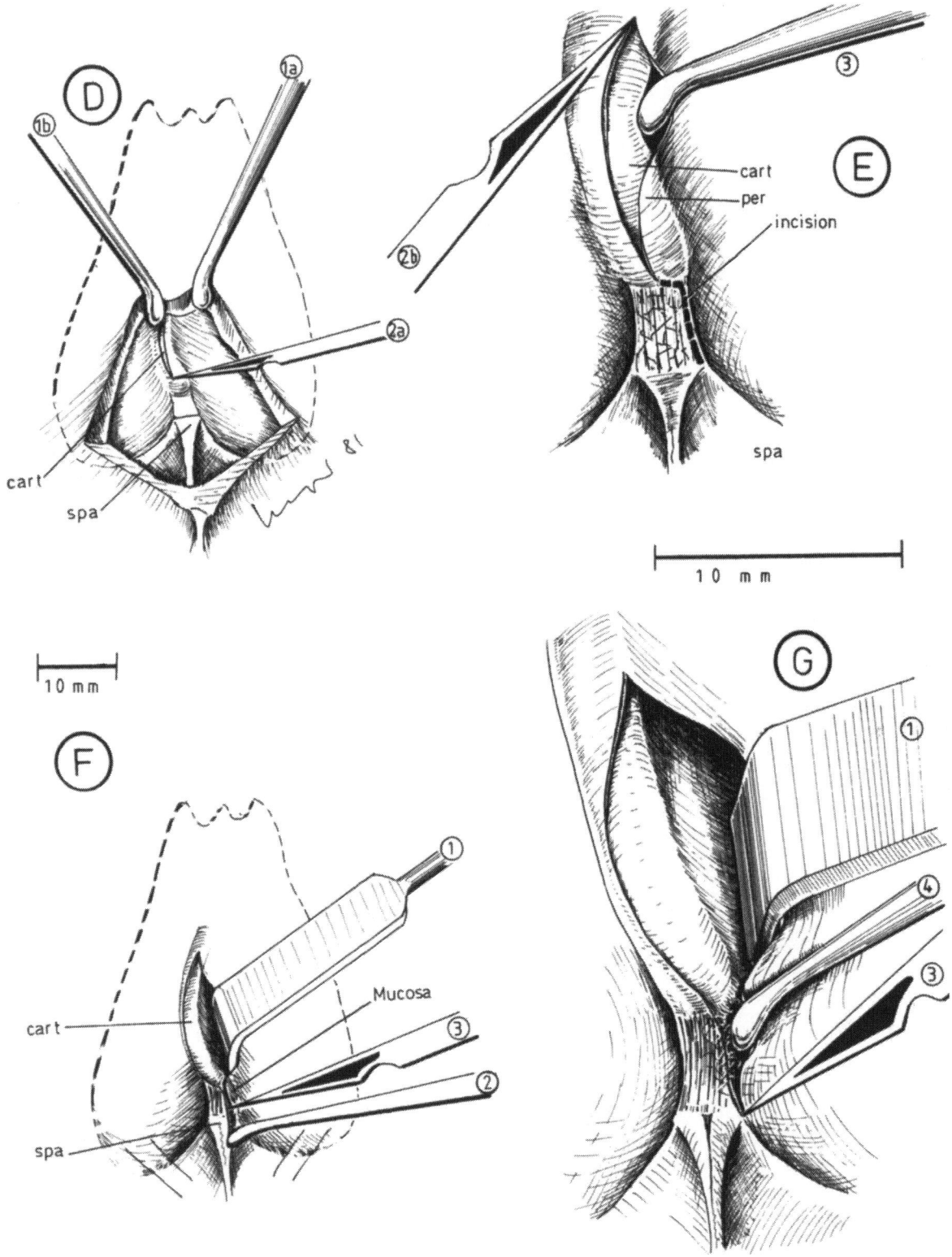
D
1a
1b
2a
cart
spa
E
3
2b
cart
per
incision
spa
10 mm
F
10 mm
1
Mucosa
3
2
cart
spa
G
1
4
3

Fig. 34. Hypophysis operation

H **Detachment of mucosa** from Apertura piriformis *–api–*

2a Position of dissector. Arrows: movements of dissector

I **1** Cutting of additional adhesions between Septum nasi and mucosa

2b Detachment of mucosa from Meatus nasi inf. and Septum nasi

H' **2a** Detachment of mucosa from floor of Meatus nasi inf.

2b Detachment of mucosa from Septum nasi. Anatomical model. S: Section plane of anatomical models **I'** and **I''**

I' + I'' Preparation in the presence of asymmetrical Septum nasi

2b, 3 Detachment of mucosa

Abbreviations:

api Apertura piriformis
cart Septum cartilagineum
lm Lamina mediana
vo Vomer

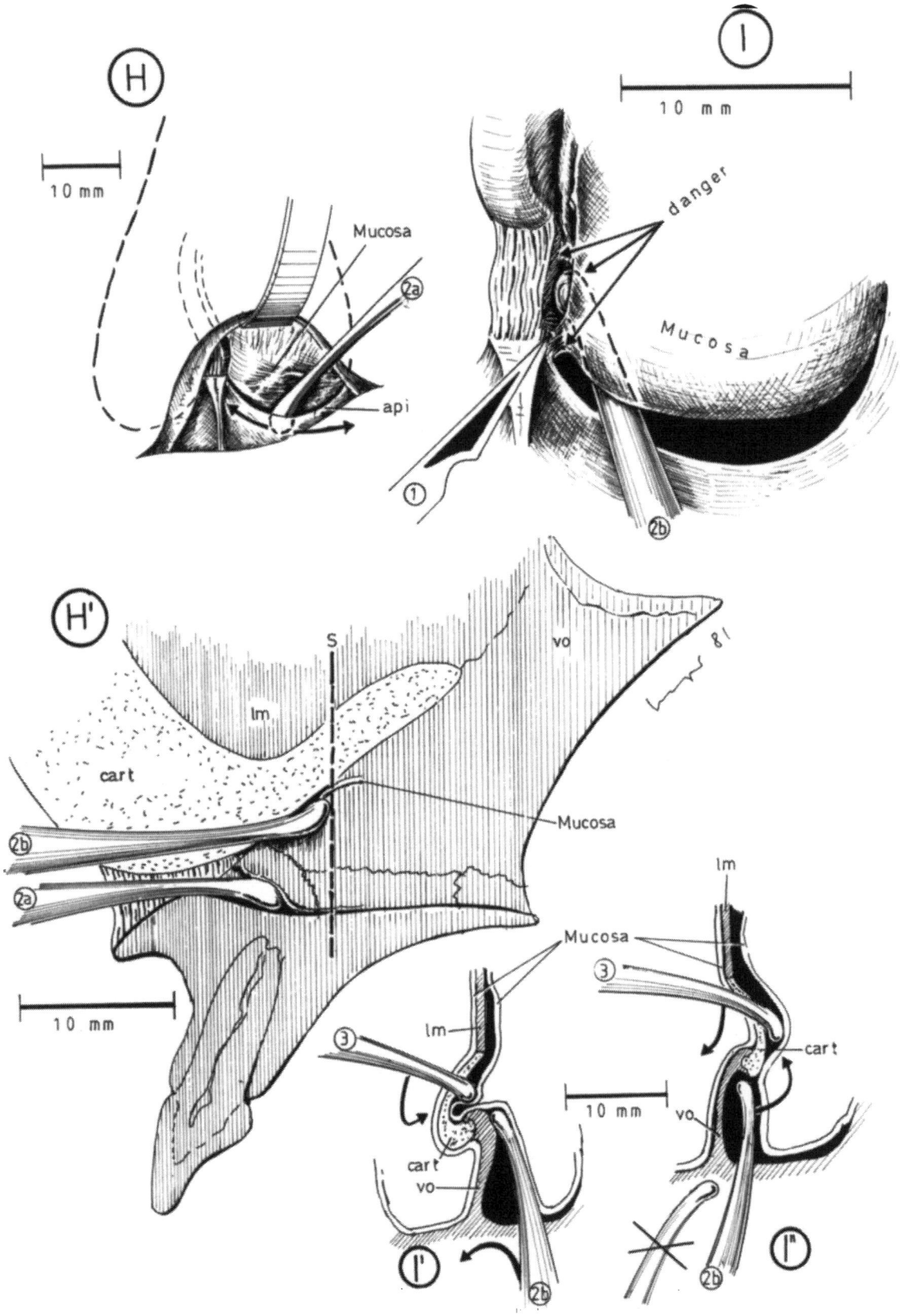
H
10 mm
Mucosa
2a
api
I
10 mm
danger
Mucosa
1
2b
H'
S
vo
lm
cart
Mucosa
2b
2a
10 mm
lm
Mucosa
3
lm
3
cart
10 mm
vo
cart
vo
I'
2b
I''
2b

Fig. 35. Hypophysis operation. Resection of Septum nasi

A X-ray ap of clinical case, Fig. 26. The deviation of Septum nasi seems slight

B Anatomical model. Cartilaginous Septum nasi – not visible by X-ray – shows considerable deviation. Arrows: possible operative approaches

C **Resection zone (broken line) of Septum nasi,** anatomical model.
For cosmetic reasons, a 10 mm strip of the anterior Septum nasi is preserved
Measurements in mm

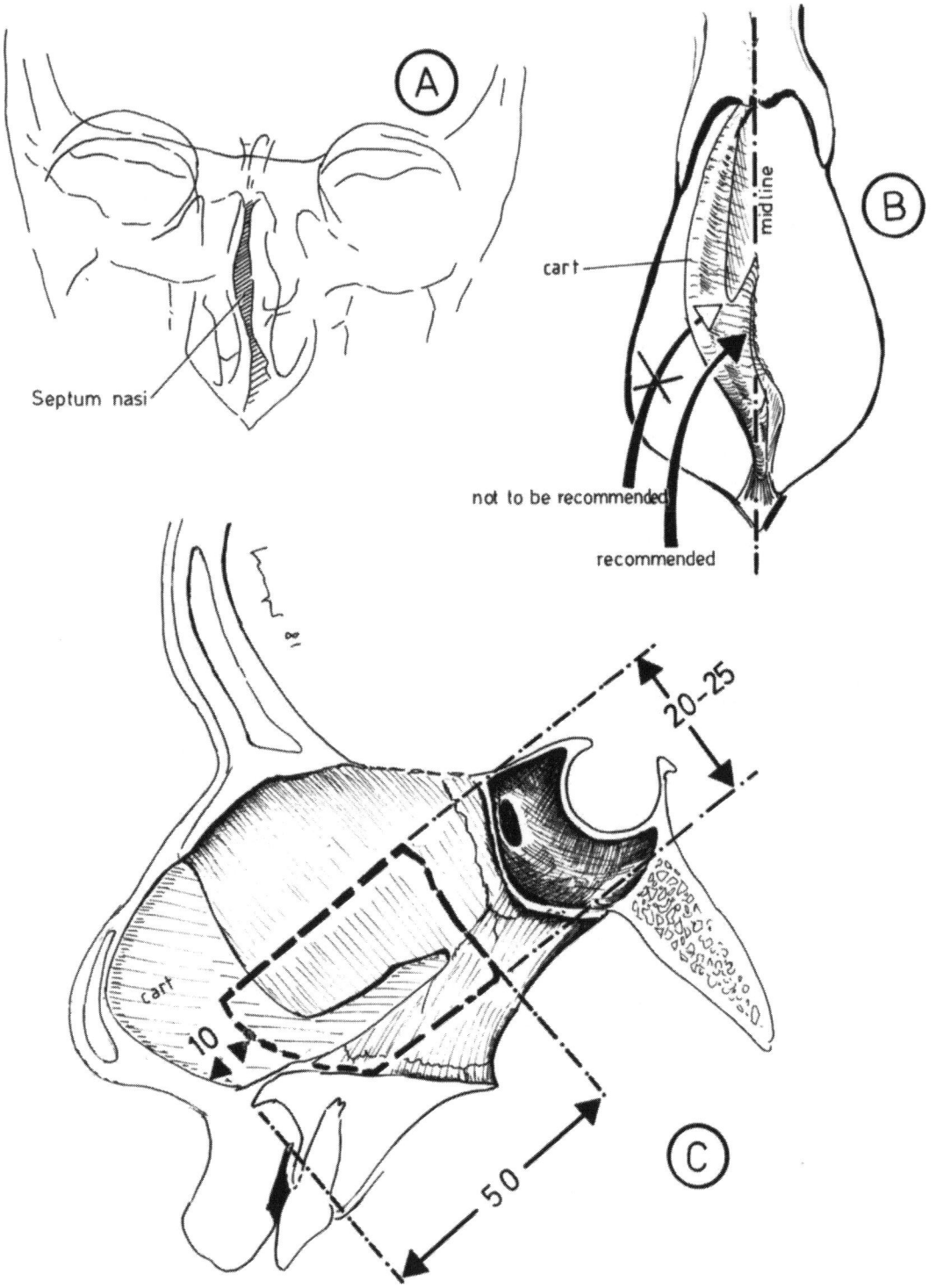
A
Septum nasi
B
midline
cart
not to be recommended
recommended
C
20-25
cart
10
50

Fig. 36. Hypophysis operation. **Resection of Septum nasi**

A – C Anterior view

A
- **1** Lifting up of upper lip and severed mucosa
- **2** Insertion of a spatula on Septum nasi
- **3** Holding back of mucosa
- **4** Incision of cartilaginous Septum nasi
  Broken line: Apertura piriformis

B Enlarged detail from **A**
- **1 – 3** As **A**
- **5** Separation of incised cartilage from contralateral mucosa with dissector. Arrows: movements of dissector. See also **C**
- **6a + 6b** Enlargement of cartilage incision, where the contralateral mucosa has been loosened.
  Dotted line: see **D**

C Model presentation of procedure **5, B'**, frontal section

D Bone resection, anatomical model
- *x:* Cartilaginous Septum nasi, already cut through (scissors **6** to be used only for resection of cartilage, not for bone resection)
- *y:* Dotted line-zone of bone resection using forceps. To begin with, resection does not extend as far as Corpus sphenoidale

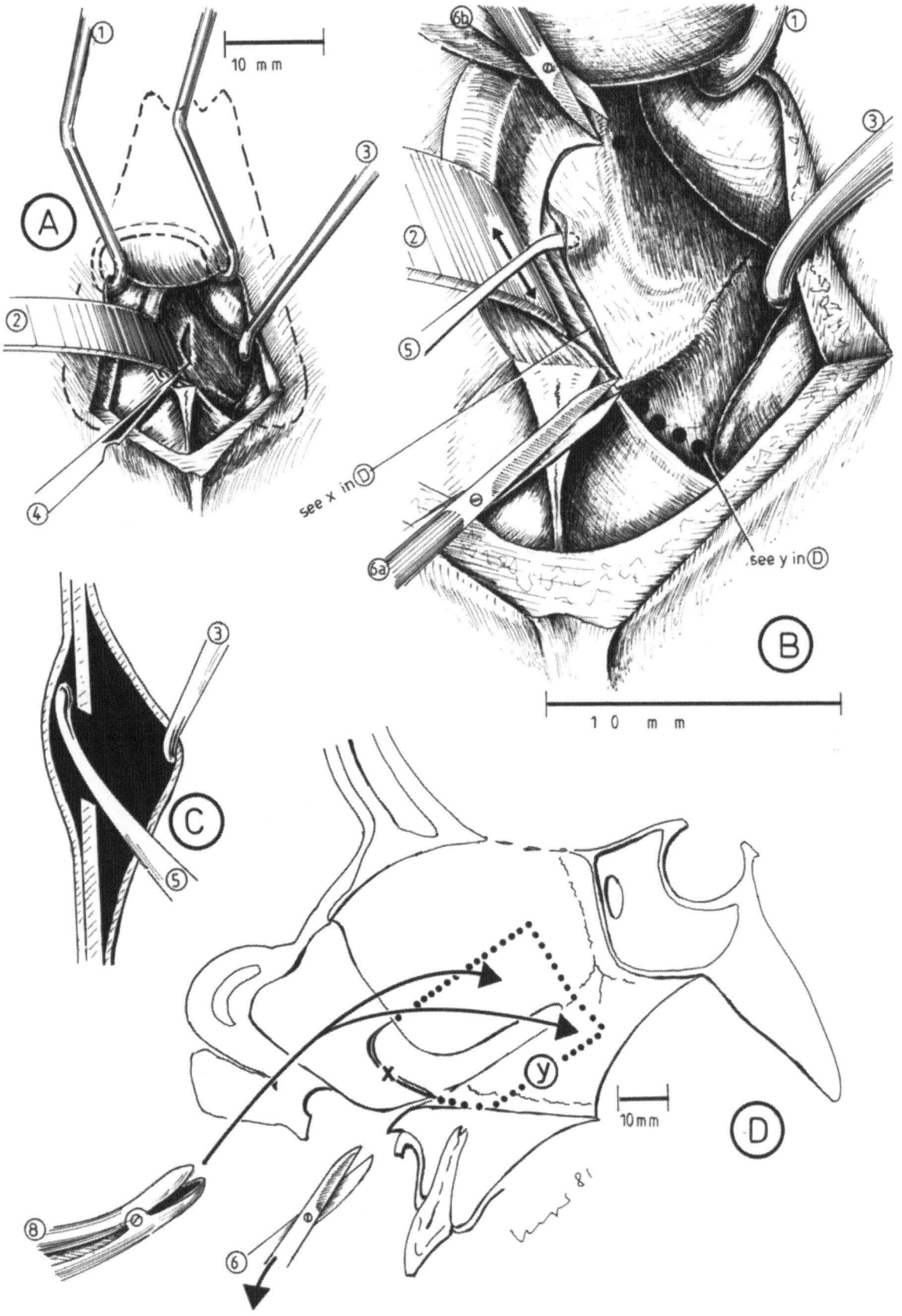
A
10 mm
B
10 mm
see x in D
see y in D
C
D
10mm

Fig. 37. Hypophysis operation. Locating **Corpus sphenoidale. Guiding structure** is **Apertura sphenoidalis**

A Anterior to Sinus sphenoidalis, a portion of Lamina mediana is preserved

B Enlarged detail from **A.** In the Apertura sinus sphenoidalis area mucosa is detached from bone surface. This mucosa continues interiorly as mucosa of Sinus sphenoidalis. Since the mucosa of Sinus sphenoidalis is removed, in the typical operative procedure, the only area where the mucosa should be opened is at Apertura sinus sphenoidalis

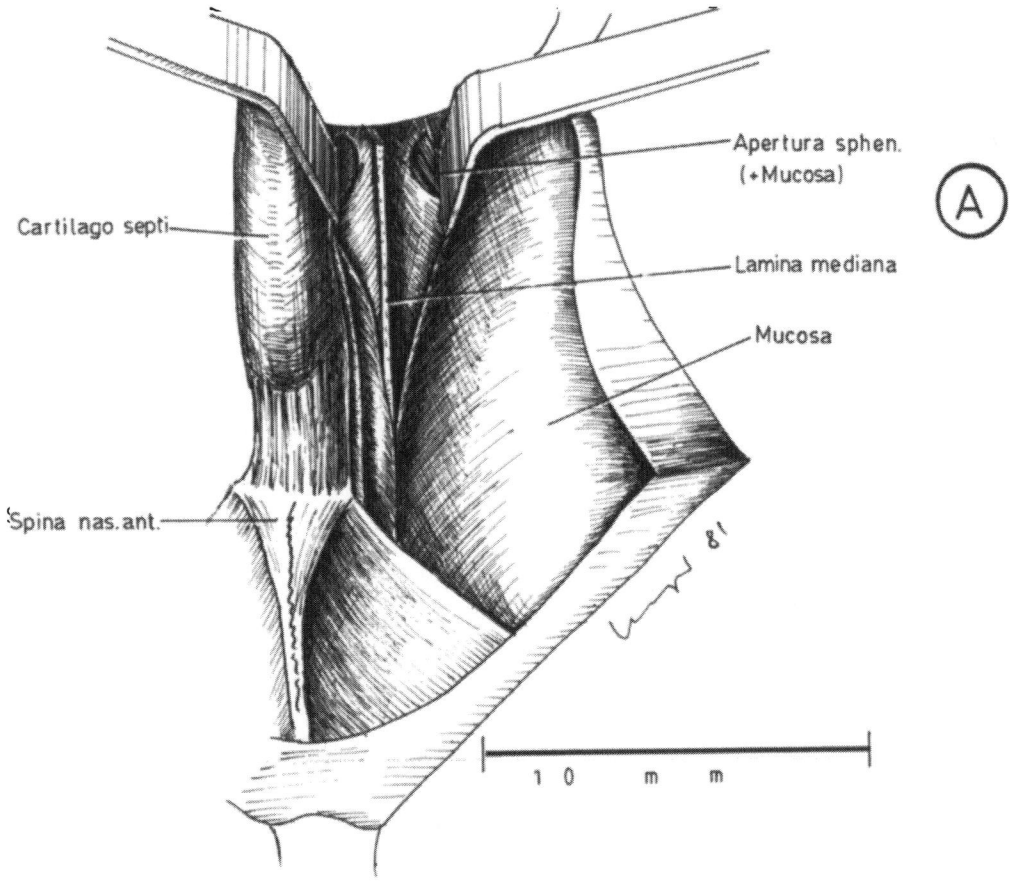
Apertura sphen.
(+Mucosa)
A
Cartilago septi
Lamina mediana
Mucosa
Spina nas. ant.
8'
1 0 m m

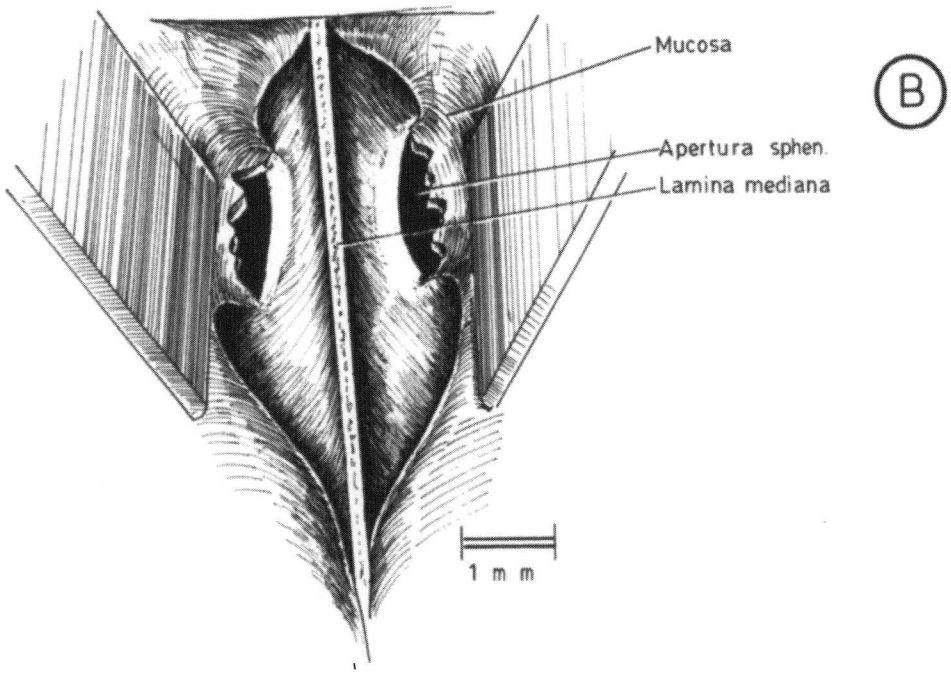
Mucosa
B
Apertura sphen.
Lamina mediana
1 m m

Fig. 38. Hypophysis operation. Microsurgical operation*

A Insertion of Hardy-speculum. Residuals of Septum nasi *–lm–* were resected previously with forceps nearly to the Os sphenoidale. Vomer and Ala vomeris are recognizable by their typical thickness

1 Resection of anterior wall of Sinus sphenoidalis, starting on both sides at Apertura sinus sphenoidalis *–asp–*

B **2b** The Sinus sphenoidalis mucosa is detached overall with dissector as thoroughly and cautiously as possible. As far as possible, leave no mucosa remnants in niches, since removal later on is difficult. Mucosa remnants mean the danger of mucocele development. Therefore forceps should not be used as yet **–2a–**

C **3** The already-detached mucosa is shrunk by electrocoagulation, in order to reach further mucosa portions easily (see **2b** in **B**)

4 Only when mucosa has been thoroughly detached should it be extracted with forceps. Slight stretching of not yet detached mucosa portions facilitates the detachment by means of dissector

Abbreviations:

asp Apertura sinus sphenoidalis
av Ala vomeris
lm Lamina mediana
vo Vomer

* Even the first part of the operation, starting with the mucosa incision, may be carried out microsurgically. Generally one uses the microsurgical technique once the Os sphenoidale is exposed.

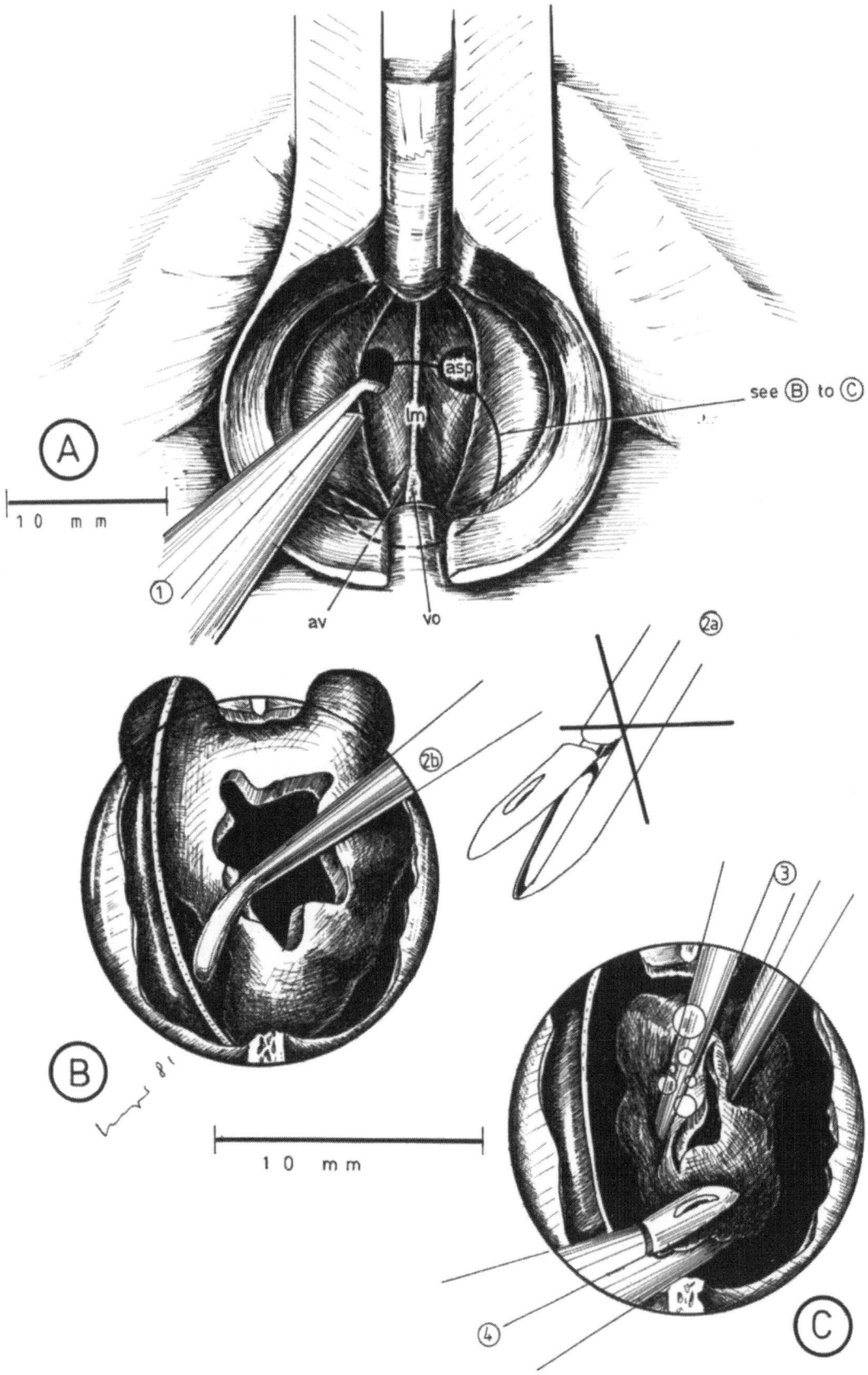
A
10 mm
asp
lm
see B to C
1
av
vo
2a
2b
B
10 mm
3
4
C

Fig. 39. Hypophysis operation. Topographical relation of **Septum sphenoidale** *–ssp–*

A Septum *–ssp–* presented in clinical example from Fig. 23

A' Anatomical model corresponding to **A.** The tumor can be reached even without septum resection (arrow)

B Another variant of Septum sphenoidale

B' Anatomical model, frontal section, corresponding to **B.** Without septum resection the tumor can be only partially removed

B'' After septum resection the tumor can be reached on both sides (arrows)

C Anatomical sketch of section planes **A', B'** and **B''**, median section plane

Abbreviation:

ssp Septum sphenoidale

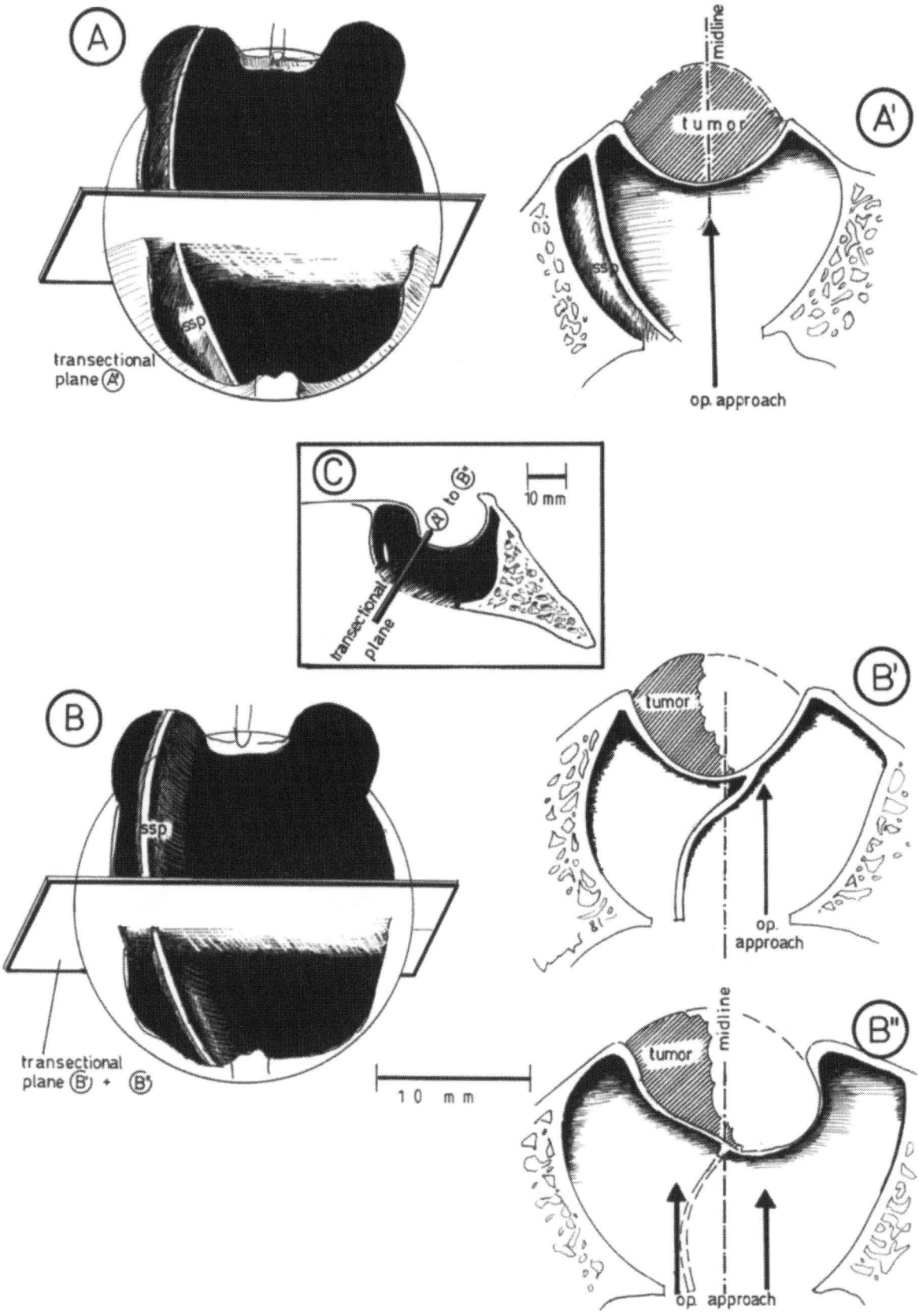
A
ssp
transectional plane A'
midline
tumor
A'
ssp
op. approach
C
A to B'
10 mm
transectional plane
B
ssp
transectional plane B' + B''
10 mm
tumor
B'
op. approach
tumor
midline
B''
op. approach

Fig. 40. Hypophysis operation. **Opening up of sella space**

A Microsurgical site

1a + 1b Chiseling of bony sella floor

2 Enlargement of opening by means of a rongeur.

Open arrow: deep posterior recessus of Sinus sphenoidalis (towards Dorsum sellae)

A' Anatomical model, sagittal section. Situation as in **A**

B Microsurgical site

1 Dura incision

2 Dura detachment with dissector

B' Anatomical model, sagittal section, corresponding to **B**

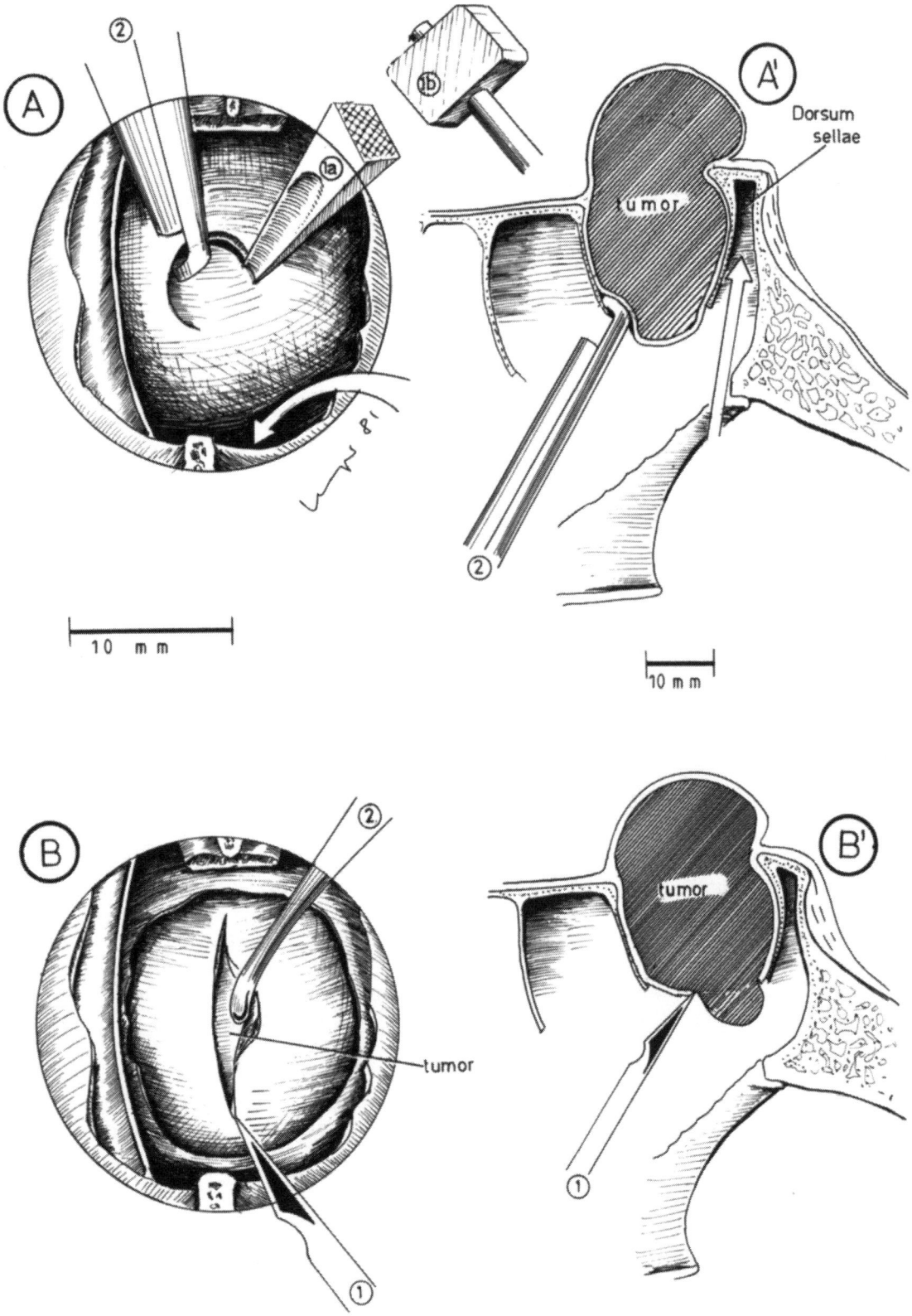
A
2
1a
1b
A'
Dorsum
sellae
tumor
2
10 mm
10 mm
B
2
tumor
1
B'
tumor
1

Fig. 41. Hypophysis operation. **Tumor extirpation**

A Microsurgical site

1a + 1b Curettage of tumor (various types of curettes see Fig. 29)
Loosening on both sides of lateral tumor portions

A' Anatomical model, sagittal section

2a + 2b Loosening of anterior and posterior tumor portions

B Main bulk of tumor is removed. Diaphragma sellae becomes visible. If Diaphragma sellae extends deeply in an inferior direction, the risk exists that marginal tumor portions remain

3a + 3b Cautious removal of lateral tumor portions

B' Anatomical model, sagittal section

4a + 4b Removal of anterior and posterior tumor remnants.
Arrows: Directions of instrument movements

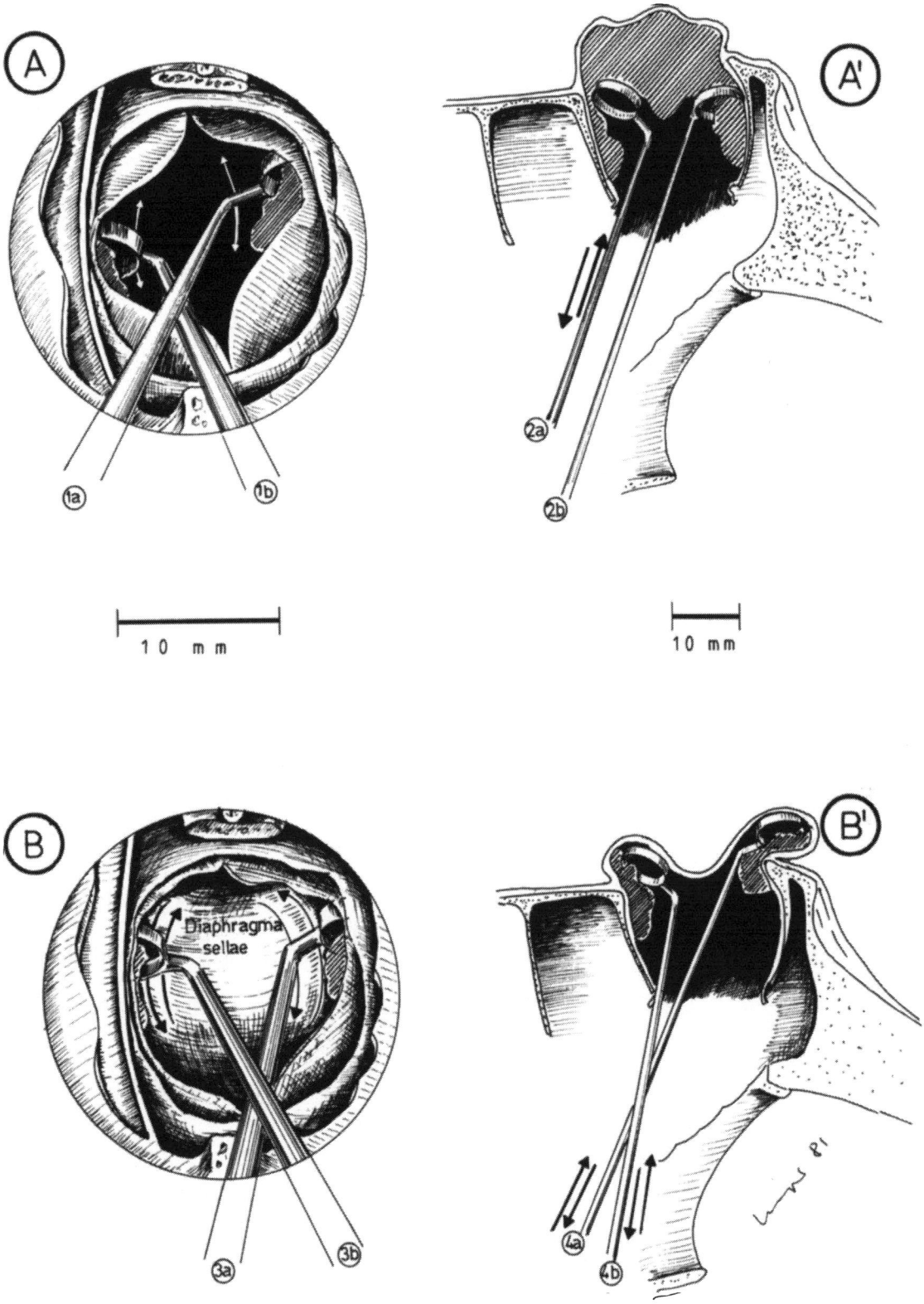
A
1a
1b
10 mm
A'
2a
2b
10 mm
B
Diaphragma sellae
3a
3b
B'
4a
4b

Fig. 42. Hypophysis operation

A Microsurgical site after tumor removal

d transverse diameter of bone defect in the sella floor

d'' transverse diameter of dura defect in the sella floor

B Disc out of cartilage, lyophilized dura (or bone). Oval piece cut from Septum nasi or from a piece of lyodura, in order to **cover dura defect in sella floor** (see **A**) from inside. Finishing of disc, see Fig. 43

C Microsurgical site. Disc is eased through dura gap to the inside. Open arrows: adjustment of disc until dura defect is completely covered from inside

C' Anatomical model of **C**, sagittal section. The properly fitted disc is fastened with tissue glue (fibrinogen concentrate)

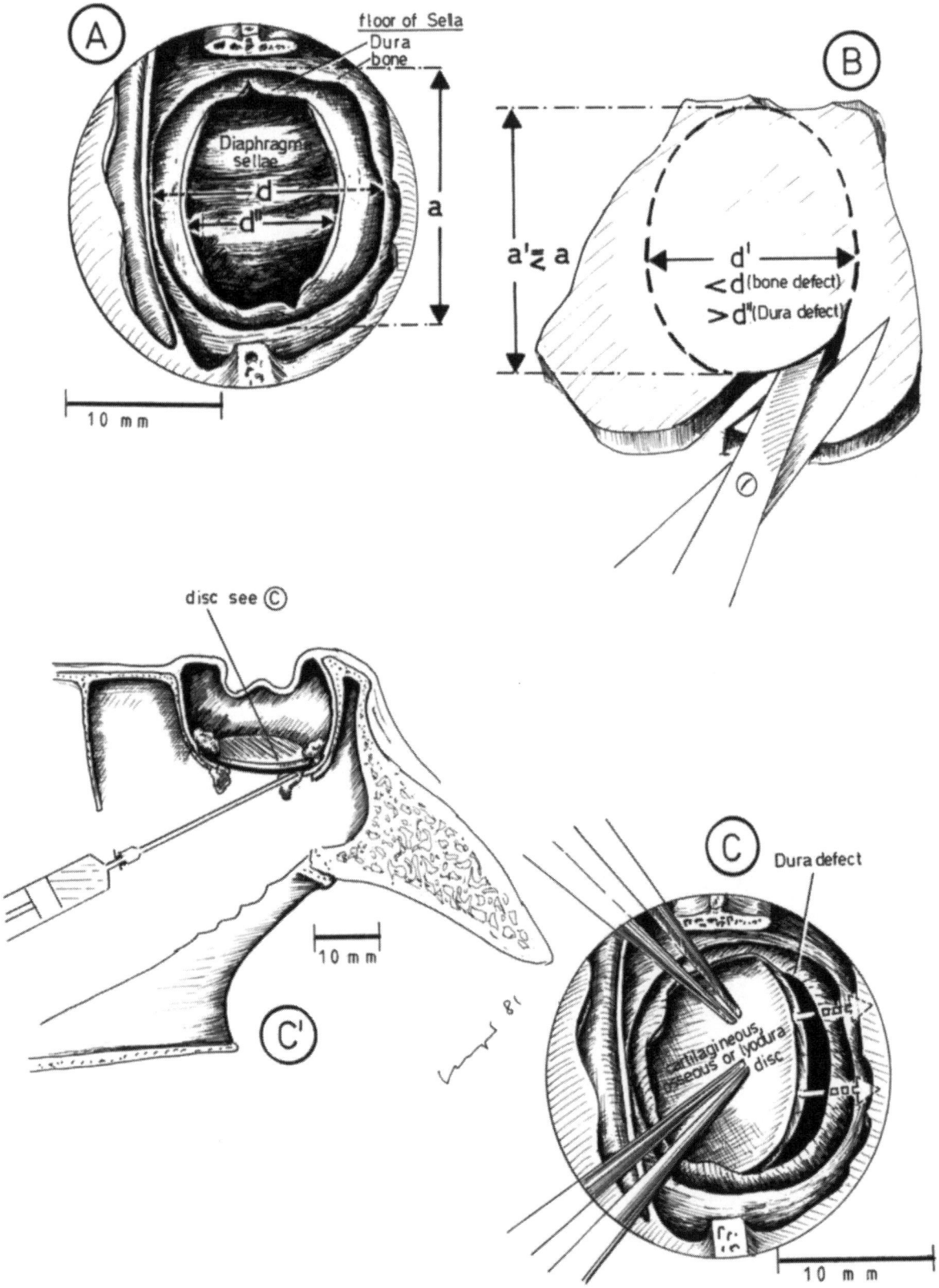
A
floor of Sella
Dura
bone
Diaphragma
sellae
d
d''
a
10 mm
B
a' ≷ a
d'
< d (bone defect)
> d'' (Dura defect)
disc see C
10 mm
C'
C
Dura defect
cartilagineous,
osseous or lyodura
disc
10 mm

Fig. 43. Hypophysis operation
Finishing of a disc flap from bone (**A**) or cartilage (**B**). Technique for **insertion of flap to the inside of dura defect**

A Finishing of flap from bone
B Cutting of cartilage
B' Slicing of cartilage if too thick
B'' Oblique trimming of the cartilage edges, in order to obtain a fine edge, which can be eased through dura opening
C Easing of disc to the inside of sella dura lining *–f–*

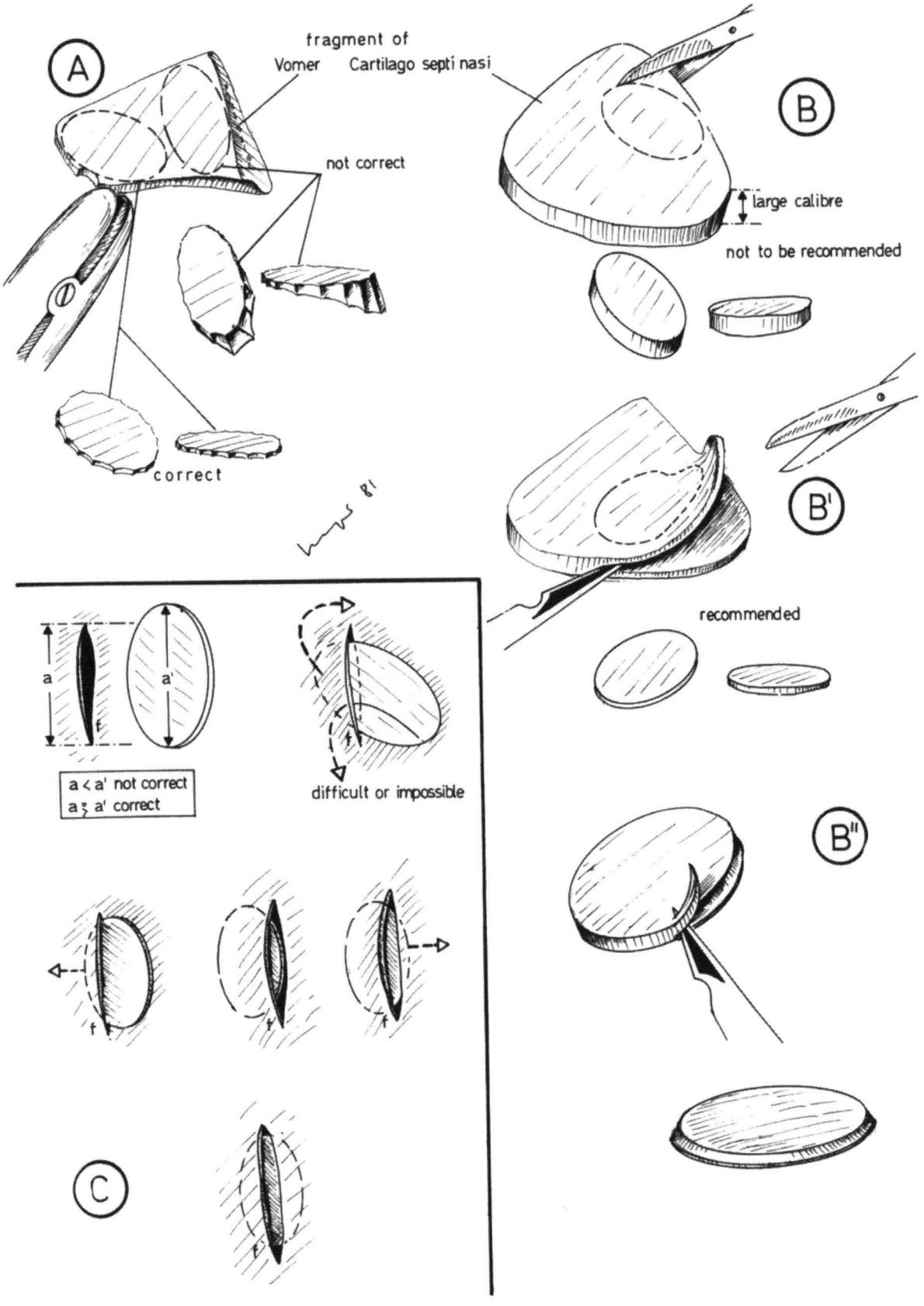
A
fragment of
Vomer
Cartilago septi nasi
not correct
correct
B
large calibre
not to be recommended
B'
recommended
a
a'
f
a < a' not correct
a ≥ a' correct
difficult or impossible
B''
C

Fig. 44. Hypophysis operation
Principle of **tamponage of Cavum nasi** with gauze

A **Correct procedure:** Using forceps, grasp gauze away from its end a; and insert it through Meatus nasi inferior

A' **Incorrect procedure:**
- Gauze gripped at its end (danger of gauze end slipping into choane area and narrowing upper respiratory tract, see **B'**)
- Insertion diagonally through Cavum nasi upwards. This prevents tamponage of the posterior portions of Cavum nasi

B Correct tamponage, by which gauze end –arrow *a*– is pressed against floor of Cavum nasi

B' **Incorrect:** Gauze end has come free, thereby narrowing the upper respiratory tract

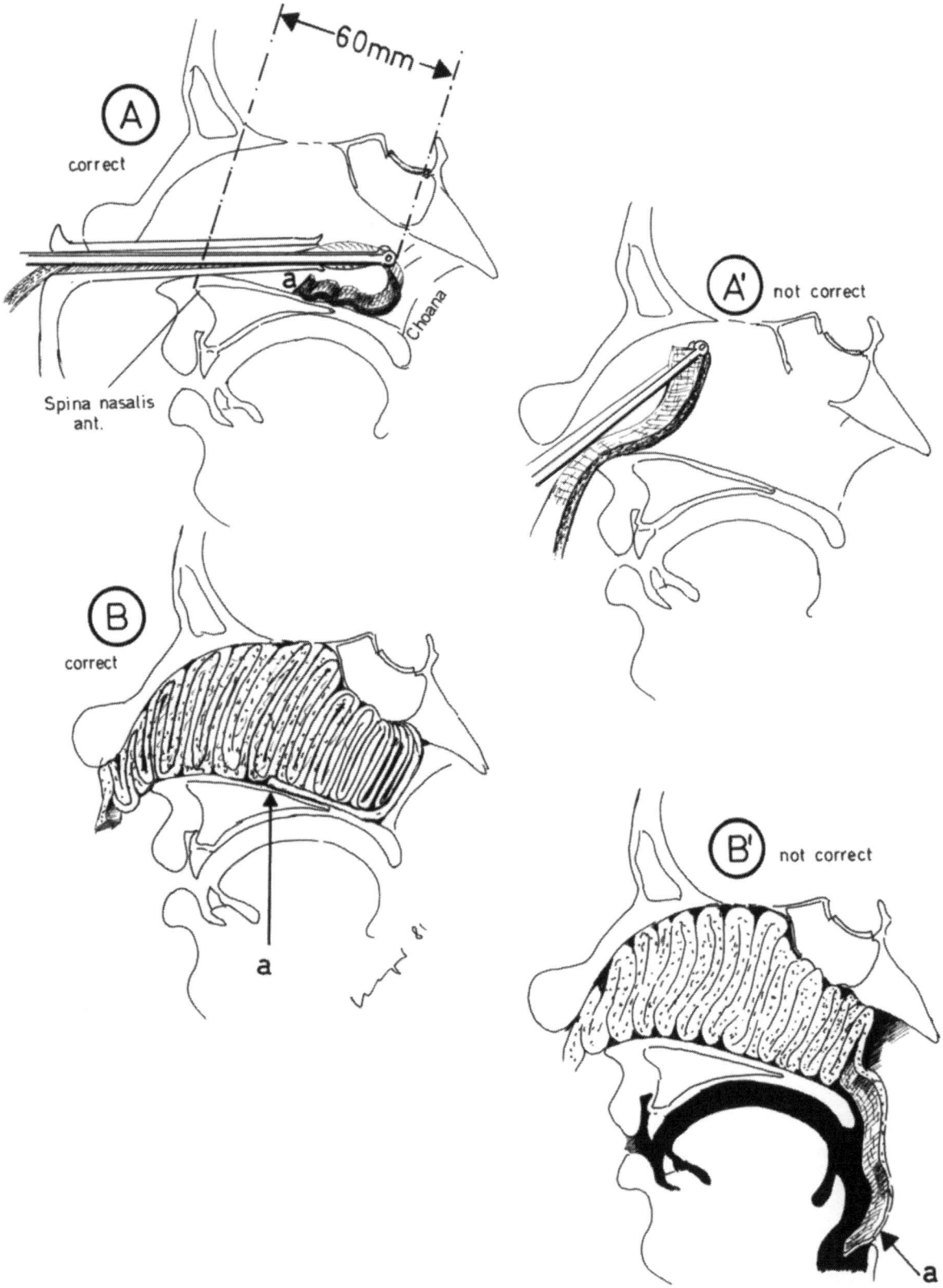
60mm
A
correct
a
Choana
Spina nasalis
ant.
A'
not correct
B
correct
a
B'
not correct
a

Fig. 45. Hypophysis operation. Tamponage with foam material. Possible mistakes (refer also to gauze tamponage)

A Correct tamponage. Measurements in mm

B Incorrect tamponage: posterior portions of Cavum nasi not packed, creating danger of blood seepage from injured mucosa of Cavum nasi or sinus into naso-pharyngeal space.

C Incorrect tamponage: packing not only Cavum nasi, but also Epipharynx with narrowing of Epi- and Mesopharynx

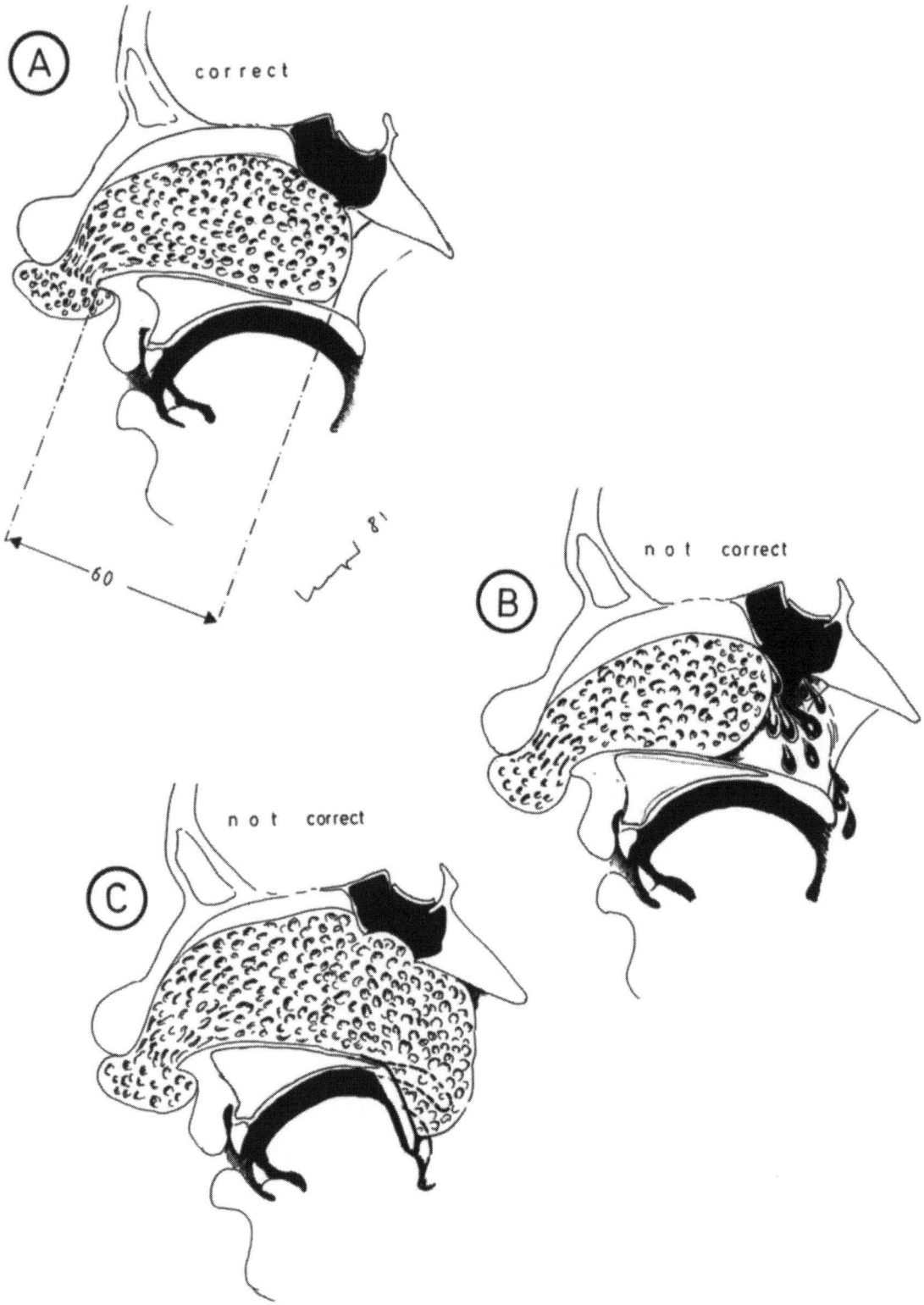
A
correct
60
81
B
not correct
C
not correct

Fig. 46. Hypophysis operation
Wound closure

A Gingiva suture

B Tamponage of Cavum nasi with foam material –*a*– or with gauze –*b*– (soakend with salve) after insertion of a speculum

C Situation after tamponage of both nasal openings

D Adhesive bandage over tamponage

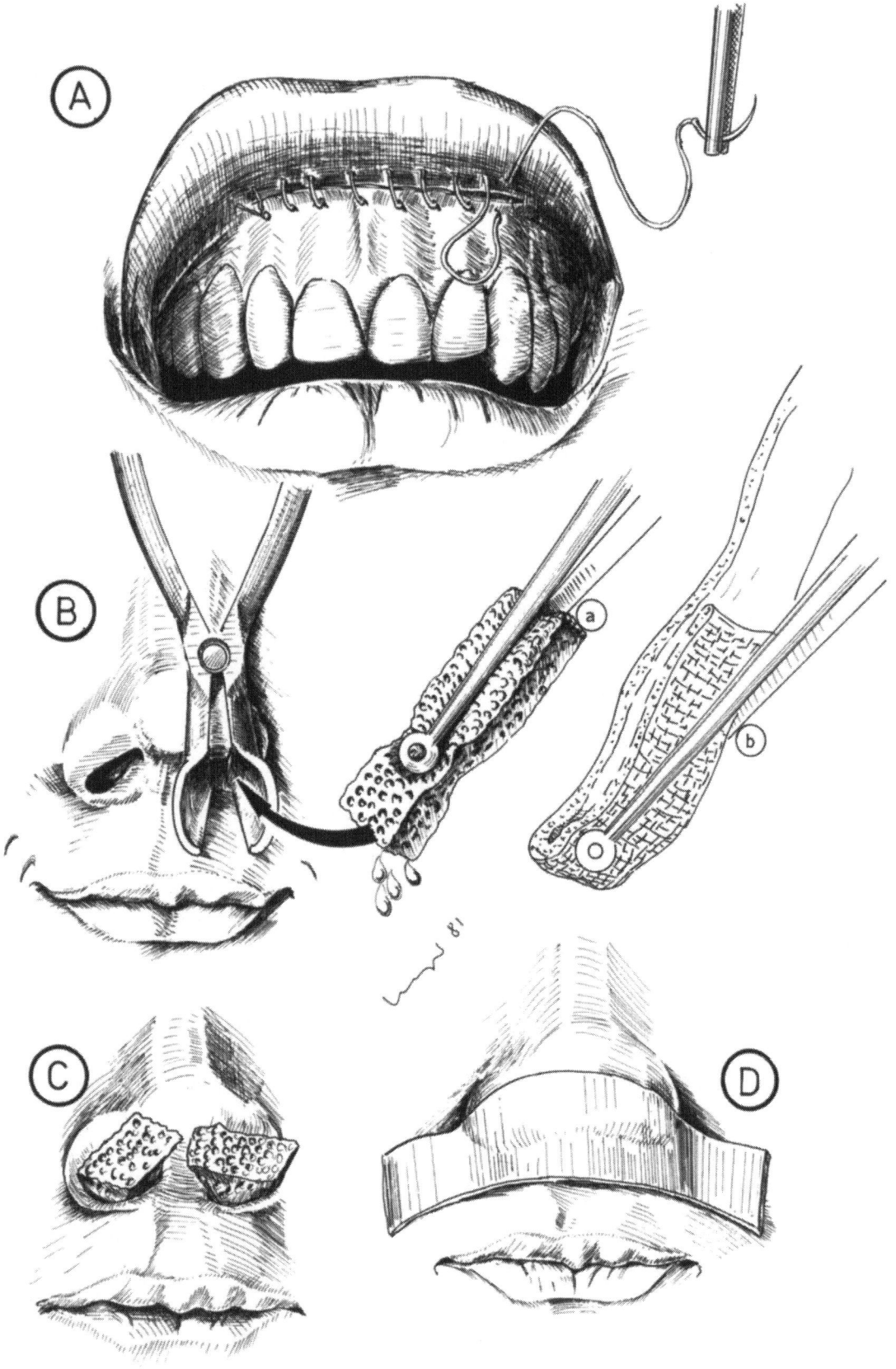
A
B
a
b
C
D

Fig. 47. Hypophysis operation

Special situations: liquorrhea through defect of Diaphragma sellae

A Microsurgical site. One sees defect in Diaphragma sellae and arachnoidea centrally located at penetration area of hypophyseal stalk

A' Anatomical model, sagittal section

B Micorosurgical site after deposition of fatty tissue into sella space

- **1** Squirting of tissue glue* (Fibrinogen and activator) around fatty tissue
- **2** Pressing of fatty tissue after introduction of tissue glue

B' Anatomical model, sagittal section

1 + 2 as in **B**

C Microsurgical site

1a + 1b Closing of sella floor with cartilagineous or osseous disc cut from Septum nasi

C' Anatomical model

2 Squirting cartilage disc with tissue glue*

---

* Immuno-Chemie, Heidelberg.

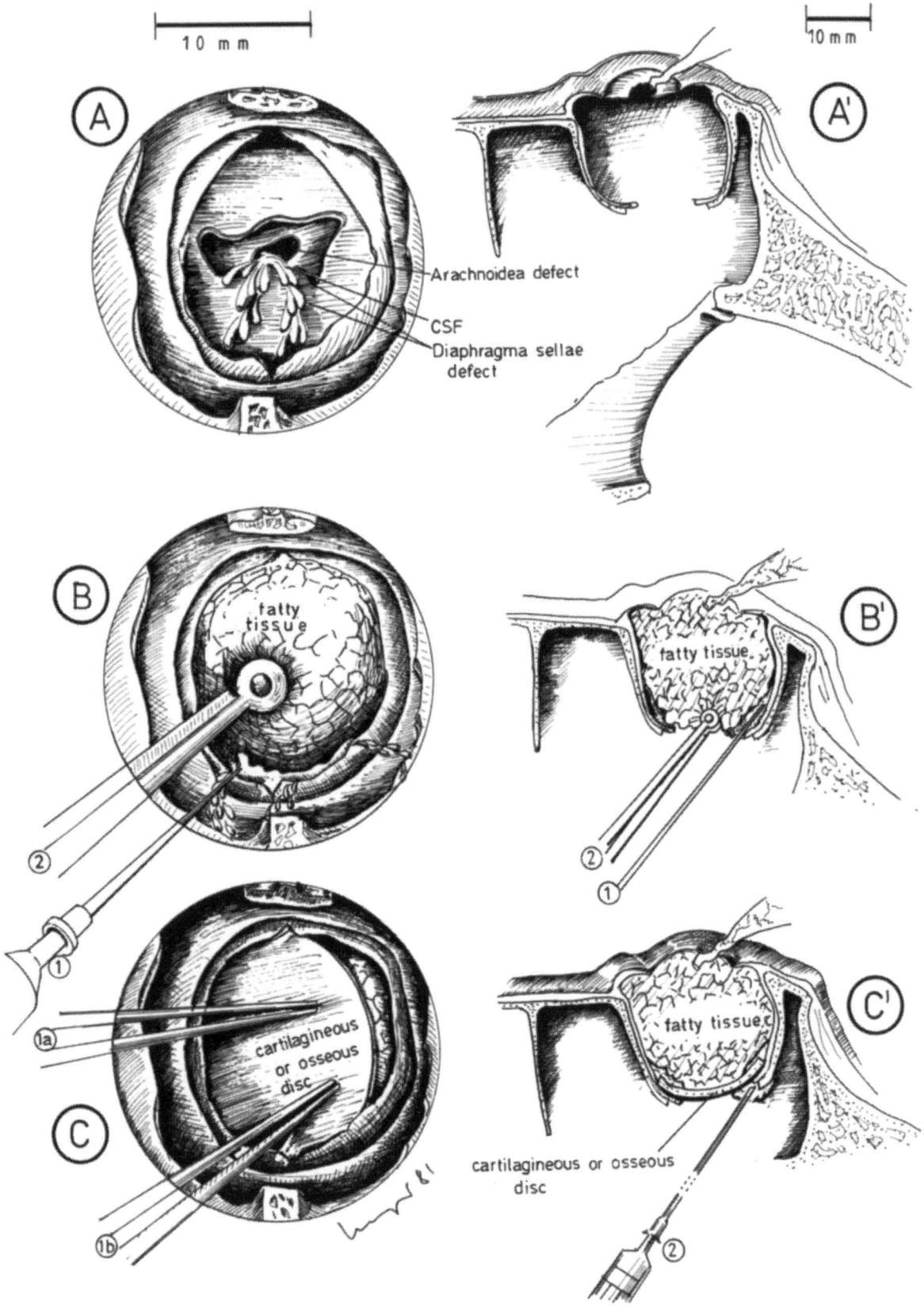
10 mm
10 mm
A
A'
Arachnoidea defect
CSF
Diaphragma sellae defect
B
B'
fatty tissue
fatty tissue
2
1
C
C'
1a
1b
cartilagineous or osseous disc
fatty tissue
cartilagineous or osseous disc
2

Fig. 48. Hypophysis operations. Special situations:
Suprasellar tumor portion without dura cover

A Anatomical model, sagittal section. Suprasellar tumor portions without dura cover. A. basilaris *–b1–*, N.II (as well as Hypothalamus, perforating arteries, Pons) lie directly against the tumor. By oro-nasal approach, the overview is not sufficiently safe to avoid injuring these structures during tumor removal

A' Anatomical model, continuation and enlargement from **A,** sagittal section

B Microsurgical site. Tumor partially removed. In spite of large residual tumor, liquorrhea shows existence of situation **A'**

If dura cover of suprasellar tumor portion is absent, this operative approach must be halted and tumor removal must be finished later by transcranial approach

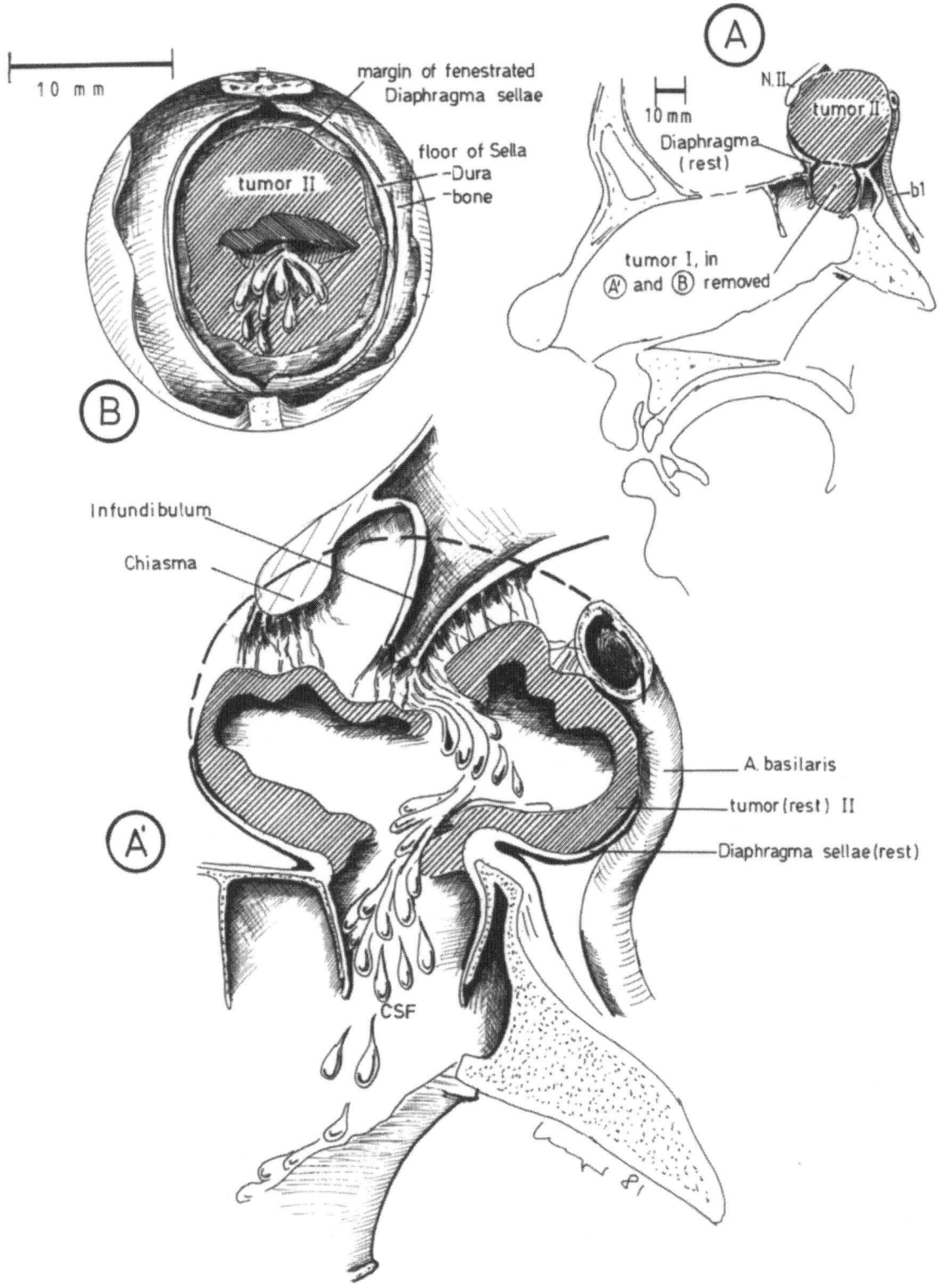
10 mm
margin of fenestrated
Diaphragma sellae
floor of Sella
-Dura
-bone
tumor II
B
A
10 mm
N.II
tumor II
Diaphragma
(rest)
bl
tumor I, in
A' and B removed
Infundibulum
Chiasma
A. basilaris
tumor (rest) II
Diaphragma sellae (rest)
A'
CSF

Fig. 49. Hypophysis operations. Special situations: Normal Diaphragma sellae, **tumor extension predominantly supradiaphragmatical without dura cover**

A Anatomical model, sagittal section

A' Enlarged detail from **A**

B Microsurgical site, corresponding to **A** and **A'**

If dura cover of suprasellar tumor portion is absent, operative approach must be halted for the same reason as in Fig. 48

Abbreviation:

ds Diaphragma sella, defect

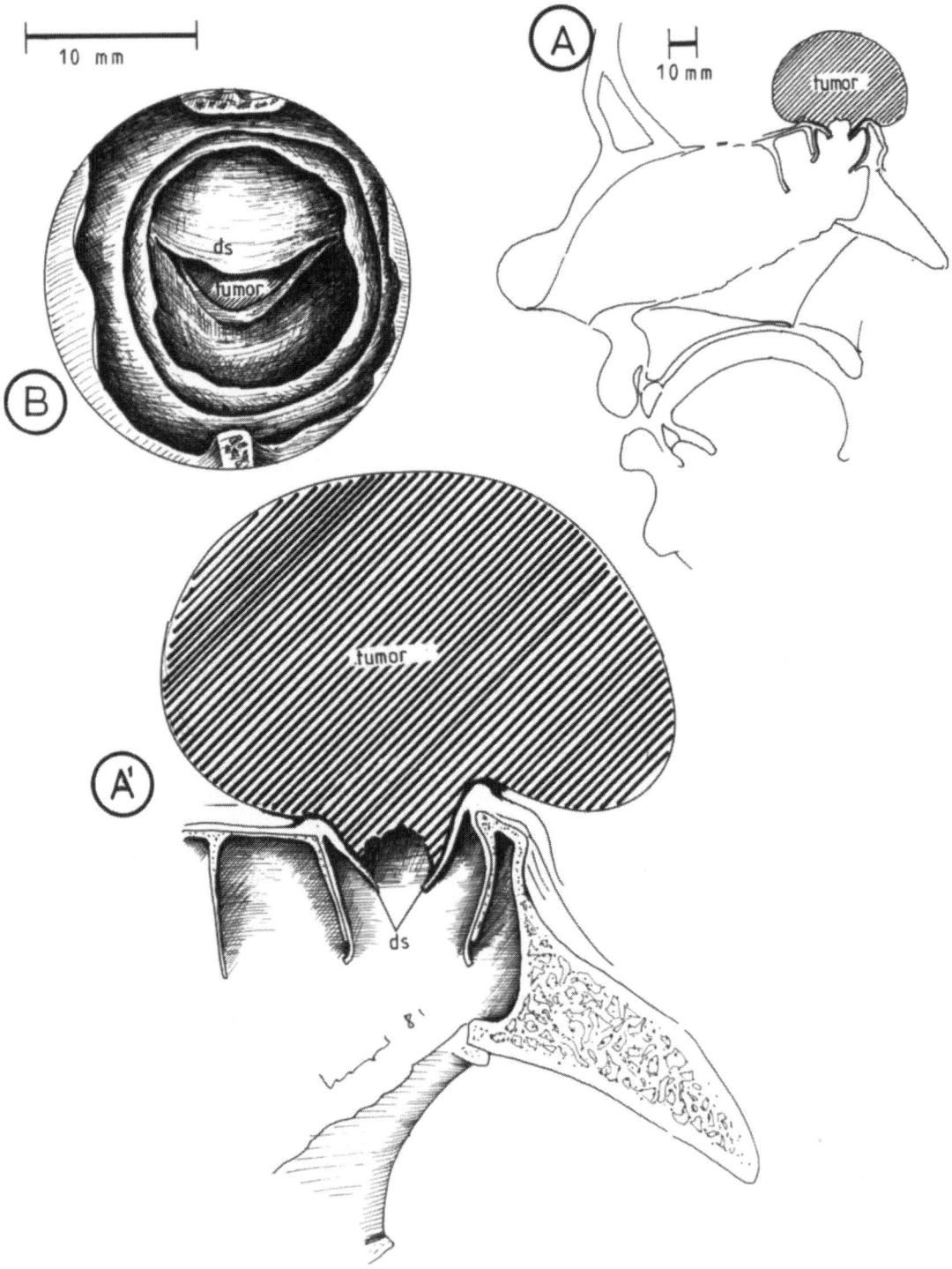
10 mm
A
10 mm
tumor
ds
tumor
B
tumor
A'
ds
8'

Chapter 2

Operations at Sinus cavernosus (Figs. 50–99)

Anatomy of Sinus cavernosus (Figs. 50 to 54)

Fig. 50. Operations in the area surrounding Sinus cavernosus.

Anatomy of **intradural path of A. carotis int.** and its branches*

A View from above: In this sketch: On the left side A. ophthalmica originates intradurally from A. carotis int; on the right side extradurally

A' + A'' A. communicans post. *–p5–* and A. chorioidea *–c5–* may originate proximally or distally from A. carotis int.; their points of origin may be close together or far apart

A''' **In the case of proximal origin of A. communicans post. and A. chorioidea ant. these vessels may be partly covered by the elongated tentorial fold. When clipping A. carotis int. at its penetration point there is danger of closing off these two arteries (especially A. communicans post.) with their perforating branches which run beneath A. carotis int.**

B Preparation similar to **A,** basal view. In addition to the typical perforating arteries from A. communicans post. and A. chorioidea ant., perforating arteries *–x–* (running to Hypothalamus) may originate directly from the A. carotis int. (according to Dawson, 1968)

Abbreviations:

c1 A. carotis int.
c5 A. chorioidea ant.
p5 A. communicans post.
te Tentorium edge
x Atypical perforating arteries

* Extensive presentation see J. Lang, 1979.

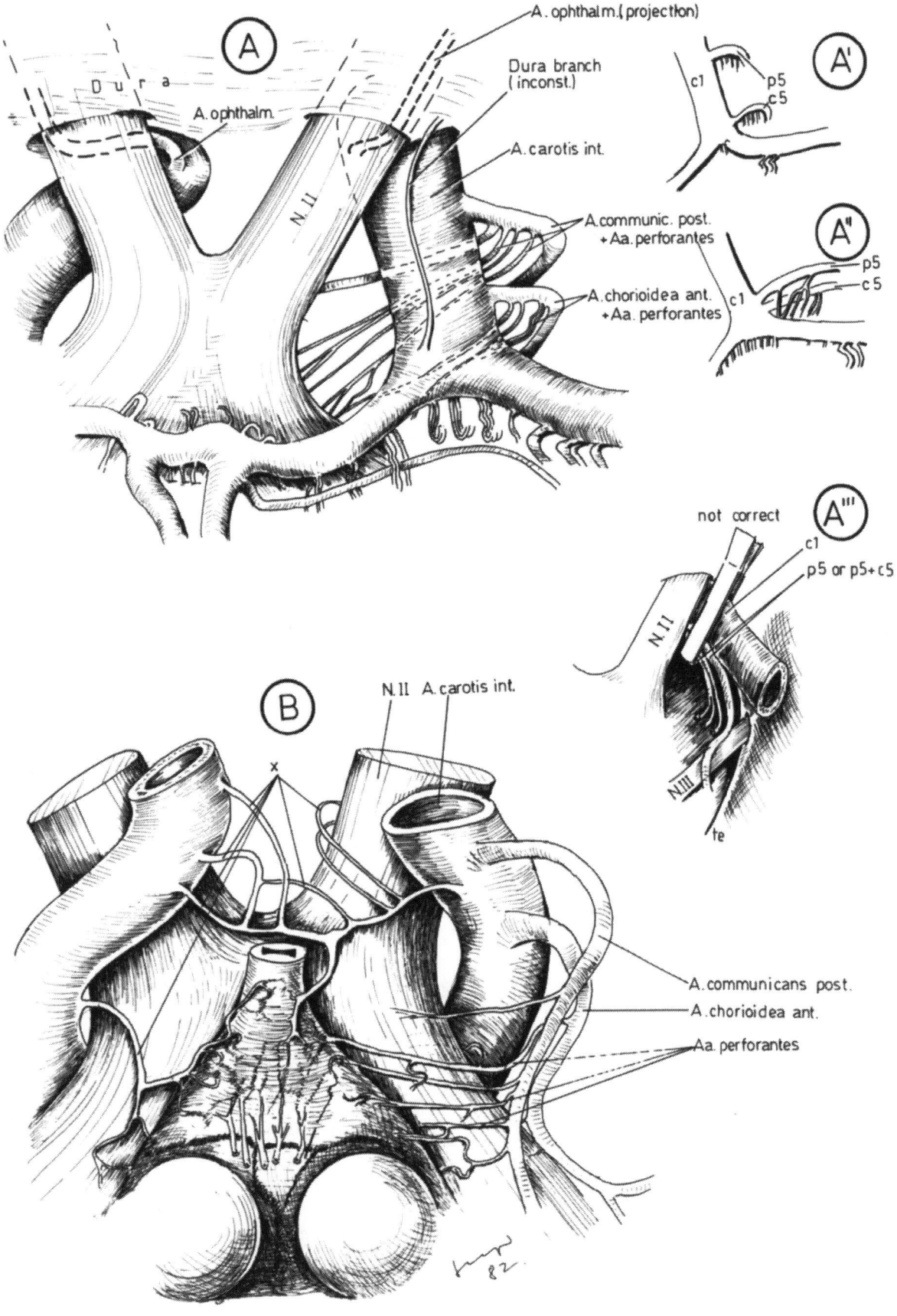
A
A. ophthalm. (projection)
Dura
A. ophthalm.
Dura branch
(inconst.)
A. carotis int.
N. II
A. communic. post.
+ Aa. perforantes
A. chorioidea ant.
+ Aa. perforantes
A'
c1
p5
c5
A''
p5
c5
c1
A'''
not correct
c1
p5 or p5+c5
N. II
N. III
te
B
N. II
A. carotis int.
x
A. communicans post.
A. chorioidea ant.
Aa. perforantes

Fig. 51. Operations in the area surrounding Sinus cavernosus.
Anatomy of the **parasellar area,** example of a skull showing senile bone atrophy
A Overview
B Enlarged detail from **A**

Abbreviations:

ca Processus clinoideus ant.
fo Foramen opticum
fos Fissura orbitalis sup.
flc Foramen lacerum
fov Foramen ovale
incl Incision of Processus clinoideus and Radix of Processus clinoideus ant. anterior to A. carotis int.
rc Radix of Proc. clin. ant.
rt Foramen rotundum
sc Sulcus caroticus
st Sella turcica
ts Tuberculum sellae

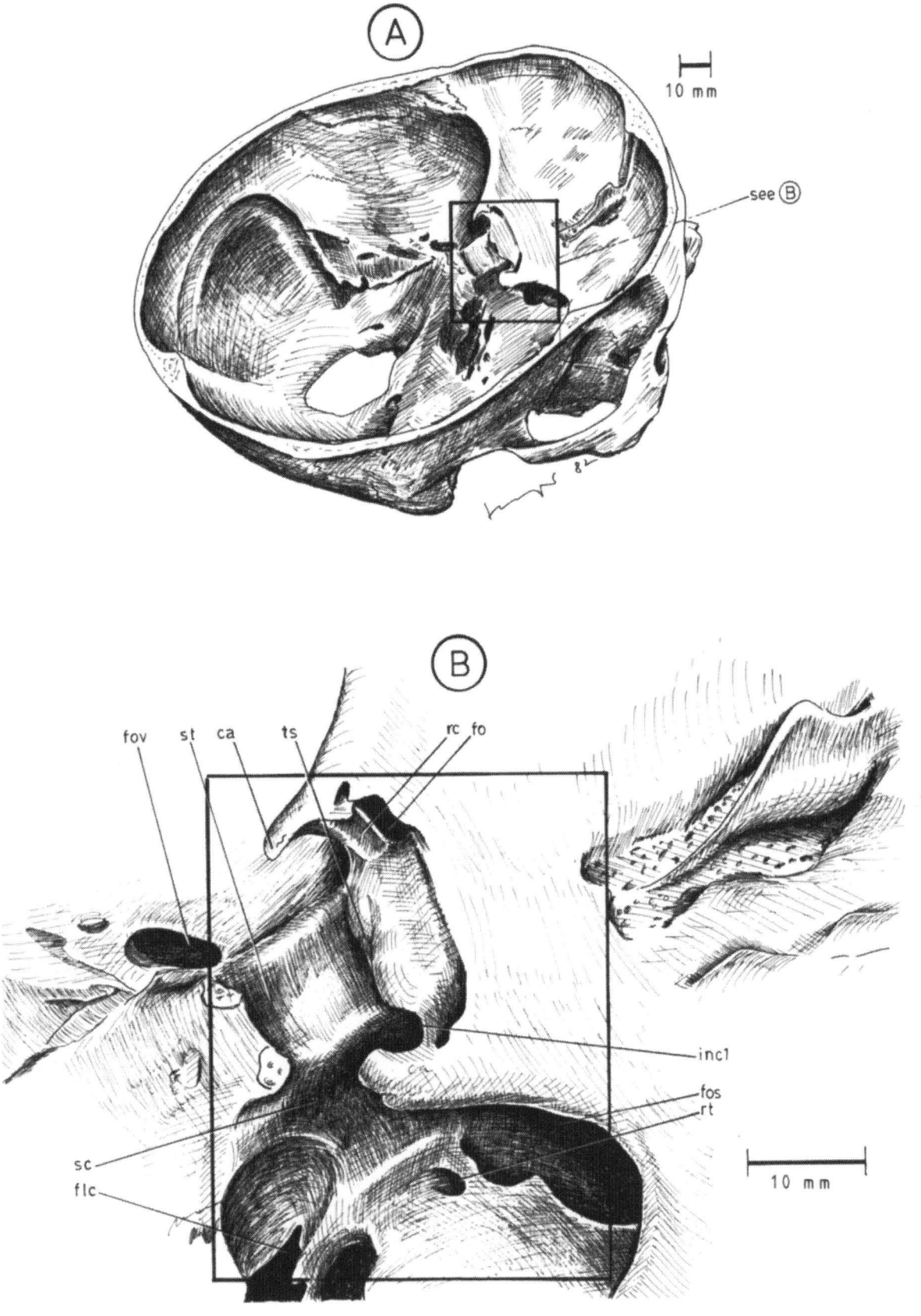
A
10 mm
see B
B
fov
st
ca
ts
rc
fo
incl
fos
rt
sc
flc
10 mm

Fig. 52. Operations in the area surrounding Sinus cavernosus.
Anatomy of the **parasellar area.** Preparation from Fig. 51, vessels and nerves sketched in. Dura structures with veins and N. maxillaris omitted
A Detail, corresponding to Fig. 51
B Enlarged detail from **A**

Abbreviations:

fos Fissura orbitalis sup.
rt Foramen rotundum
st Sella turcica
ts Tuberculum sellae

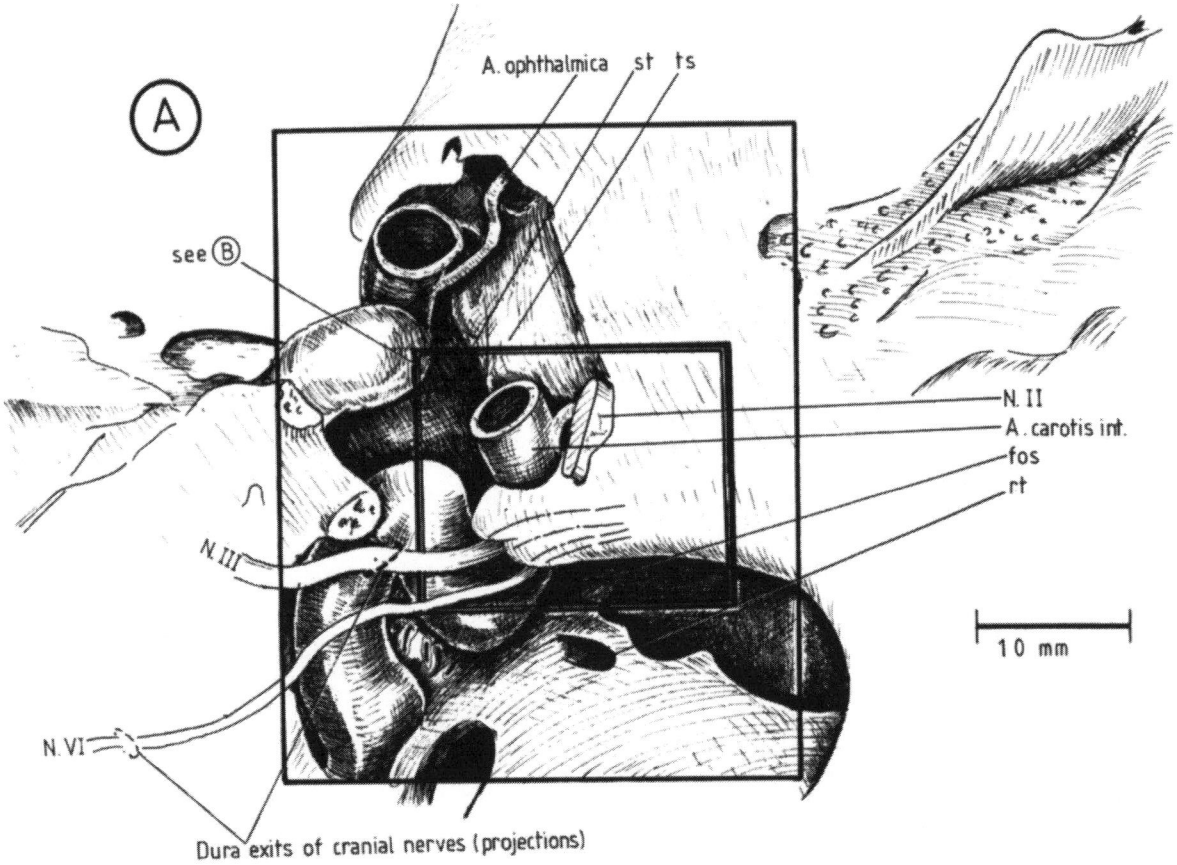
A
A. ophthalmica
st
ts
see B
N. II
A. carotis int.
fos
rt
N. III
10 mm
N. VI
Dura exits of cranial nerves (projections)

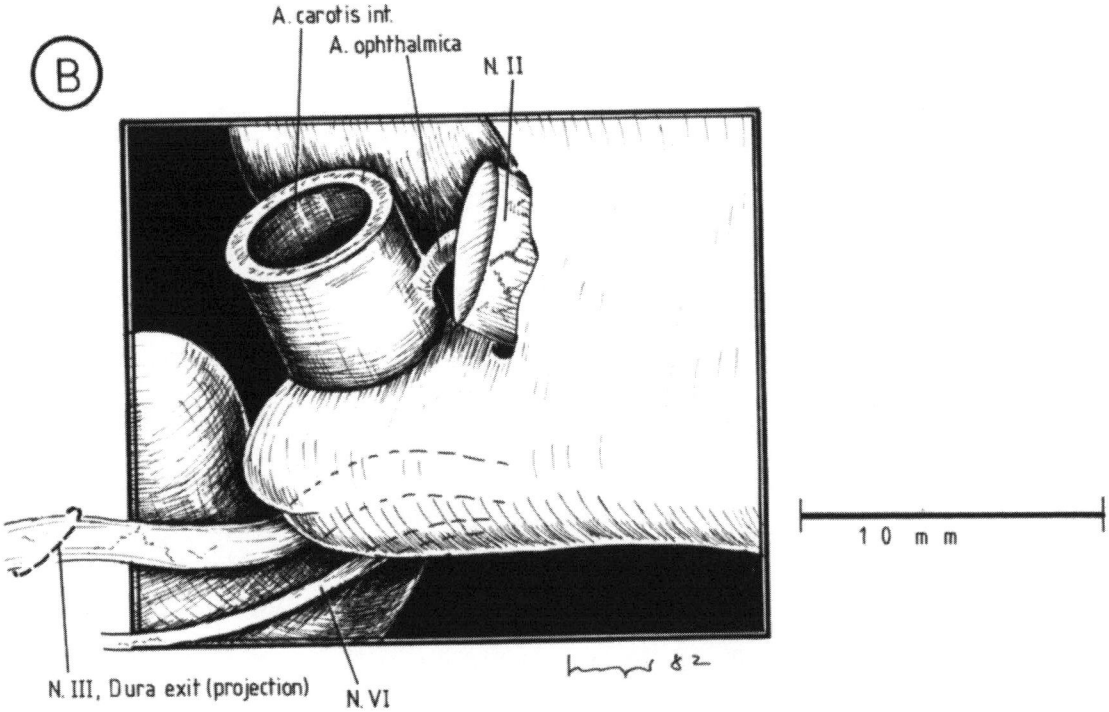
B
A. carotis int.
A. ophthalmica
N. II
10 mm
N. III, Dura exit (projection)
N. VI

Fig. 53. Operations in the area surrounding Sinus cavernosus.

Anatomy of path of A. ophthalmica, variants* (frequency percentage)

Path of A. ophthalmica after resection of Canalis opticus roof (**A, C** and **D**) with additional resection of Processus clinoideus ant. and its covering dura (**A' + B**)

A Typical path of A. ophthalmica

A' Same preparation as **A,** N.III and N.VI sketched in

B Rare variant: A. ophthalmica with its own bony canal. N.III and N.VI sketched in

C Second most frequent variant

D Rare variant: A. ophthalmica is replaced by branch of A. meningea media.

The typical path of A. ophthalmica (see A) is thus characterized: origin *–o–* is medial anterior from the point where A. carotis int. penetrates dura; path continues laterally behind N. opticus with a loop *–an–*forward then to leave dura sheath of N. opticus –penetration point *p* –

Abbreviations:

c1 A. carotis int.

c2 A. ophthalmica

---

* After S. S. Haydreh and R. Dass (1962), modified.

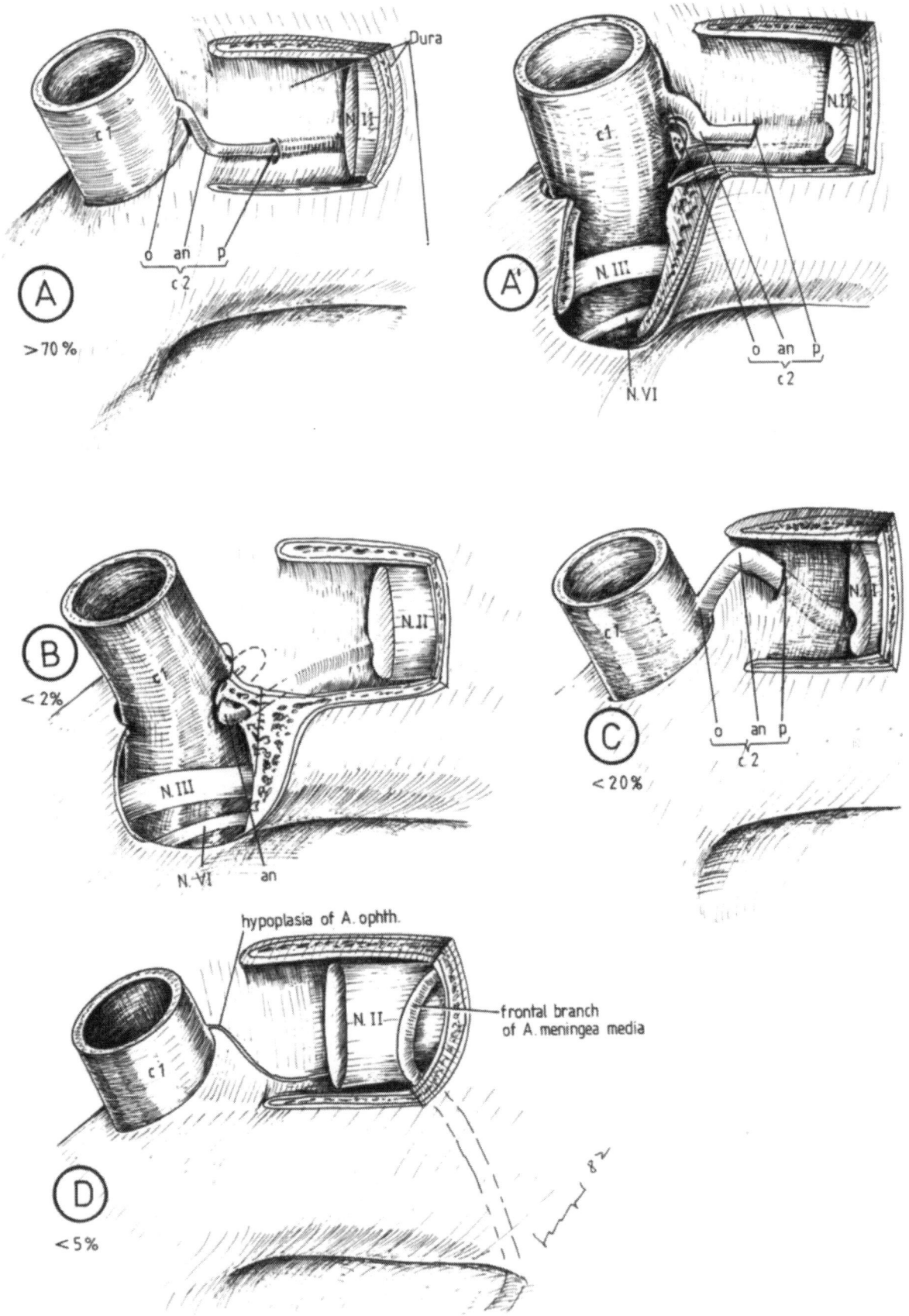
Dura
c1
N. II
o an p
c2
A
>70 %
A'
N. III
N. VI
B
<2%
C
<20%
hypoplasia of A. ophth.
frontal branch
of A. meningea media
D
<5%

Fig. 54. Operations in the area surrounding Sinus cavernosus.

Anatomical topographical relation of **A. carotis int. penetration point** to adjoining structures

A Anatomical sketch, similar to Fig. 52 **B,** dura sketched in. Structures covered by dura are sketched in with broken lines

B Anatomical sketch as in **A,** dura and bone partially removed

Abbreviations:

ca Processus clinoideus ant.
(ca) Processus clinoideus ant. (projection)
cl A. carotis int.
(cl) A. carotis int. (projection)
(N.VI) N. abducens (projection)
rca Pneumosinus in the area of Radix processus clinoidei (protrusion of Sinus sphenoidalis)
ts Tuberculum sellae

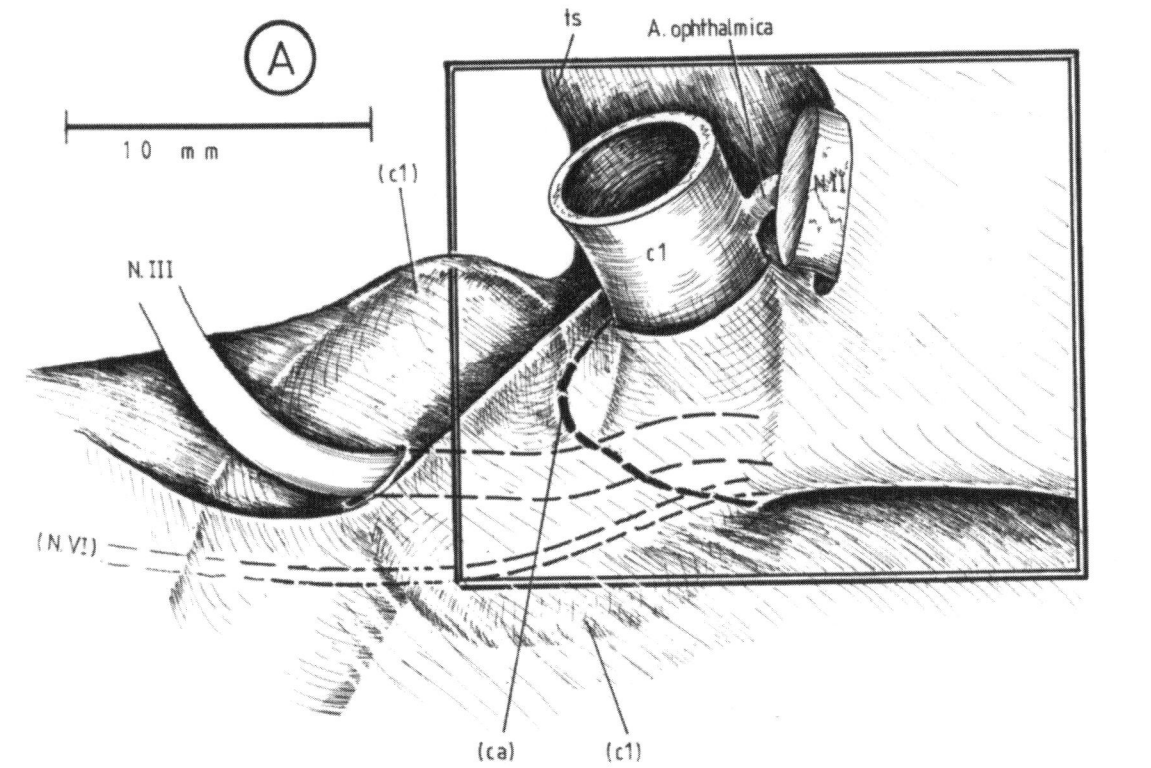
A
10 mm
ts
A. ophthalmica
(c1)
N. II
c1
N. III
(N. VI)
(ca)
(c1)

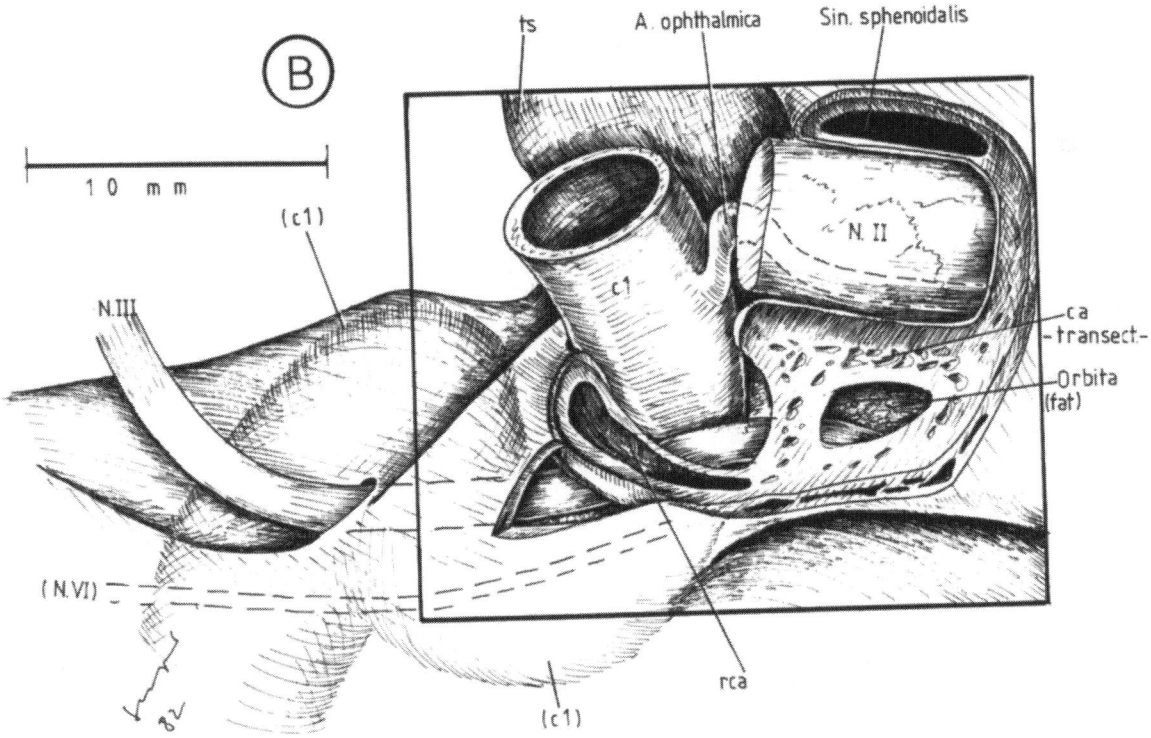
B
10 mm
ts
A. ophthalmica
Sin. sphenoidalis
(c1)
N. II
c1
N. III
ca
-transect.-
Orbita
(fat)
(N. VI)
rca
(c1)

Ophthalmic aneurysms (Figs. 55 to 60)

Fig. 55. Operations in the area surrounding Sinus cavernosus.
Clinical example of an **A. ophthalmica aneurysm** *
Subarachnoidal hemorrhage 6 days prior to operation with slight leftsided hemiparesis, meningism, psychical slowing; oriented. Quick regression of pathological symptoms postoperatively**.
Secondary finding: Aneurysm of A. communicans ant.

A + A' Preoperative angiogram
B + B' Angiography immediately after operation. Both aneurysms are clipped

---

* I am grateful to Prof. Dr. K. Kendel and PD Dr. G. Reinshagen (Neurological Clinic, District Hospital Lahr) for the preoperative angiogram.
** Operation performed by Dr. J. Gilsbach, author's coworker.

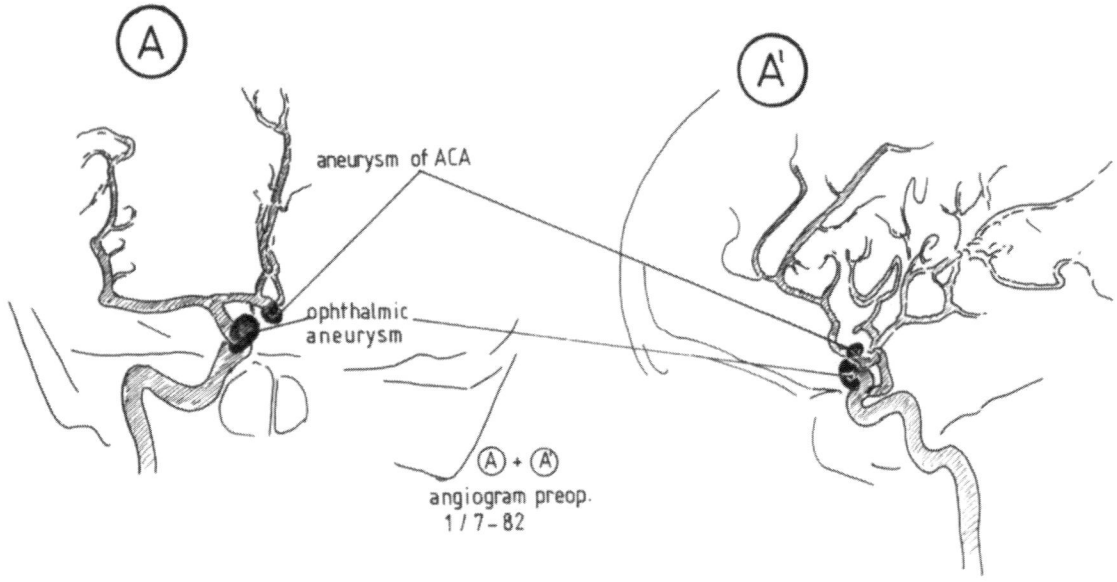

Oe, V, ♂, 6 / 20 - 53
op. 1 / 8 - 82

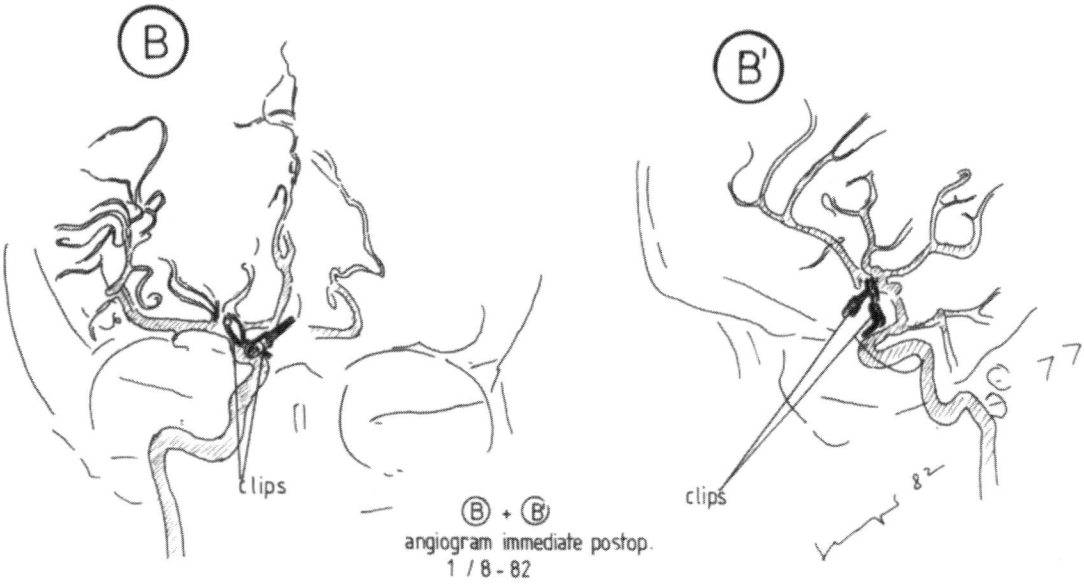

Fig. 56. Operations in the area surrounding Sinus cavernosus.

A. ophthalmica aneurysm. Operation

A Location of skin incision and **pterional trepanation**

B Location of trepanation, skull preparation, microsurgical site **C** sketched in

C Microsurgical site after **opening of dura**

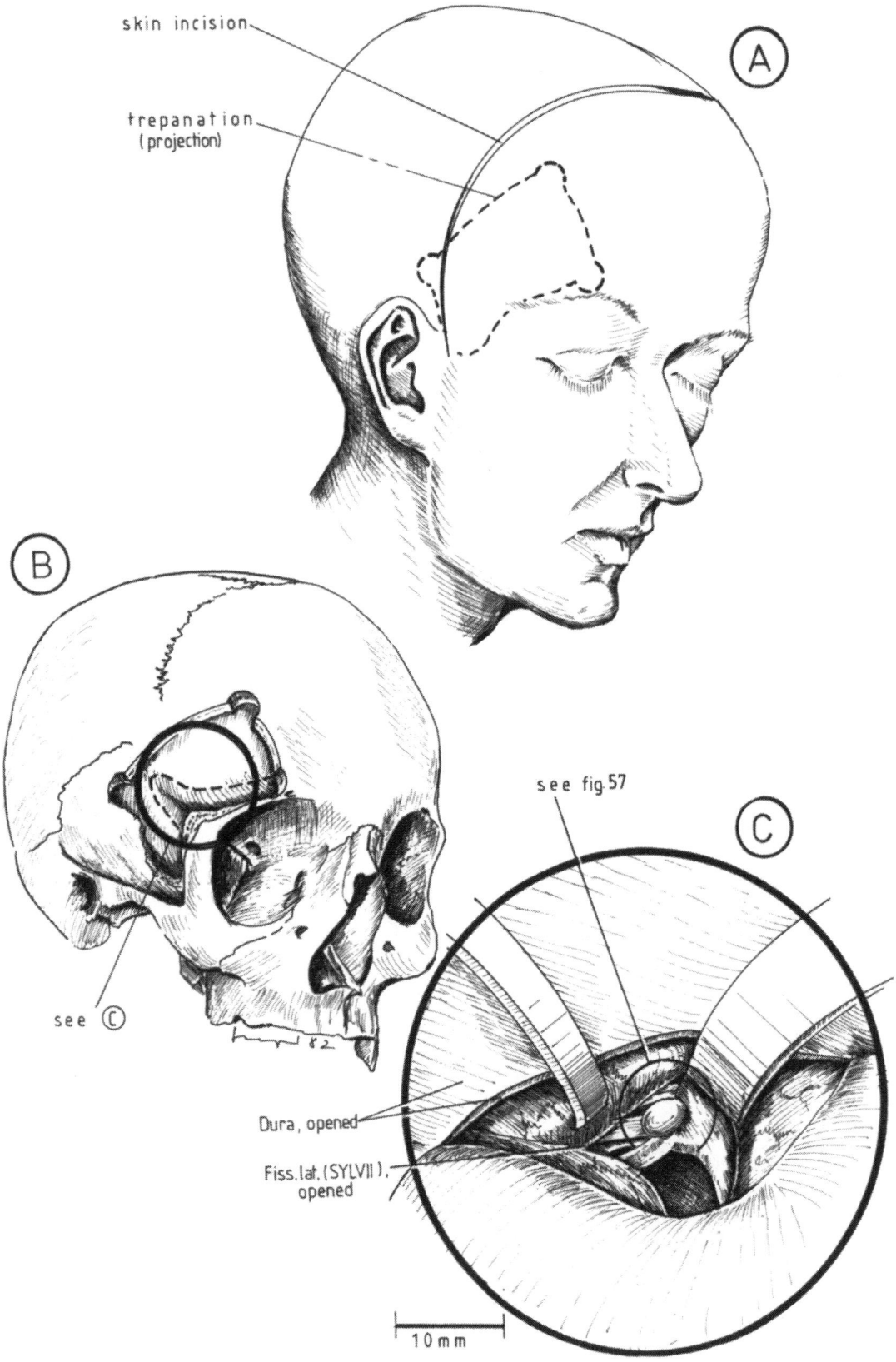
skin incision
trepanation
(projection)
A
B
see C
see fig. 57
C
Dura, opened
Fiss. lat. (SYLVII),
opened
10 mm

Fig. 57. Operations in the area surrounding Sinus cavernosus.

A. ophthalmica aneurysm, operation

A Enlarged microsurgical site from Fig. 56 **C**, rotated 90°

- **1** Dura incision in front of A. ophthalmica aneurysm
- **2** Dura pulled back from Processus clinoideus ant.

B **1** Separation of dura bridge which lies over N.II and aneurysm

- **2** **Drilling of Processus clinoideus ant. and osseous roof of N.II**

C **1** Separation of adhesions from neck of aneurysm

- **2** Since clipping is not yet possible, aneurysm is shrunk by bipolar electrocoagulation

Abbreviations:

ap Ala minor
ca Processus clinoideus ant.
cl A. carotis int.
fcm Fossa cranii media
gr Gyri recti
ts Tuberculum sellae

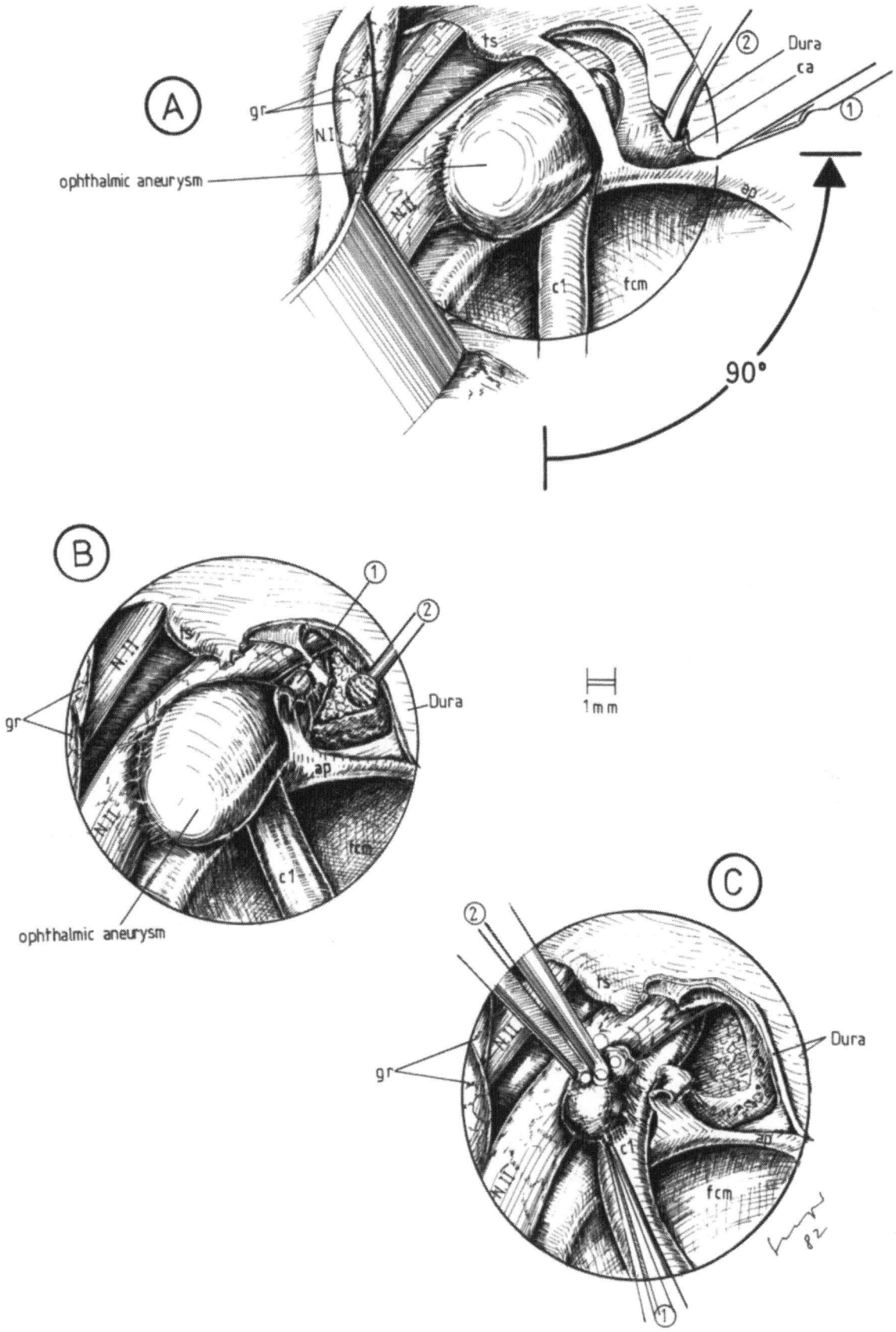
A
gr
N.I
ts
②
Dura
ca
①
ophthalmic aneurysm
N.II
ap
c1
fcm
90°
B
①
②
ts
N.II
gr
Dura
1mm
ap
N.III
fcm
c1
ophthalmic aneurysm
C
②
ts
Dura
gr
c1
ap
N.III
fcm
①

Fig. 58. Operations in the area surrounding Sinus cavernosus.

A **A. ophthalmica aneurysm** is clipped

B Aneurysm with clip is folded back laterally. Arrows: neck of aneurysm only partially eliminated. **Clip correction** in direction of arrows

C Situation of final aneurysm clipping.
On A. communicans ant., a second aneurysm was found and eliminated immediately after with the typical technique

Abbreviations:

ap Ala minor
ca Processus clinoideus ant. (residual)
cl A. carotis int.
fcm Fossa cranii media
gr Gyri recti
ts Tuberculum sellae

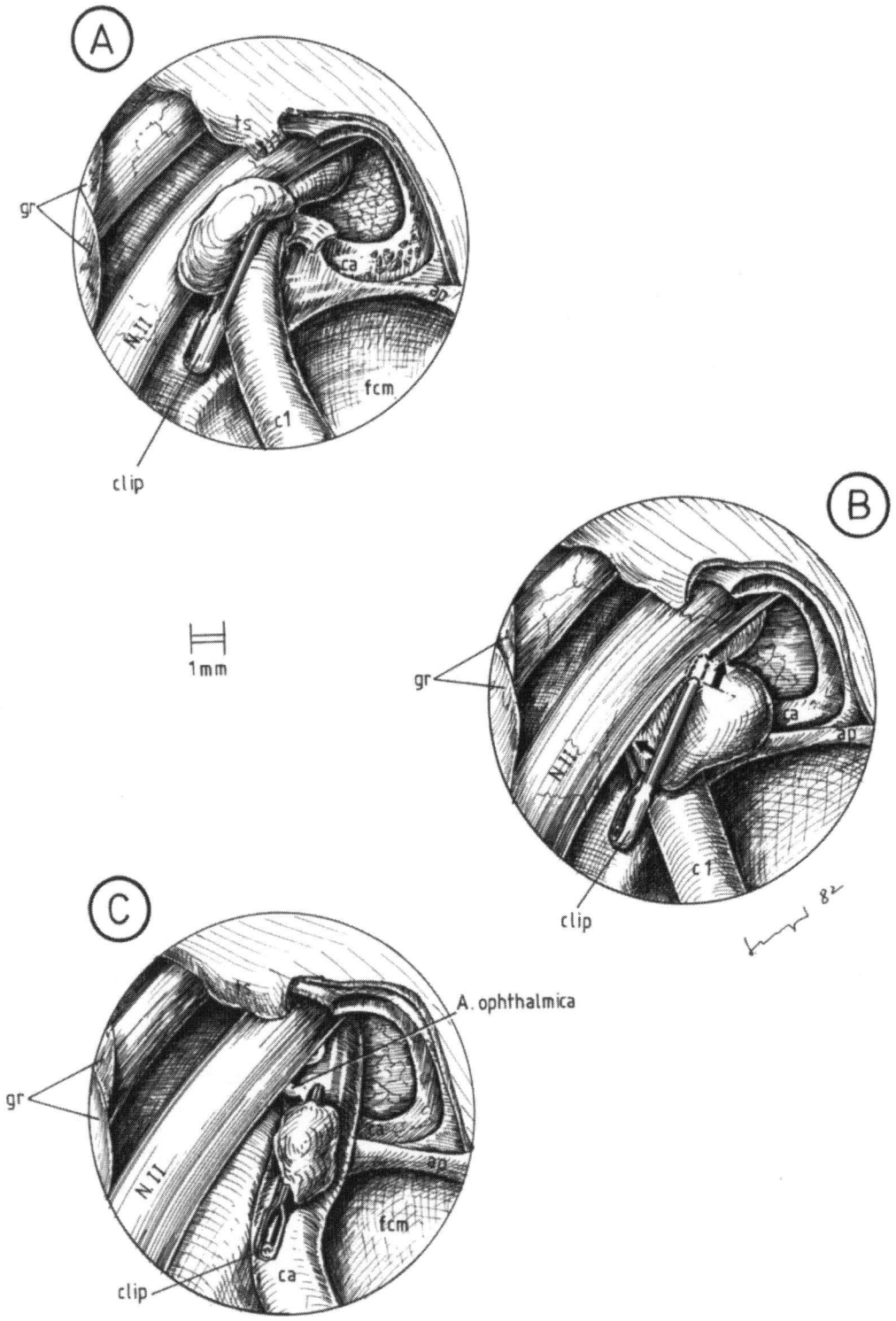
A
gr
ts
ca
ap
N II
fcm
c1
clip
1mm
B
gr
ca
ap
N II
c1
clip
C
A. ophthalmica
gr
N II
ap
fcm
ca
clip

Fig. 59. Operations in the area surrounding Sinus cavernosus.

Various types of A. ophthalmica aneurysms, anatomical sketches of clinical examples.

Broken lines: path of A. carotis int. in the area of Sinus cavernosus (projection)

A – B' After subarachnoidal hemorrhage, blind in both eyes; two weeks later, after angiography, acute left hemiplegia, psychical slowing; shortly before operation visual improvement on the left side, on the right side complete nasal hemianopsia, mixed aphasia. Postoperative recession of left arm pareses, partial leg paresis remains, improvement of right visual field, speech and behavior normalized within several weeks*

A + A' Anatomical presentation of preoperative status

B + B' Anatomical presentation of postoperative status

C + D Anatomical presentation of pre- and postoperative status of Fig. 55 to 58**

E + F No actual clinical example available

---

* Operation performed by author during his time at the Neurosurgical Clinic, University of Giessen, Director Prof. Dr. Dr. h. c. H. W. Pia.

** Operation performed by Dr. J. Gilsbach, author's coworker.

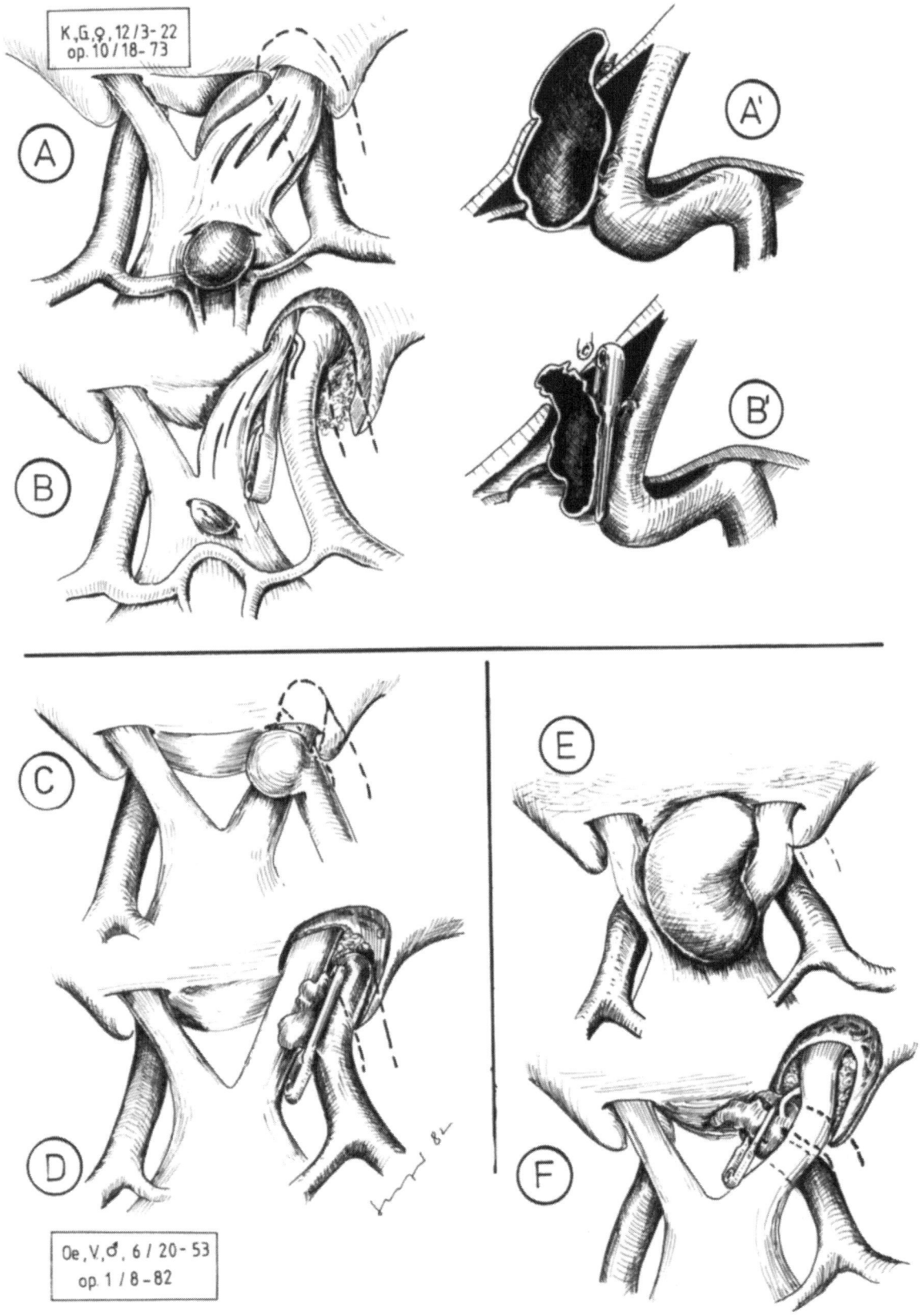
K.G.♀, 12/3-22
op. 10/18-73
A
A'
B
B'
C
D
E
F
Oe.V.♂, 6/20-53
op. 1/8-82

Fig. 60. Operations in the area surrounding Sinus cavernosus.

Various types of A. ophthalmica aneurysms, anatomical sketches of clinical examples

A – B' For several months gradual diminishing visual acuity and mydriasis on left side, no postoperative worsening*

A + A' Anatomical presentation of preoperative status

B + B' Anatomical presentation of postoperative status

C – D' Within 6 months gradual diminishing of left side visual acuity with temporal visual field defect*. Postoperative visual acuity improvement from 0,6 to 0,8, visual field defects no longer demonstrable

C + C' Anatomical presentation of preoperative status

D + D' Anatomical presentation of postoperative status

---

* Operation performed by Dr. J. Gilsbach, author's coworker.

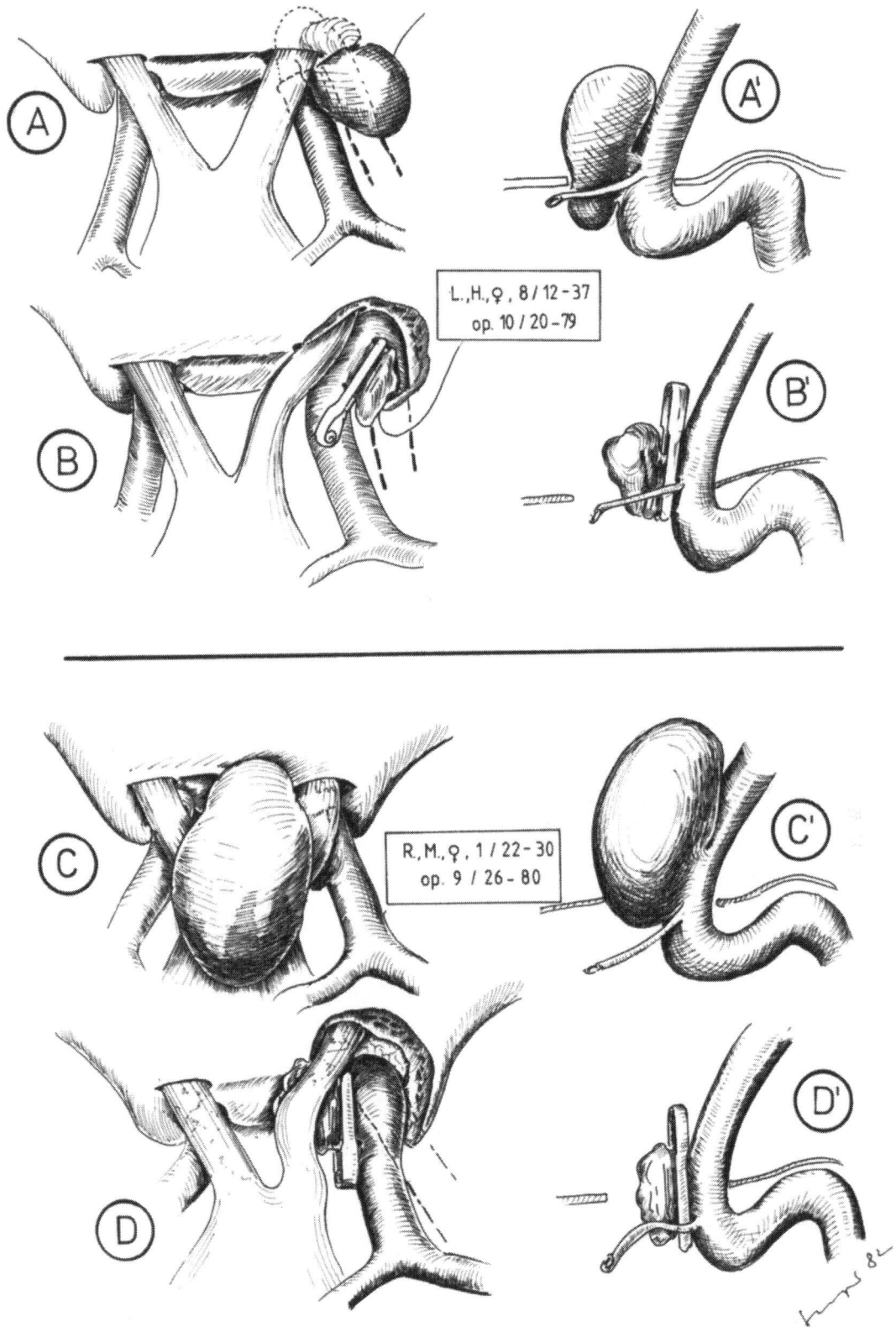
A
A'
L.,H.,♀, 8/12-37
op. 10/20-79
B
B'
C
R.,M.,♀, 1/22-30
op. 9/26-80
C'
D
D'

Pneumosinus dilatans (Figs. 61 to 68)

Fig. 61. Operations in the area surrounding Sinus cavernosus.

Pneumosinus dilatans (of Processus clinoideus ant.), anatomy

A Position of Sinus sphenoidalis and Canales optici (broken line). Processus clinoideus ant. not pneumatized. Position of Sinus sphenoidalis beneath Planum sphenoidale, Tuberculum sellae, Sella turcica, and Sulcus caroticus, and reaching Foramen rotundum

B + B' Bone preparation with Pneumosinus dilatans*

B Preparation, view as in **A**

B' Sagittal section, medial posterior view. Tuberculum sellae and posterior portion of medial wall of Canalis opticus are removed. The remaining portion of Canalis opticus medial wall frequently protrudes into Sinus sphenoidalis. Arrows show that Sinus sphenoidalis extends around Canalis opticus into Processus clinoideus ant., and here surrounds Canalis opticus laterally as well = Pneumosinus dilatans

---

* Skull preparation of Neurosurgical Clinic, University of Freiburg.

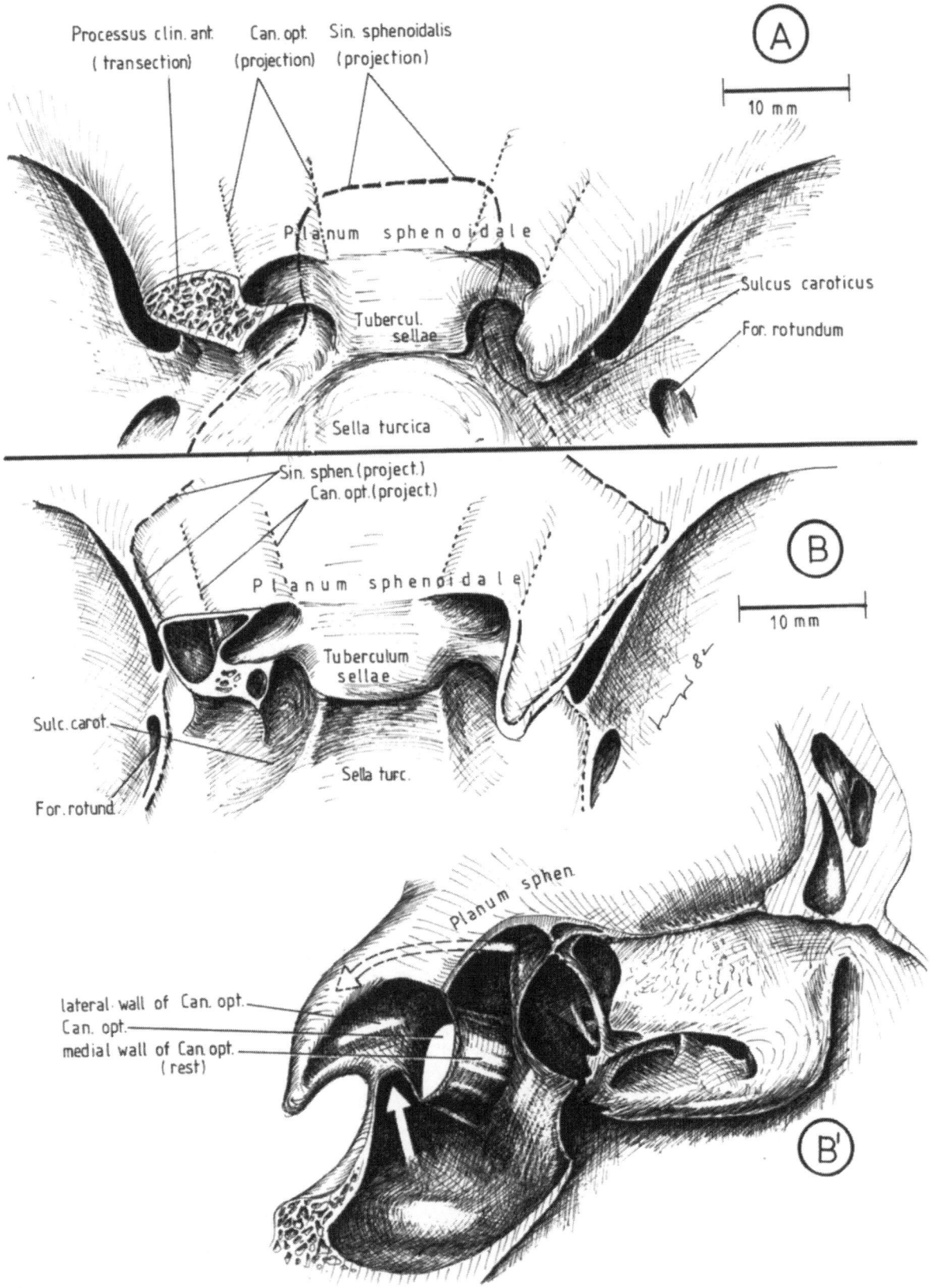
Processus clin. ant.
(transection)
Can. opt.
(projection)
Sin. sphenoidalis
(projection)
A
10 mm
Planum sphenoidale
Tubercul.
sellae
Sulcus caroticus
For. rotundum
Sella turcica
Sin. sphen. (project.)
Can. opt. (project.)
B
Planum sphenoidale
10 mm
Tuberculum
sellae
Sulc. carot.
Sella turc.
For. rotund.
Planum sphen.
lateral wall of Can. opt.
Can. opt.
medial wall of Can. opt.
(rest)
B'

Fig. 62. Operations in the area surrounding Sinus cavernosus.

Pneumosinus dilatans (of Processus clinoideus ant.), anatomy

A Skull preparation (detail), superior view, section planes **B – D'** sketched in

B Normal finding: Topographical relation of Processus clinoideus ant., Canalis opticus and Sinus sphenoidalis

C Pneumosinus dilatans. Arrows mark the connection of Sinus sphenoidalis into Pneumosinus dilatans, here formed by two recesses of Sinus sphenoidalis *–a + b–*

D Pneumosinus dilatans. Arrows mark connection of Sinus sphenoidalis into Pneumosinus, here consisting of **one** recess only, corresponding to *b* in **C. Pneumosinus** has a **thick wall,** especially **in the presence of Canalis opticus meningiomas**

B' – D' Section plane somewhat more rostral compared to **B – D (see A)**

B' Processus clinoideus ant. not pneumatized, Canalis opticus of normal size protruding *–c–* into Sinus sphenoidalis

C' Pneumosinus dilatans *–a–* and *–b–* corresponding to **C.** Arrows show connection of Sinus sphenoidalis into Pneumosinus dilatans. **Narrowed Canalis opticus** is almost completely surrounded by Pneumosinus, thus lies nearly free in Sinus sphenoidalis

D' Pneumosinus dilatans *–b–*. Arrow shows connection of Sinus sphenoidalis into Pneumosinus. Canalis opticus very narrow, protruding freely into Sinus sphenoidalis

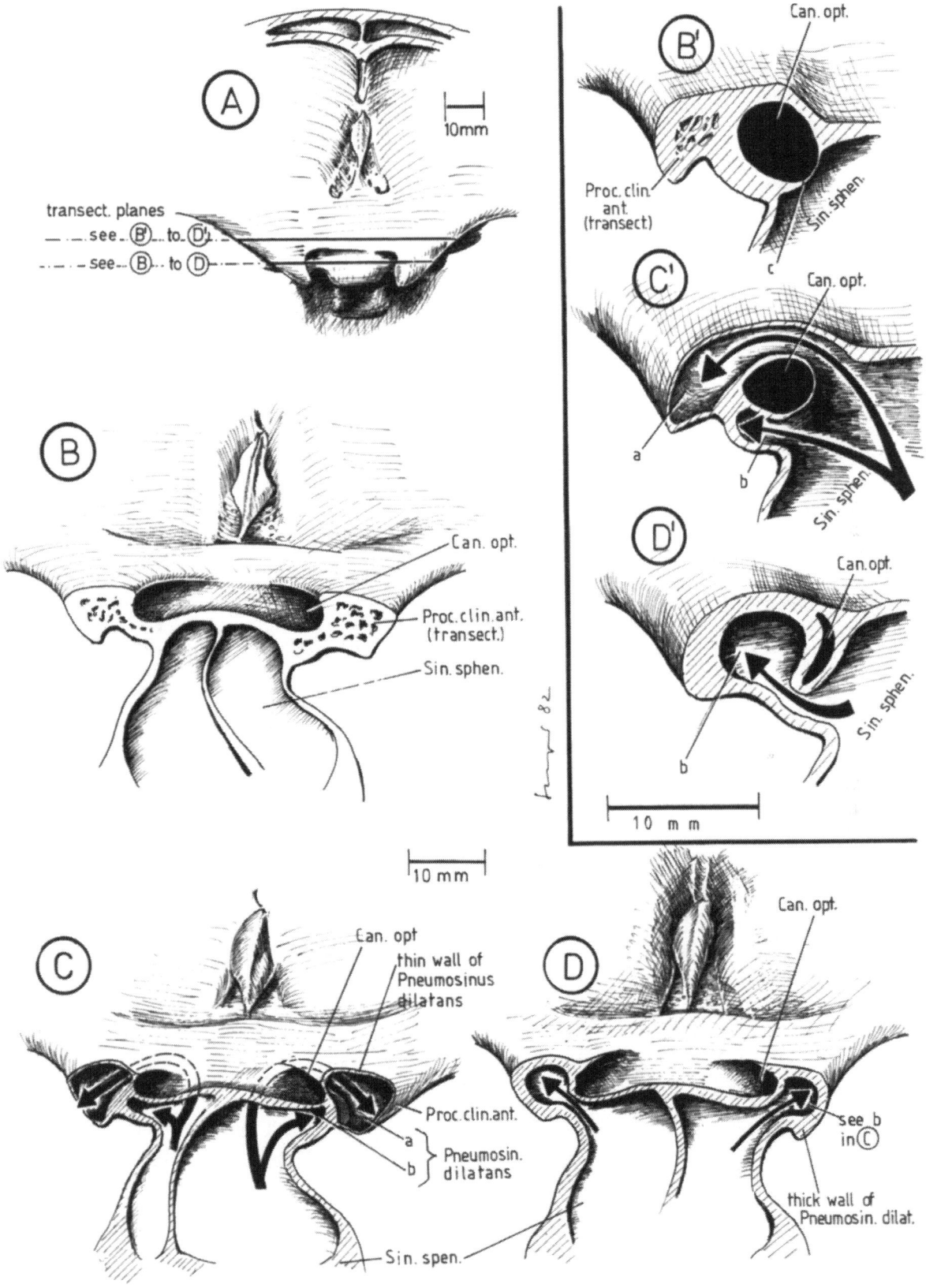
A
10mm
transect. planes
see B' to D'
see B to D
B
Can. opt.
Proc. clin. ant. (transect.)
Sin. sphen.
10 mm
B'
Can. opt.
Proc. clin. ant. (transect)
Sin. sphen.
c
C'
Can. opt.
a
b
Sin. sphen.
D'
Can. opt.
Sin. sphen.
b
10 mm
C
Can. opt
thin wall of Pneumosinus dilatans
Proc. clin. ant.
a
b
Pneumosin. dilatans
Sin. spen.
D
Can. opt.
see b in C
thick wall of Pneumosin. dilat.

Fig. 63. Operations in the area surrounding Sinus cavernosus.

Clinical example of **Pneumosinus dilatans.** Visual acuity preoperatively diminishing, postoperatively improved from 0,8 to 1,2, color perception improvement on right side; irreversible N. opticus damage on the left*, therefore no operation here**

A – A'	Preoperative X-ray findings (oblique views). Open arrow: Pneumosinus dilatans. Canalis opticus greatly narrowed on both sides
B – C'	CT, preoperative. Open arrows: Pneumosinus dilatans
B	*s:* Section plane of reconstruction **B'**
C	*s:* Section plane of reconstruction **C'**
D	Postoperative X-ray, oblique view. Open arrows: Pneumosinus dilatans. Bony wall of Canalis opticus removed
E – F'	CT, postoperative
E	Reconstruction from **E'.** Defect of Processus clinoideus ant. recognizable
E'	*s:* Section plane of reconstruction **E**
F	Bone defect, after removal of the osseous surrounding of Canalis opticus, recognizable
F'	Enlarged detail from **F.** Black arrow: operative approach for bone resection. Open arrow: N. opticus path

---

* I am grateful to Dr. Unsöld, ophthalmol. Clinic, Univ. Freiburg/Br. (Director: Prof. Dr. Mackensen) for the preop. and postop. findings.

** Operation performed by Dr. W. Hassler, author's coworker.

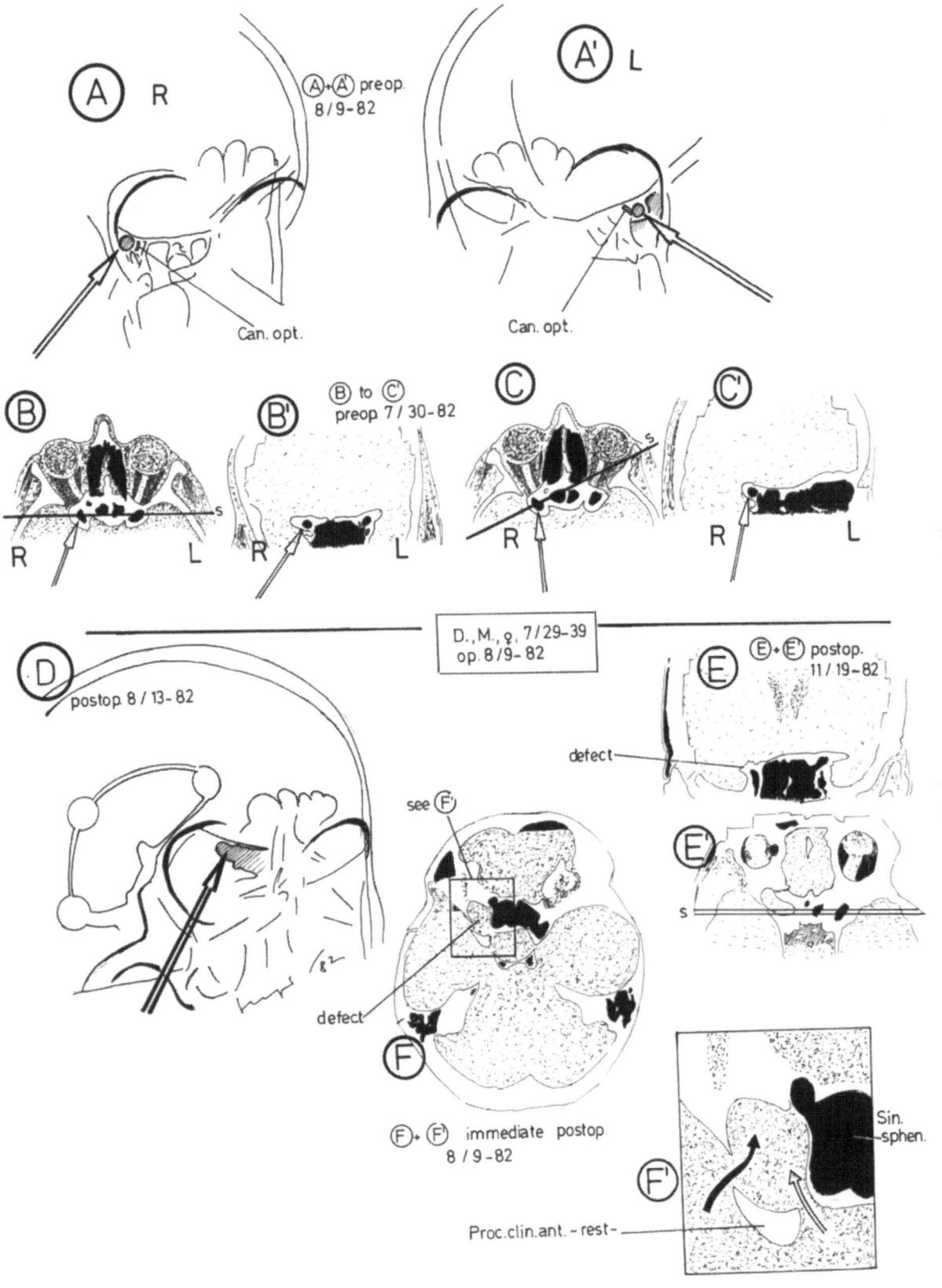
A
R
A+A' preop.
8/9-82
Can. opt.
A'
L
Can. opt.
B
R
L
s
B'
B to C'
preop. 7/30-82
R
L
C
s
R
C'
R
L
D.,M., ♀, 7/29-39
op. 8/9-82
D
postop. 8/13-82
E
E+E' postop.
11/19-82
defect
E'
s
see F'
defect
F
F+F' immediate postop.
8/9-82
F'
Sin.
sphen.
Proc.clin.ant. - rest -

Fig. 64. Operations in the area surrounding Sinus cavernosus.
Pneumosinus dilatans oblique view of skull preparation (detail). Operative approach along Ala minor sketched in

A Projection (broken lines) on bone surface of **Pneumosinus dilatans,** narrowed Canalis opticus and portion of Sinus sphenoidalis wall

B Preparation as **A** after resection of Canalis opticus wall. Open arrow: path of Canalis opticus. Broken arrow: Connection of Sinus sphenoidalis to still remaining portions of Pneumosinus dilatans

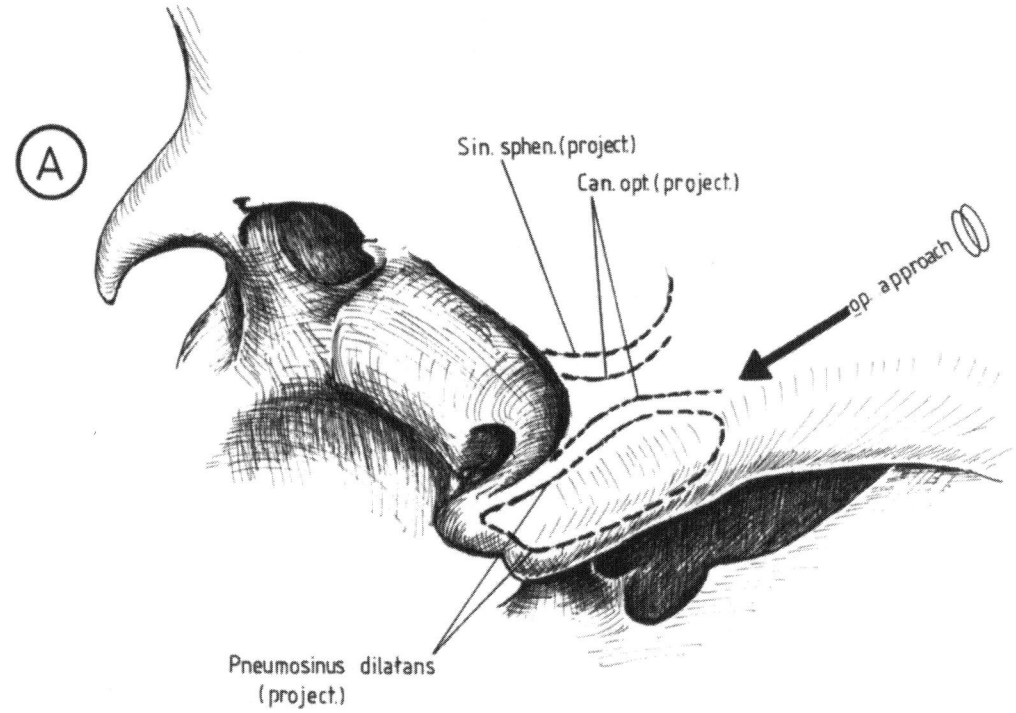
A
Sin. sphen. (project.)
Can. opt. (project.)
op. approach
Pneumosinus dilatans
(project.)

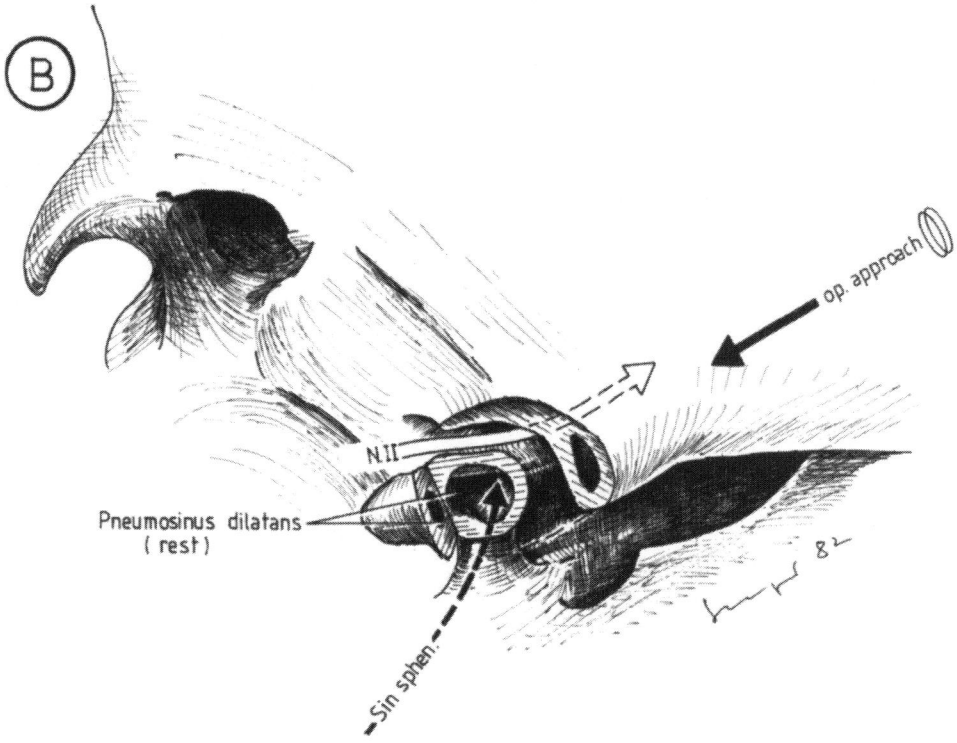
B
op. approach
N.II
Pneumosinus dilatans
(rest)
Sin sphen.

Fig. 65. Operations in the area surrounding Sinus cavernosus.

Pneumosinus dilatans

A Both Nn. optici and right A. carotis int. sketched on skull preparation

B Situation after bone resection. Canalis opticus and Fissura orbitalis sup. form a common space after removing bony walls of N. opticus

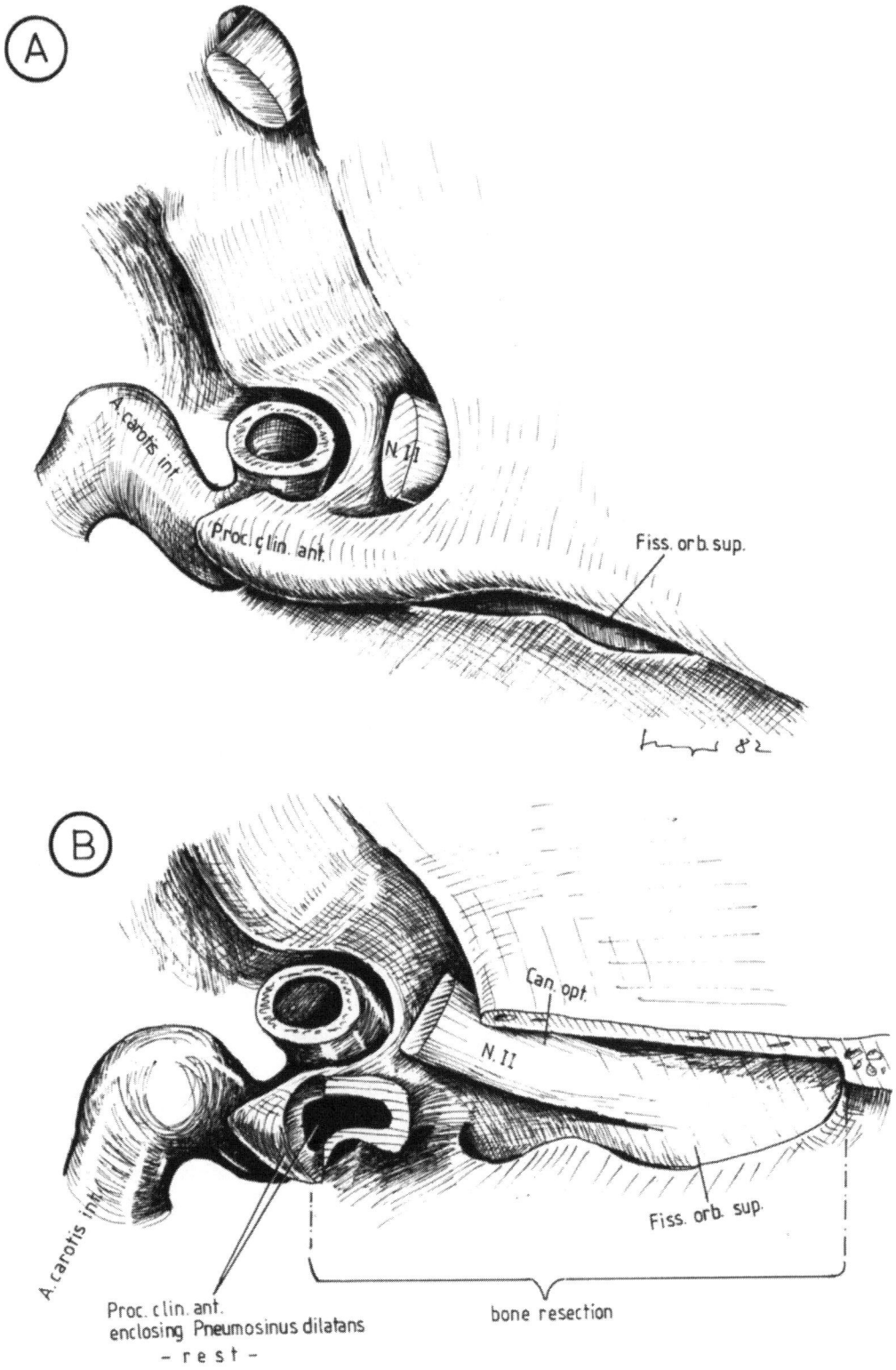
A
A. carotis int.
N. III
Proc. clin. ant.
Fiss. orb. sup.
B
Can. opt.
N. II
A. carotis int.
Fiss. orb. sup.
Proc. clin. ant.
enclosing Pneumosinus dilatans
- r e s t -
bone resection

Fig. 66. Operations in the area surrounding Sinus cavernosus.

Pneumosinus dilatans

Microsurgical site

A Pterional trepanation, sketched on skull preparation

A' Various microsurgical views (arrows), sketched on skull preparation

B Microsurgical site after dura exposure. Because of oblique perspective, Ala minor appears foreshortend. Drilling into Ala major and Ala minor

C After drilling Ala minor, roof of Fissura orbitalis sup. is opened

D Enlarged detail from **C.** Drilling at juncture of Processus clinoideus ant. and Ala minor remnant. Lateral wall of Canalis opticus partially removed, Pneumosinus dilatans opened in several places

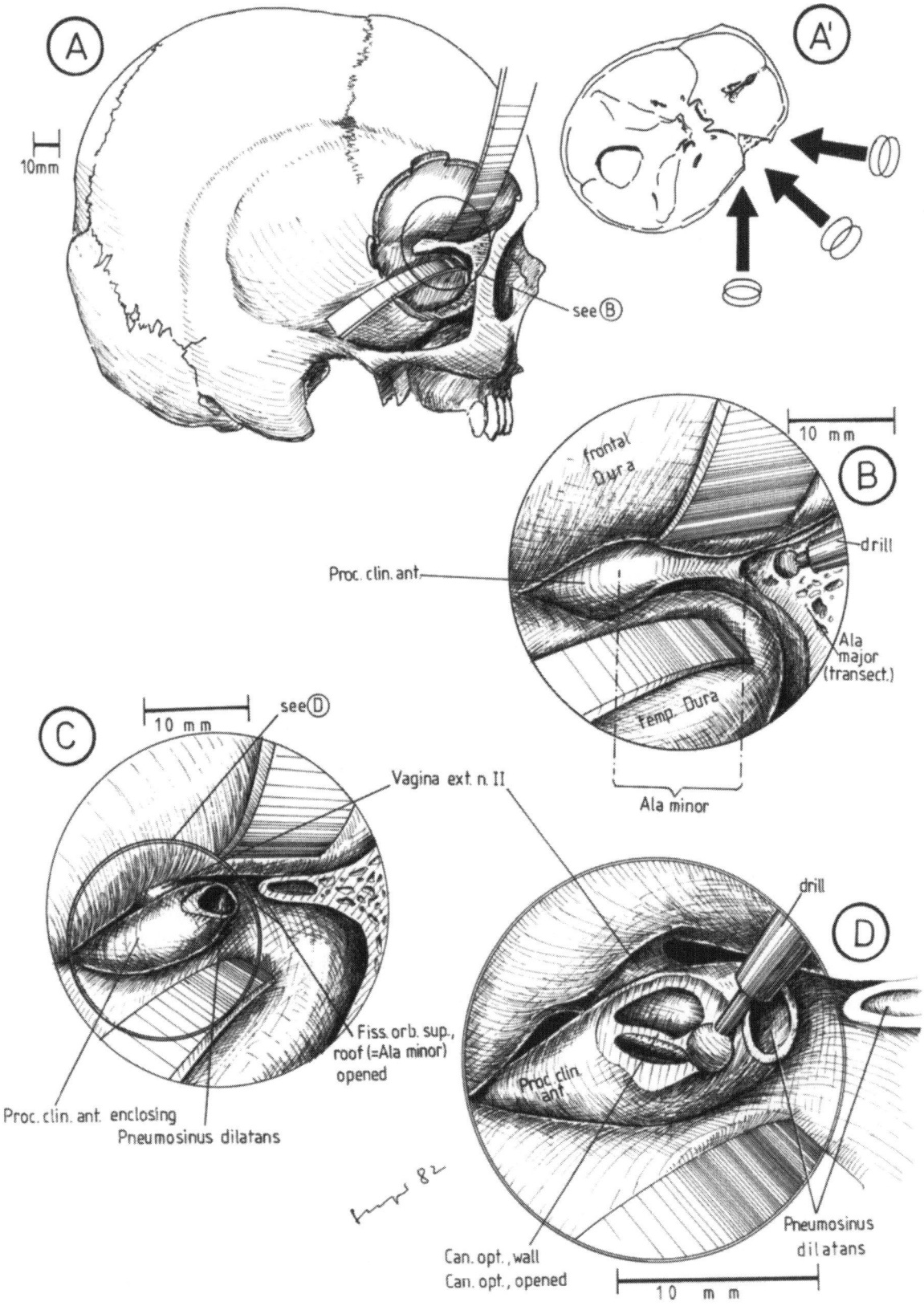
A
10mm
see B
A'
10 mm
B
frontal Dura
drill
Proc. clin. ant.
Ala major (transect.)
Temp. Dura
Ala minor
C
10 mm
see D
Vagina ext. n. II
Fiss. orb. sup., roof (=Ala minor) opened
Proc. clin. ant. enclosing Pneumosinus dilatans
D
drill
Proc. clin. ant.
Pneumosinus dilatans
Can. opt., wall
Can. opt., opened
10 mm

Fig. 67. Operations in the area surrounding Sinus cavernosus.

Pneumosinus dilatans

A Drilling of Canalis opticus wall must be carried out very cautiously (low drill speed, extensive irrigation) in order to prevent negative mechanical and thermal effects to N. opticus already damaged by compression

B Lateral wall of Canalis opticus removed. Stenosed N.II recognizable

1 Resection of Canalis opticus formed by Planum sphenoidale

2 Detachment of mucosa in Pneumosinus dilatans

C After mucosa removal from Pneumosinus dilatans, fatty tissue (from abdominal wall) is placed on decompressed N. opticus. Fatty tissue closes entrance of Pneumosinus dilatans, thus preventing communication of Sinus sphenoidalis and epidural space

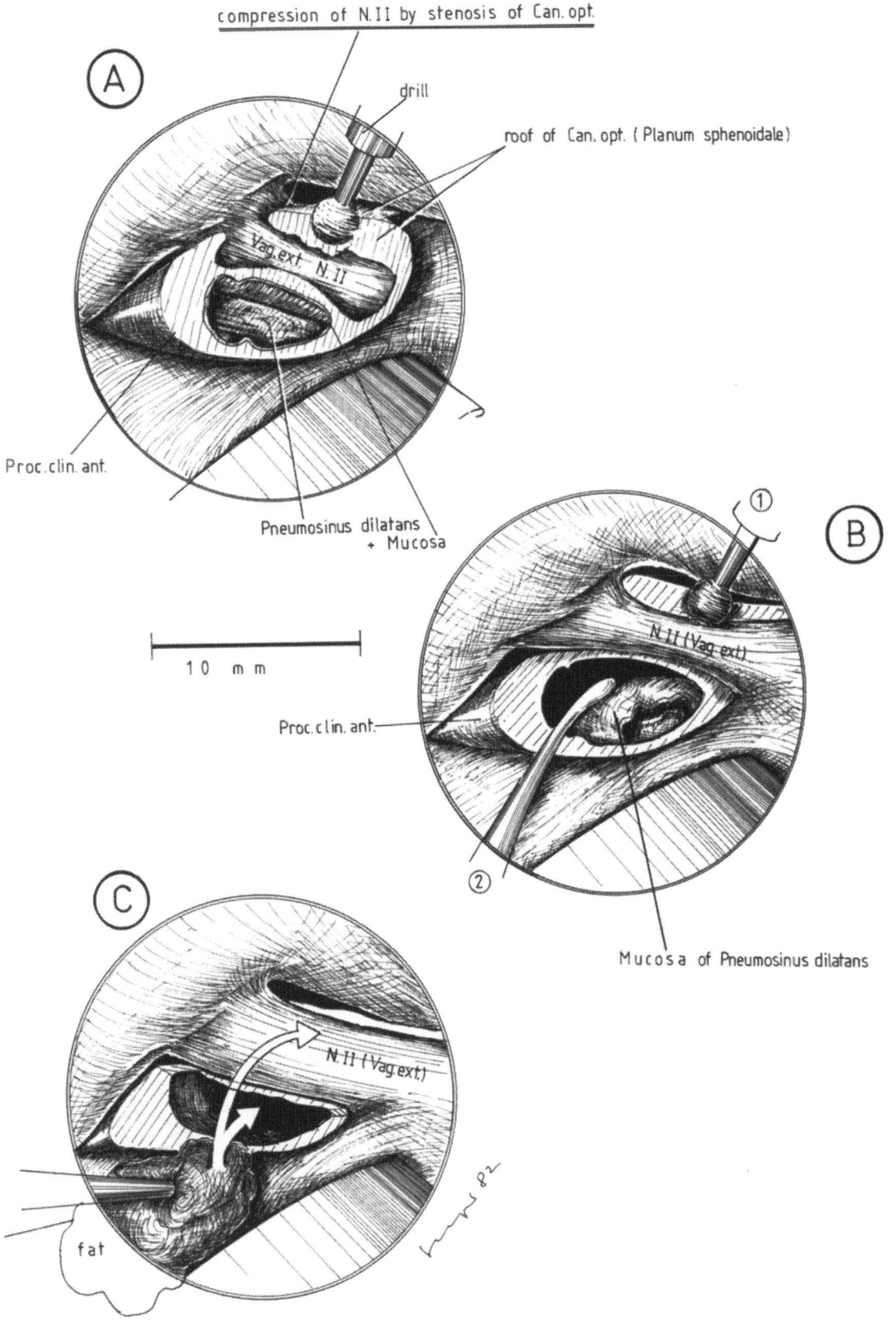
compression of N.II by stenosis of Can. opt.
A
drill
roof of Can. opt. (Planum sphenoidale)
Vag. ext.
N. II
Proc. clin. ant.
Pneumosinus dilatans
+ Mucosa
B
1
N. II (Vag. ext.)
10 mm
Proc. clin. ant.
2
Mucosa of Pneumosinus dilatans
C
N. II (Vag. ext.)
fat

Fig. 68. Operations in the area surrounding Sinus cavernosus.

Pneumosinus dilatans

A **1** Squirting of fatty tissue with tissue glue (fibrinogen + activator)*

2 Cautions pressing of fatty tissue against the stump of Pneumosinus dilatans

B Anatomical model. N. opticus –(N.II)– and A. carotis int. –*(c1)*– projected on dura surface. One sees that the opened up Canalis opticus and Fissura orbitalis sup. form a common cavity separated only by the Processus clinoideus ant.

---

* Immuno-Chemie, Heidelberg.

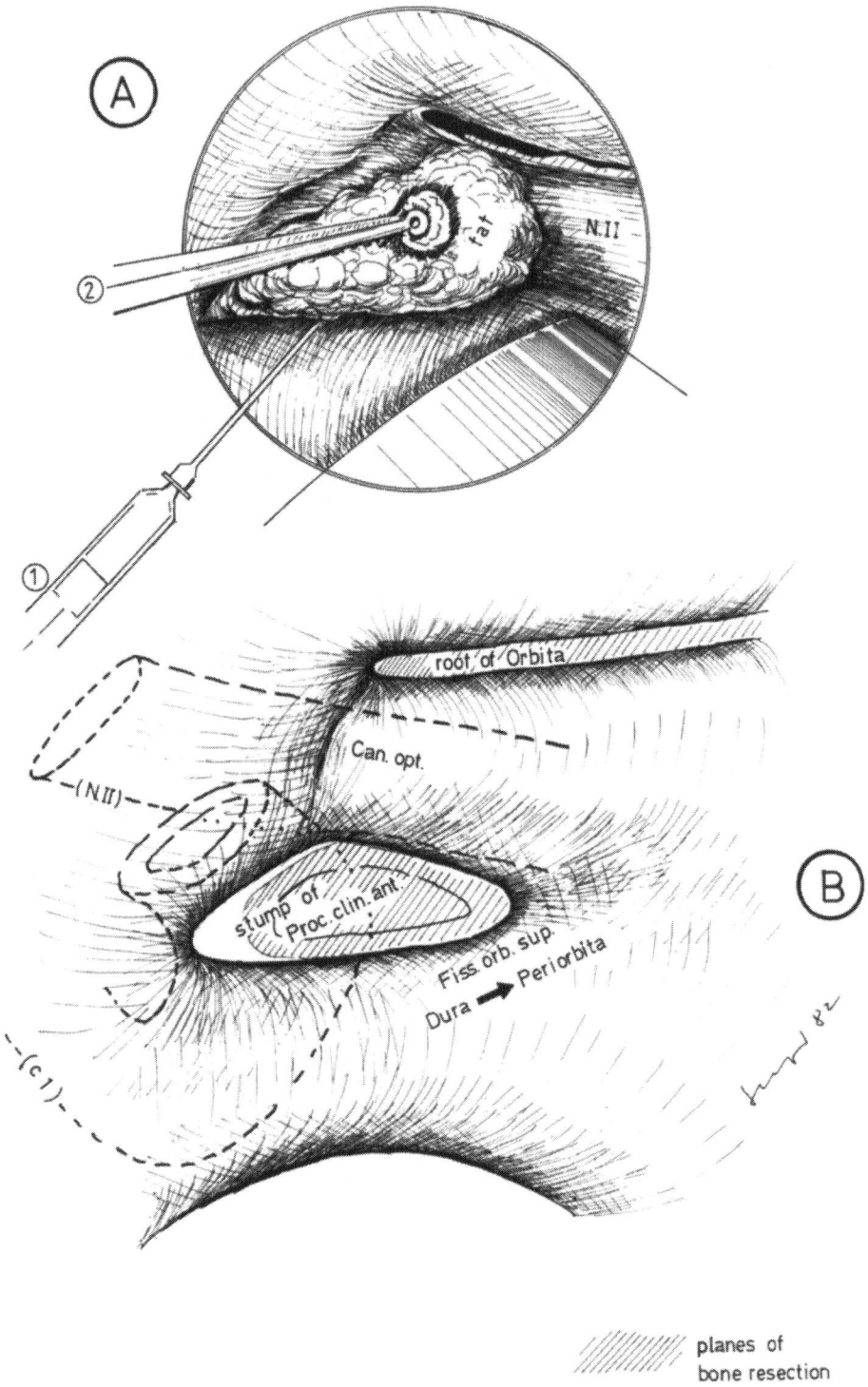
A
fat
N.II
2
1
root of Orbita
Can. opt.
(N.II)
stump of
Proc. clin. ant.
Fiss. orb. sup.
Dura
Periorbita
(c I)
B
planes of
bone resection

Tumors (Figs. 69 to 99)

Fig. 69. Operations in the area surrounding Sinus cavernosus.
Flat **meningioma in Sinus cavernosus area** with considerable **bone reaction** of Ala major and minor. Dorso-superior view, right side. Preliminary anatomical remarks

A Skull preparation, **resection line** sketched in (broken line)

B Enlarged detail from **A.** One sees that Canalis opticus, Fissura orbitalis sup. and lateral wall of Foramen rotundum will form a common space

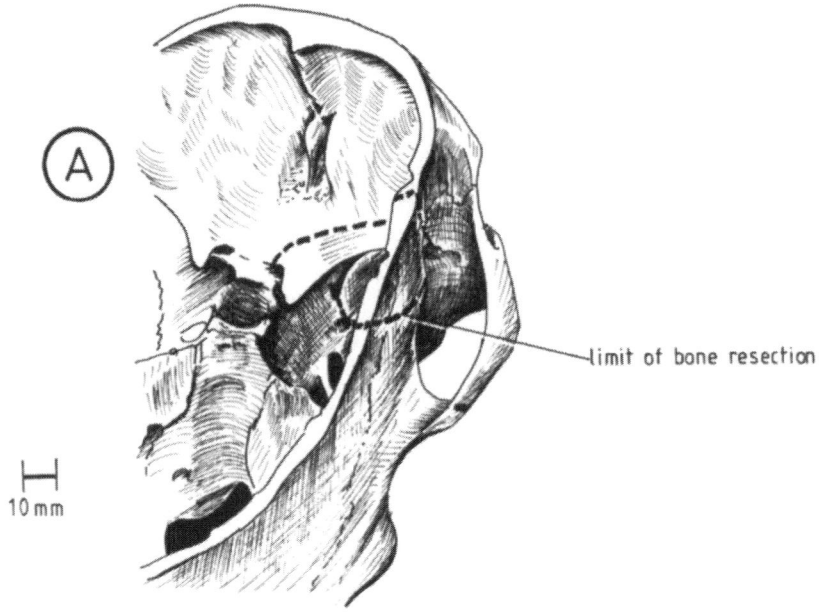
A
limit of bone resection
10 mm

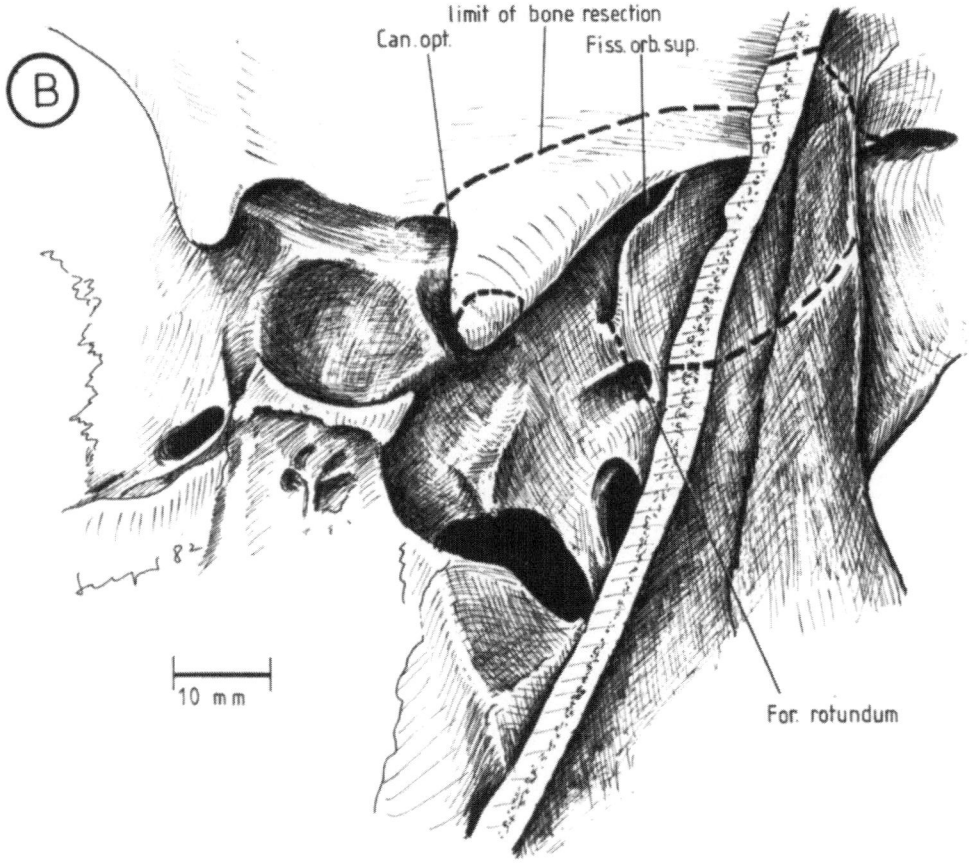
B
limit of bone resection
Can. opt.
Fiss. orb. sup.
10 mm
For. rotundum

Fig. 70. Operations in the area surrounding Sinus cavernosus.
Flat meningioma in Sinus cavernosus area with extensive bone reaction of Ala major and Ala minor
Preliminary anatomical remarks
Topographical **relation of A. carotis int. to bone structures,** from skull preparation; **variants**

A Sulcus caroticus and surrounding structures in skull preparation. Projection of lateral A. carotis int. wall on bone structures (broken line). Medial side of Processus clinoideus ant. shows a deep impression *–imp–* resulting from A. carotis int. siphon

B Another example, sketched on larger scale. As in **A,** wall of A. carotis int. lies close against Canalis rotundus. Medial side of Processus clinoideus ant. root *–ra–* shows bone impressions *–imp–* resulting from A. carotis int. siphon

C In this example one sees that the impression of A. carotis int. is quite deeply sculpted. It impresses Processus clinoideus ant. medially; radix of Processus clinoideus ant. *–ra–*, Tuberculum sellae *–ts–* and lateral wall of Sella turcica *–st–* become impressed too

D Typical bone connection *–co1–* between Processus clinoideus ant. and Tuberculum sellae *–ts–*. Thus A. carotis int. siphon is surrounded by bony ring behind Canalis opticus. In this case one could not move A. carotis int. to the side during bone resection

E Similar to **D.** However, sella bridge *–co2–* is also present here, that is, a connection between Processus clinoideus ant. and Processus clinoideus post., or Dorsum sellae *–cp–* also

Abbreviations:

ca Processus clinoideus ant.
cop Canalis opticus
cp Processus clinoideus post.
co1 Connection between Processus clinoideus ant. and Tuberculum sellae
co2 Connection between Processus clinoideus ant. and Processus clinoideus post.
imp Impressions by A. carotis int.
lac Foramen lacerum
ov Foramen ovale
ra Radix of Processus clinoideus ant.
rt Foramen rotundum
st lat. wall of Sella
ts Tuberculum sellae

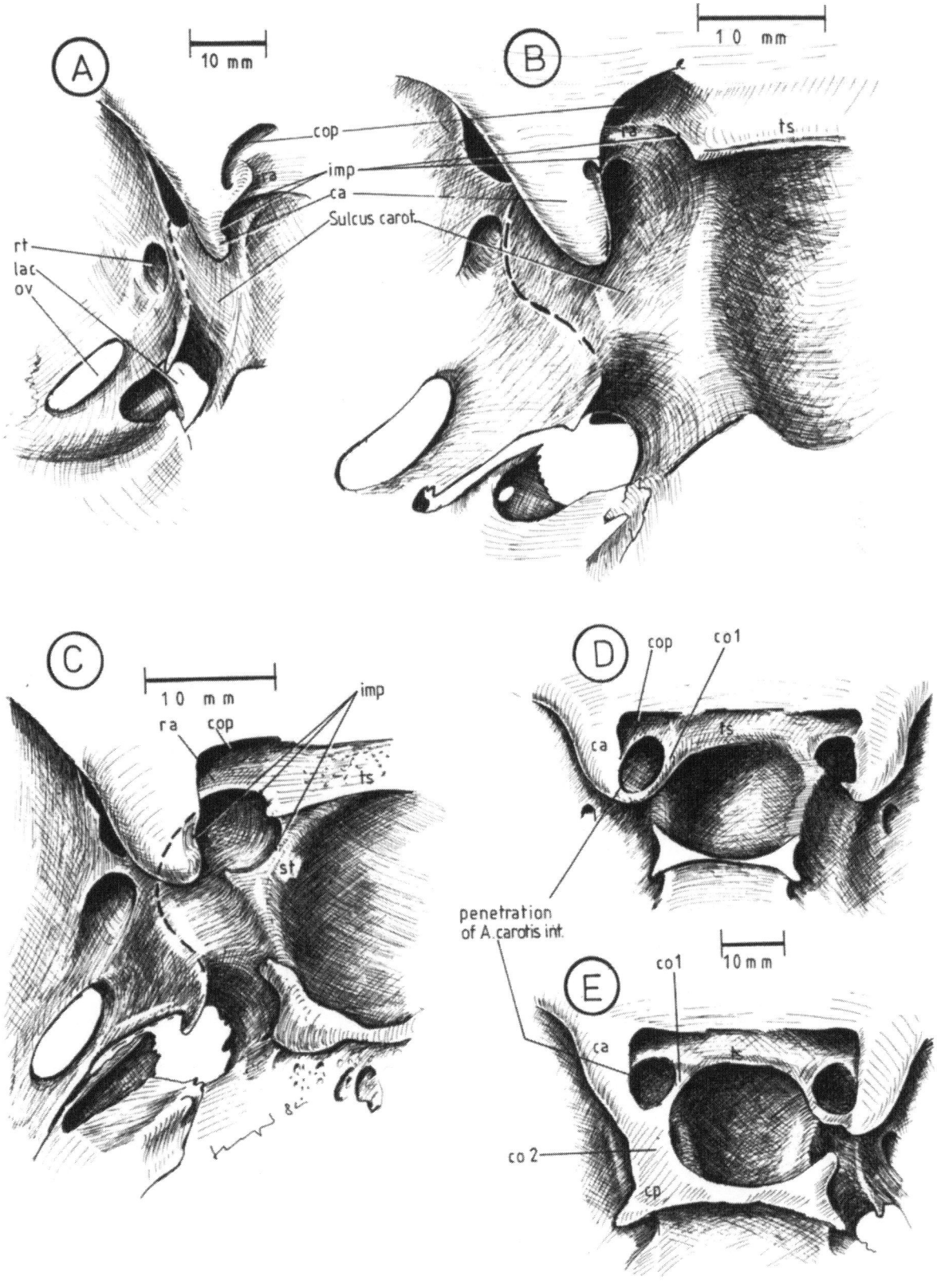
A
10 mm
cop
ra
imp
ca
Sulcus carot.
rt
lac
ov
B
10 mm
ra
ts
C
10 mm
imp
ra
cop
ts
st
D
cop
co1
ca
ts
penetration
of A. carotis int.
E
10 mm
co1
ca
co 2
cp

Fig. 71. Operations in the area surrounding Sinus cavernosus.
Flat meningioma in Sinus cavernosus area with extensive bone reaction of Ala major and Ala minor
Anatomical preparation after bone resection

A **Bone preparation.** Arrow: Path of N. maxillaris after opening up Canalis opticus, Fissura orbitalis sup. and Foramen rotundum

B As in **A,** A. carotis int. and nerve structures sketched in. Dura and veins omitted
In the area of Fissura orbitalis sup. and nearby bone passages for nerves and vessels is a dura sheath, masking nerves and vessels. At these bone passages vessels and nerves are greatly endangered when bone is drilled. Low drill speed with extensive irrigation is required

Abbreviation:

Ggl G Ganglion semilunare (Gasseri)

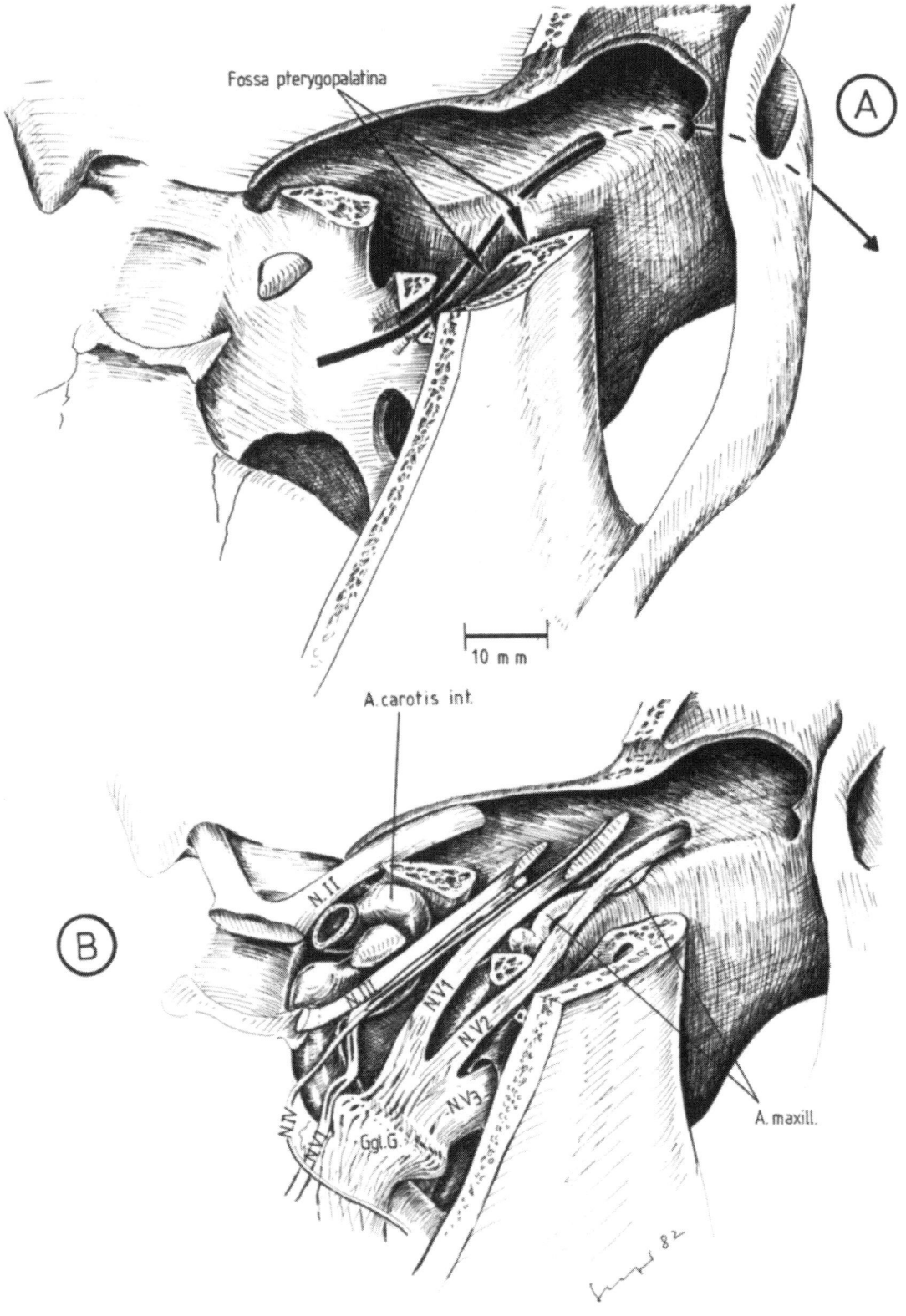
Fossa pterygopalatina
A
10 mm
A. carotis int.
B
N. II
N. III
N. V1
N. V2
N. V3
N. IV
N. VI
Ggl. G.
A. maxill.

Fig. 72. Operations in the area surrounding Sinus cavernosus.

Anatomical preparation showing vessels and nerves in the area of **Sinus cavernosus.** Dura and veins omitted

A Skull sketch with A. carotis int. N. abducens is the cranial nerve in closest contact to A. carotis int. in Sinus cavernosus area

B As **A.** Superficial nerves additionally sketched in, *s1, s2:* Section plane –*s*– of Fig. 73 sketches

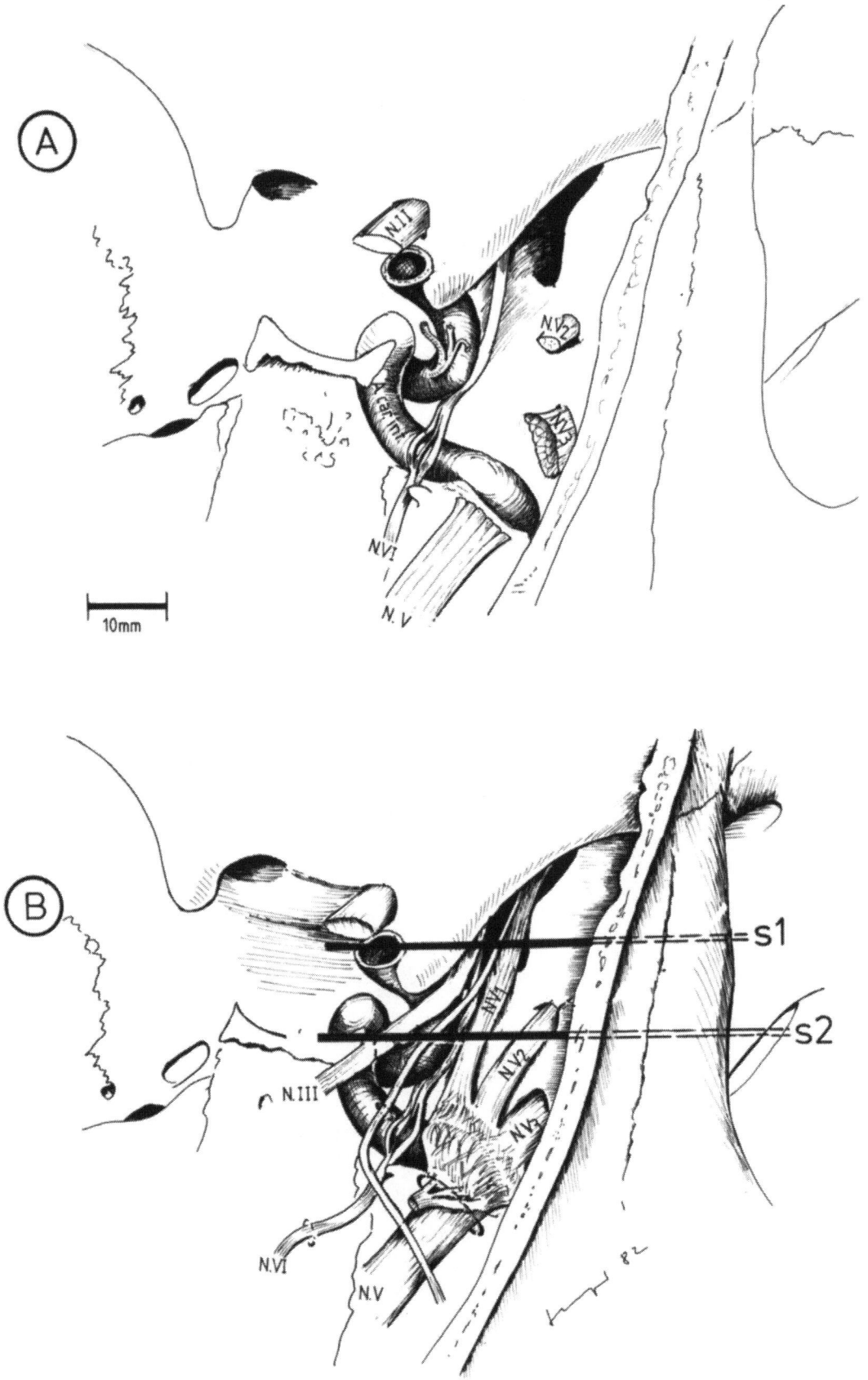
A
N.II
N.V2
N.V3
N.VI
N.V
10mm
B
s1
s2
N.III
N.V1
N.V2
N.V3
N.VI
N.V

Fig. 73. Operations in the area surrounding Sinus cavernosus.

Frontal section of anterior and posterior **Sinus cavernosus** area (section planes see Fig. 72)

A One sees the close topographical relation of A. carotis int. to N. abducens and N. oculomotorius (deep nerve layer), and to the superficial nerve layer with N. trochlearis, N. ophthalmicus –N.V1– and N. maxillaris –N.V2– in Foramen rotundum. A. carotis int. is sectioned twice in the Curvatura ant. of A. carotis int.

B Section plane at level of Dorsum sellae (Processus clinoideus post.). Here also the close relation between A. carotis int. and N. abducens is seen. Just after dura entry N. oculomotorius still lies in a superficial position. Superficial nerve layer –N. trochlearis and both N. trigeminus branches– lie close under superficial dura layer as in **A**

Sinus cavernosus lies predominantly medial to A. carotis int.

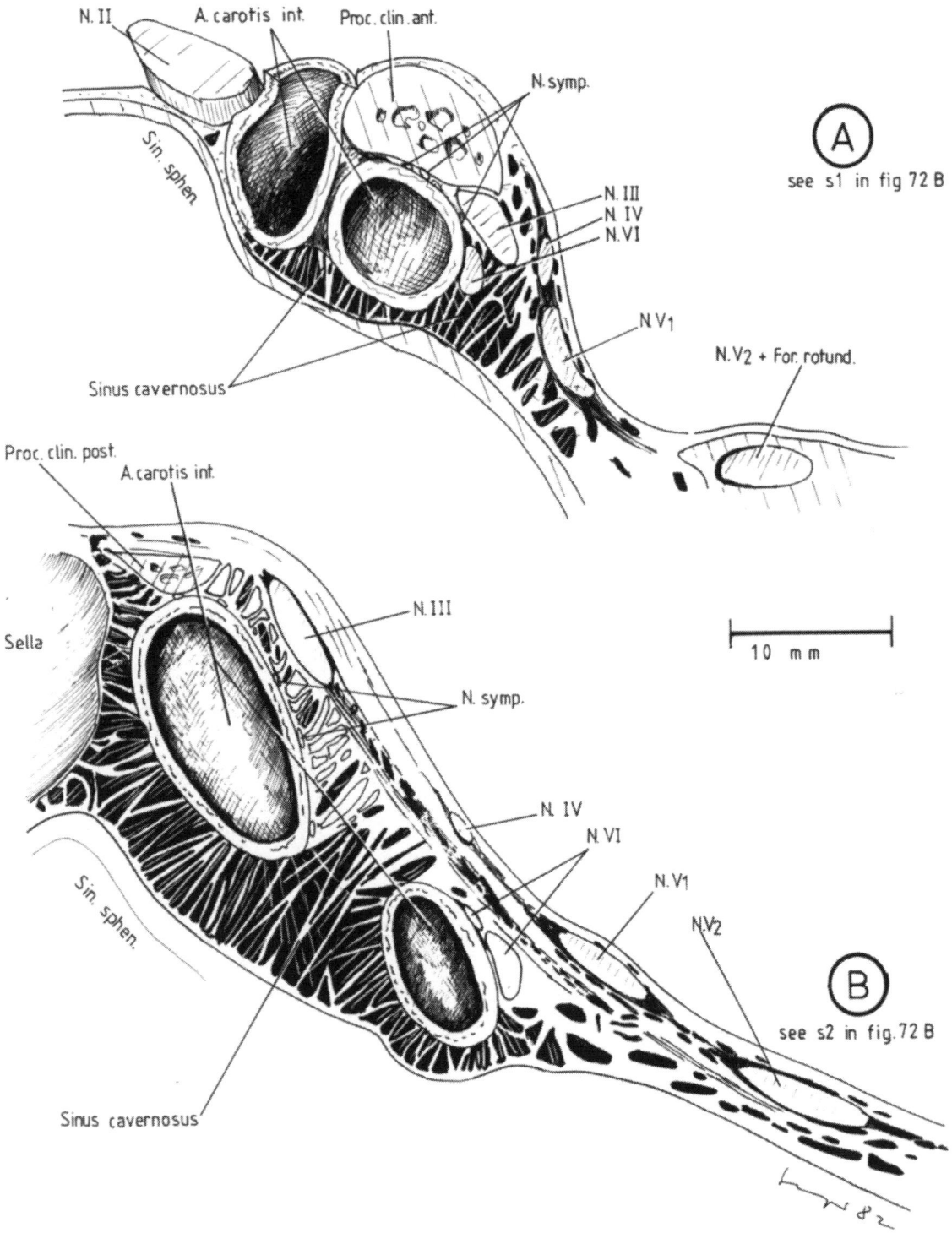
N. II
A. carotis int.
Proc. clin. ant.
N. symp.
Sin. sphen.
A
see s1 in fig 72 B
N. III
N. IV
N. VI
N. V1
N. V2 + For. rotund.
Sinus cavernosus
Proc. clin. post.
A. carotis int.
Sella
N. III
10 mm
N. symp.
N. IV
N. VI
N. V1
N. V2
Sin. sphen.
B
see s2 in fig. 72 B
Sinus cavernosus

Fig. 74. Operations in the area surrounding Sinus cavernosus.
Flat **meningioma in Sinus cavernosus** area with extensive **bone reaction** of Ala major and Ala minor*.
For three weeks Protrusio bulbi on the right with swelling of upperlid. No additional postoperative abnormalities. (Histological finding: Meningioma)
Diagnostic procedures

A	**Preoperative** X-ray of skull, ap. Bone reaction in Ala minor and Ala major area
A'	Preoperative angiography of right A. carotis int.: no displacement
B, B', B''	Black arrows: bone reaction in orbital area (**B**) and Ala major with protrusion of Facies orbitalis alae majoris in posterior orbital area (**B** to **B''**)
C + C'	**Postoperative** findings. Open arrows: bone defect in orbital area, Ala minor (**C**) and in Ala major (**C'**)
D	Lateral skull sketch with CT-planes **B – C'**

* Operation performed by Dr. W. Hassler, author's coworker.

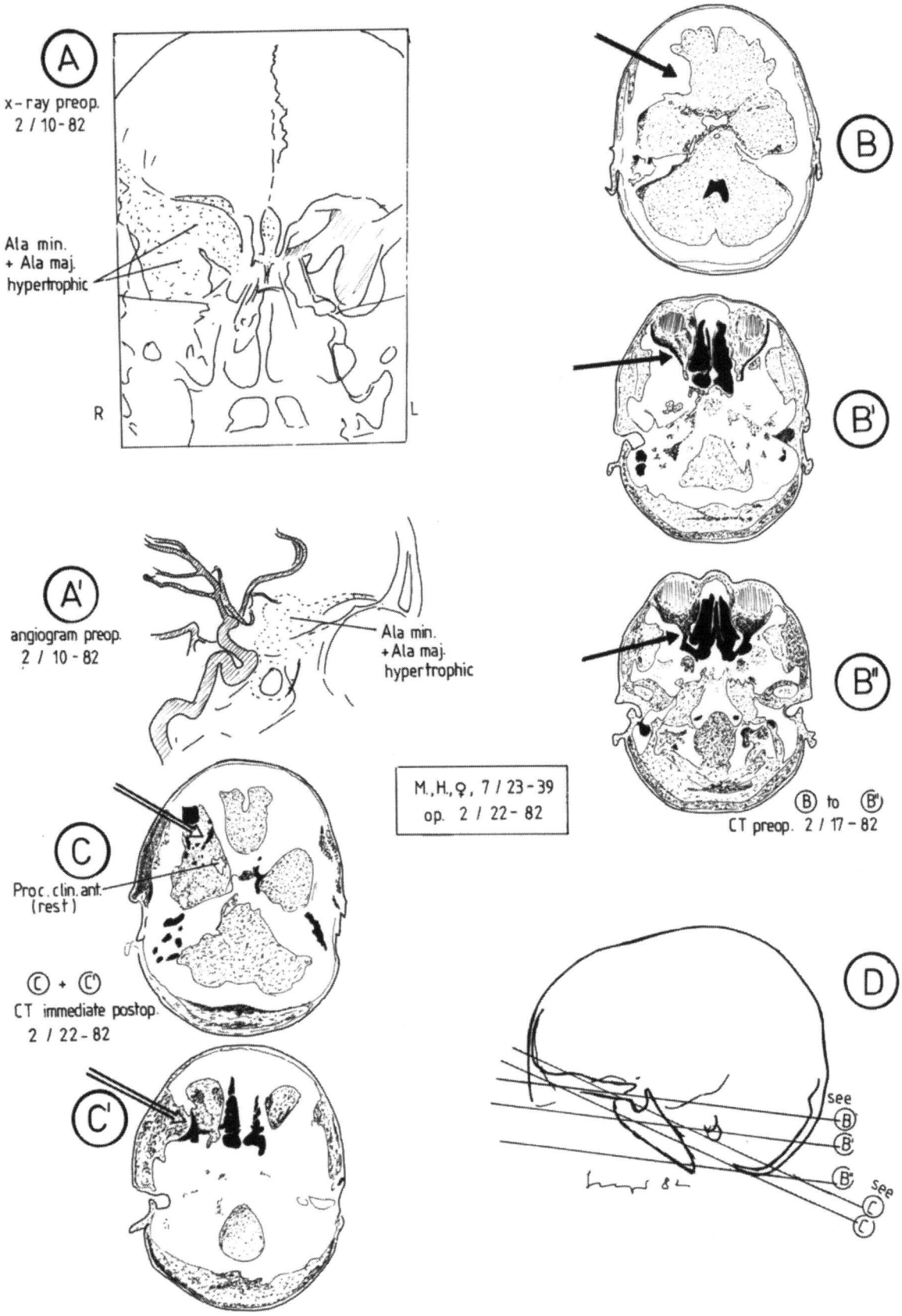
A
x-ray preop.
2 / 10-82
Ala min.
+ Ala maj.
hypertrophic
R
L
B
B'
B''
B to B''
CT preop. 2 / 17-82
A'
angiogram preop.
2 / 10-82
Ala min.
+Ala maj.
hypertrophic
M.,H.,♀, 7 / 23-39
op. 2 / 22-82
C
Proc. clin. ant.
(rest)
C + C'
CT immediate postop.
2 / 22-82
C'
D
see
B
B'
B''
see
C
C'

Fig. 75. Operations in the area surrounding Sinus cavernosus.
Flat meningioma in Sinus cavernosus area with extensive **bone reaction** of Ala major and Ala minor.
Postoperative X-ray findings

A Arrow: bone defect in area of orbital roof, Ala major and Ala minor. Normal contralateral findings

B + C X-ray, oblique projection

B Site of operation. Arrow: Defect in Canalis opticus wall

C Normal contralateral findings

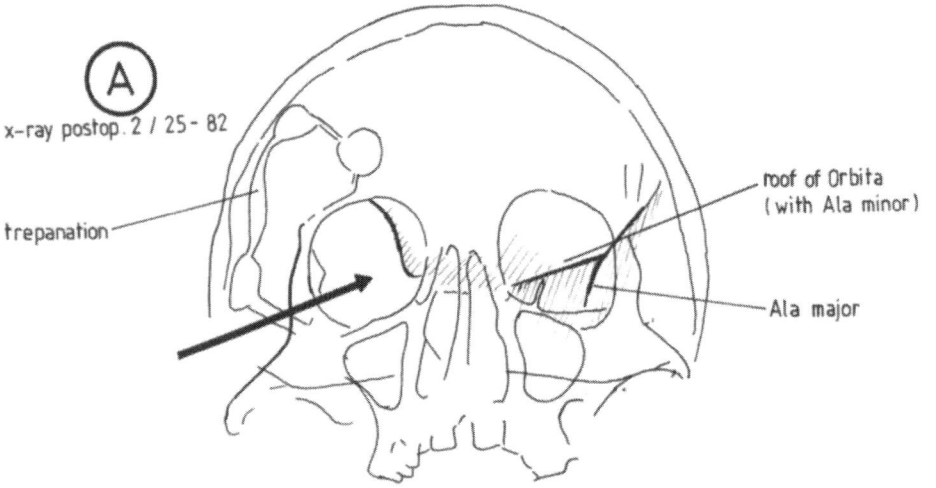

M., H., ♀, 7 / 23 - 39
op. 2 / 22 - 82

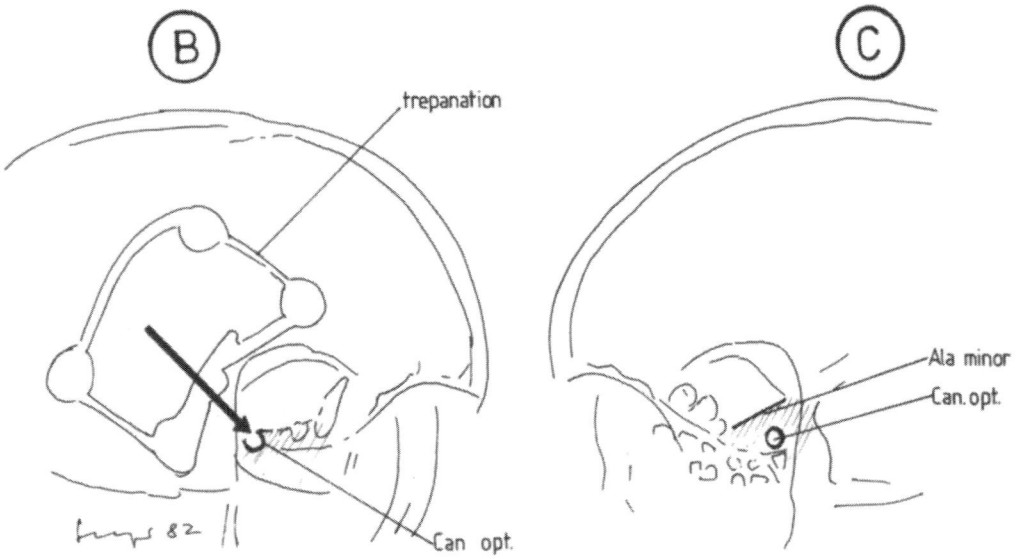

Ⓑ + Ⓒ x-ray postop. 2 / 25 - 82

Fig. 76. Operations in the area surrounding Sinus cavernosus.

Flat meningioma in Sinus cavernosus area with extensive bone reaction of Ala major and Ala minor.

Principles of bone resection

A Skull preparation, skin incision, immediately in front of Meatus acusticus externus sketched in (broken line)

B Situation after pterional trepanation, after drilling of Ala major and Ala minor. Periorbita (continuation of dura within orbita) exposed

B' Enlarged skull preparation, without dura sketched in, corresponding to anatomical sketch **B**

Arrow *a:* path of N. opticus

Arrow *b:* path of nerves and vessels, surrounded by Fissura orbitalis sup.

Arrow *c:* path of N. maxillaris

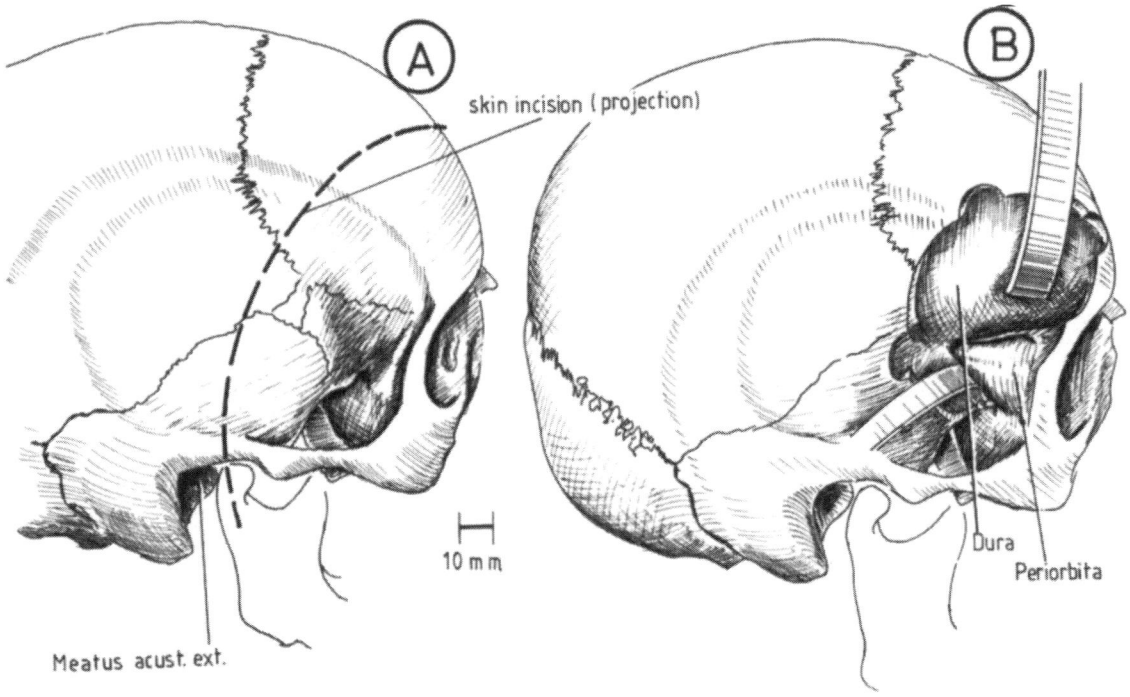
A
B
skin incision (projection)
10 mm
Meatus acust. ext.
Dura
Periorbita

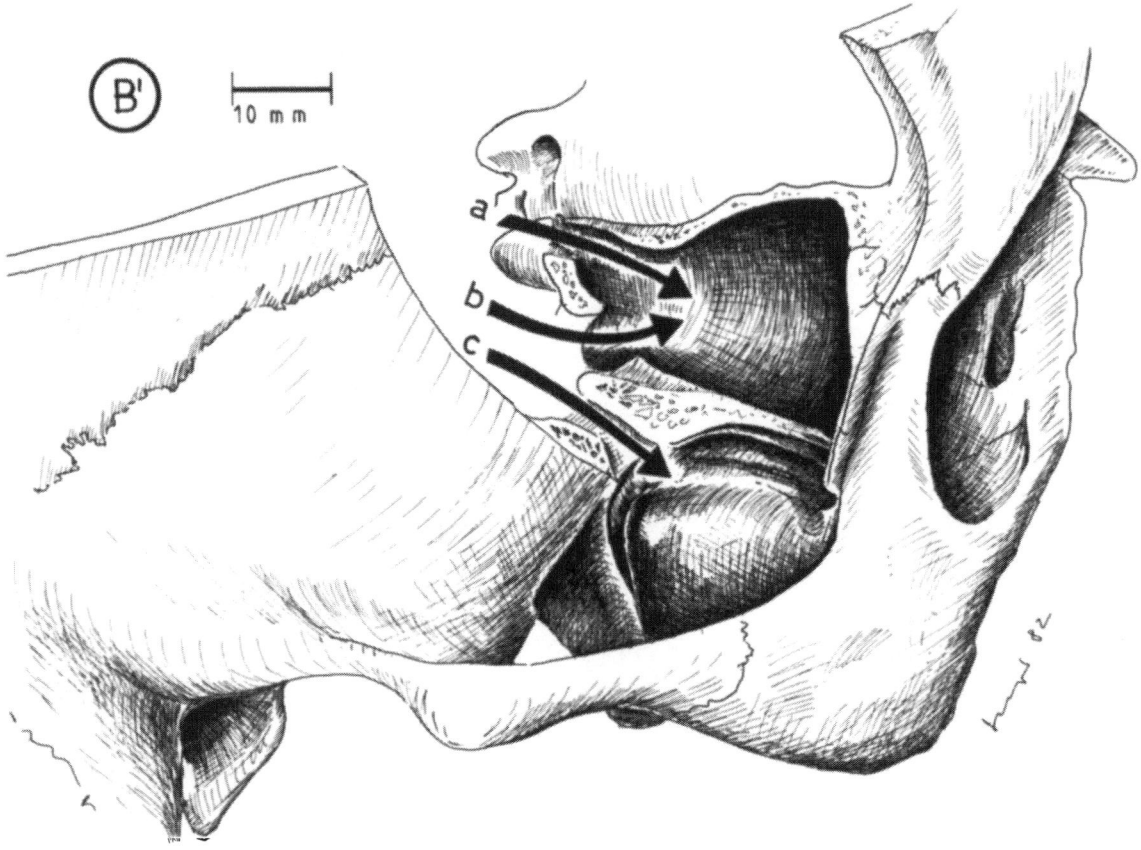
B'
10 mm
a
b
c

Fig. 77. Operations in the area surrounding Sinus cavernosus.
Flat meningioma in Sinus cavernosus area with extensive bone reaction of Ala major and Ala minor.

Principles of bone resection

A Anatomical sketch showing area of cranio-orbital juncture. Nerves and vessels shown through transparent Dura layer. Dura and Periorbita sketched in; structures enveloped by them are projected upon Dura and periorbital surface. Note close topographical relation of Vagina ext. n.II, Radix processus clinoideus ant., N.III to Curvatura cavernosa ant. of A. carotis int.
–.–.–: level of Fissura orbitalis sup.
Arrows: Topographical relation of Fissura orbitalis sup., Orbita, Fossa cranii media and Fossa pterygopalatina

A' Anatomical skull sketch, view from **A**

B Microsurgical site corresponding to anatomical sketch **A.** Due to altered direction of view, orbital roof appears greatly foreshortened. View direction see **B'**

B' View direction for **B**

Abbreviations:

(ch)	Chiasma (projection)
(Gsem)	Ganglion semilunare Gasseri (projection)
(N.III)	N.III (projection)
(N.V1)	N.V1 (projection)
tr	Transition between Dura mater and Periorbita
x	Bone remnant between N.V2 and juncture of Dura to Periorbita, as well as between Orbita (and Fossa pterygopalatina) and Fossa cranii media

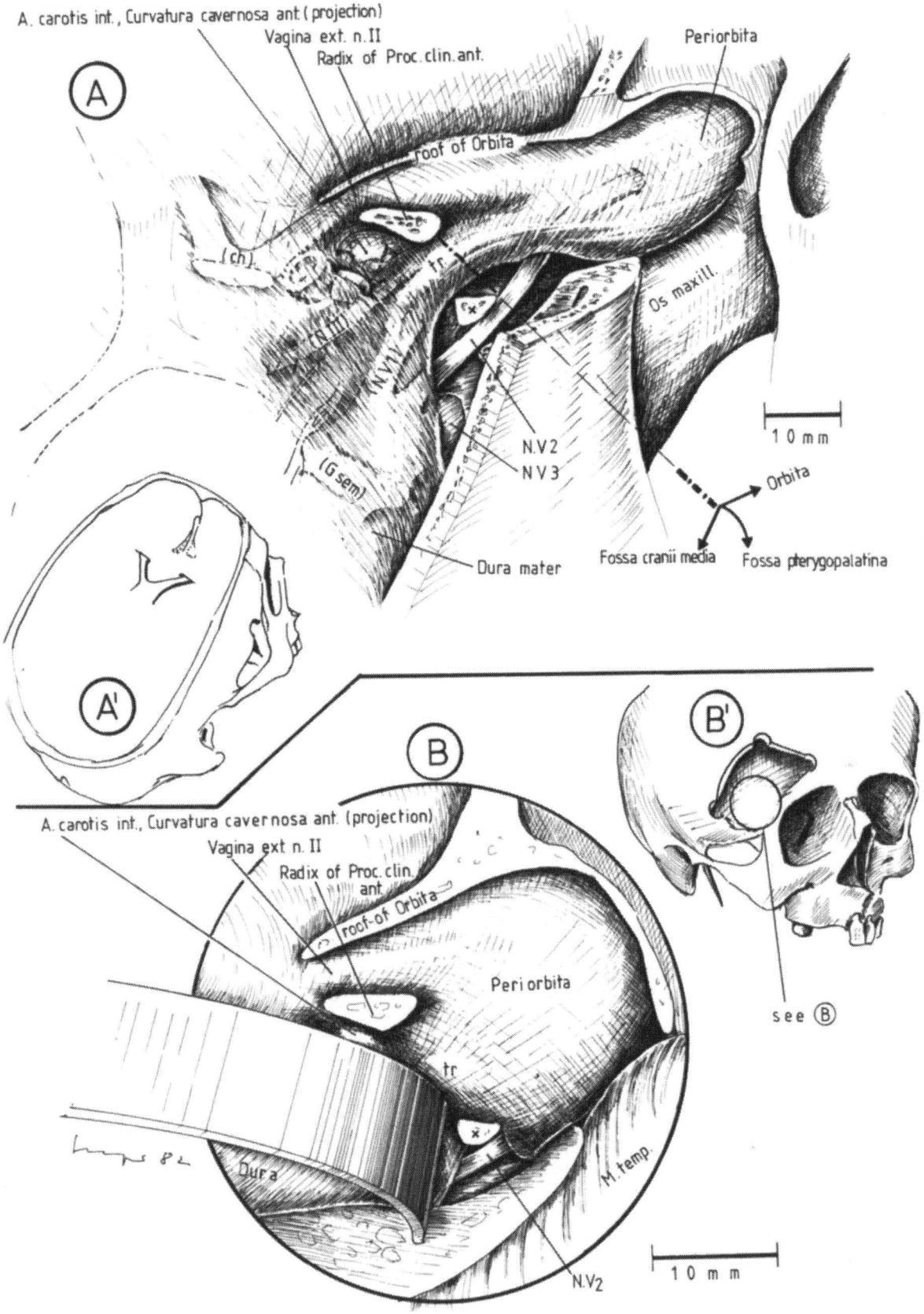
A
A. carotis int., Curvatura cavernosa ant. (projection)
Vagina ext. n. II
Radix of Proc. clin. ant.
Periorbita
roof of Orbita
(ch)
tr
Os maxill.
N.V1
(G sem)
N.V2
N.V3
10 mm
Orbita
Dura mater
Fossa cranii media
Fossa pterygopalatina
A'
B
B'
A. carotis int., Curvatura cavernosa ant. (projection)
Vagina ext. n. II
Radix of Proc. clin. ant.
roof of Orbita
Periorbita
see B
tr
Dura
M. temp.
N.V2
10 mm

Fig. 78. Operations in the area surrounding Sinus cavernosus.
Flat meningioma in Sinus cavernosus area with extensive bone reaction of Ala major and Ala minor.
Microsurgical site
Broken lines = projections

A **Opening up Dura** and posterior portions of Periorbita at the site of opened Fissura orbitalis sup.

B After opening of Fissura Sylvii:
- **1** Lifting of frontal lobe
- **2** Drawing back of temporal pole. Exposure of small meningioma which lies over Sinus cavernosus area; projection on Dura and meningioma of more deeply lying structures

Abbreviations:

(c1)	A. carotis int. (projection)
ra	Radix of Processus clinoideus ant.
(ra)	Radix of Processus clinoideus ant. (projection)
roo	Resection surface of Orbota roof
(N.III)	N.III (projection)
(N.V1)	N.V1 (projection)
(N.V2)	N.V2 (projection)
(N.V3)	N.V3 (projection)

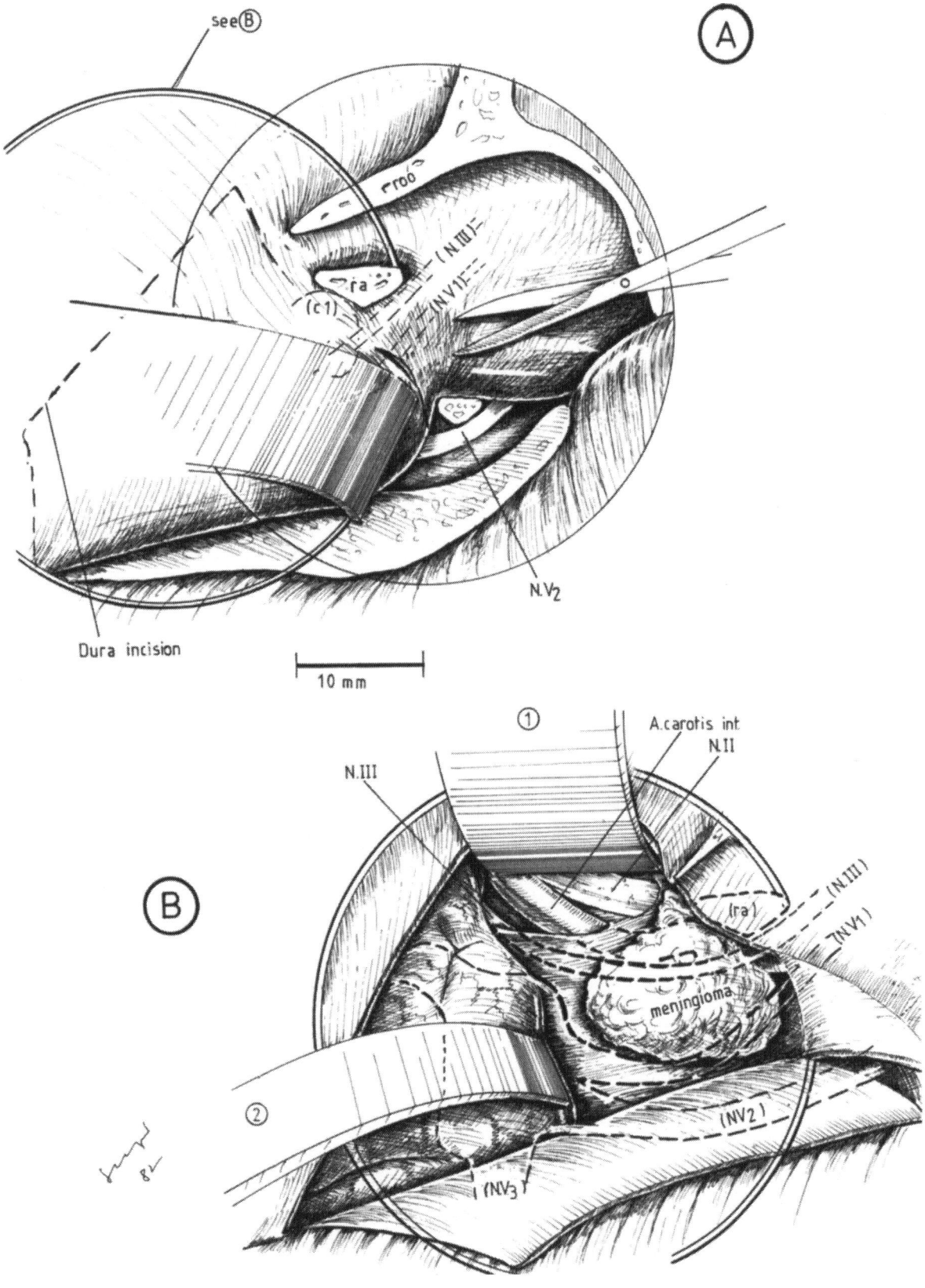
see B
A
roo
(N.III)
ra
(c1)
(N.V1)
N.V2
Dura incision
10 mm
1
A.carotis int.
N.II
N.III
B
(ra)
(N.III)
(N.V1)
meningioma
2
(NV2)
(NV3)

Fig. 79. Operations in the area surrounding Sinus cavernosus.
Flat meningioma in Sinus cavernosus area with extensive bone reaction of Ala major and Ala minor.
Meningioma is removed, its dura insertion scraped out, with sharp dissector.
Measurements in mm

A **1** Tumor-cleared dura surface is coagulated by means of low amperage
2 Excision of dura insertion of meningioma except for 5 mm wide remnant lateral to N. opticus and A. carotis int.

B Enlarged detail from **A.** After dura fenestration over Sinus cavernosus area, one sees the superficial nerve layer –N.V1 and N.IV–, and then somewhat deeper N.III shimmering through, and A. carotis int. with N. abducens, covered by loose connective tissue. Veins lateral to Sinus cavernosus area normally are less developed than veins medial to A. carotis int. In the case presented, the lateral veins were scarcely bleeding, nearly obliterated by tumor pressure

Abbreviations:

cl	A. carotis int.
(clcc)	A. carotis int., Curvatura cavernosa ant. (projection)
(ggsG)	Ganglion Gasseri (projection)
(N.III)	N.III (projection)
(N.IV)	N.IV (projection)
(N.V1)	N.V1 (projection)
(N.V2)	N.V2 (projection)
(N.V3)	N.V3 (projection)
(N.VI)	N.VI (projection)
(ra)	Radix of Processus clinoideus ant. (projection)

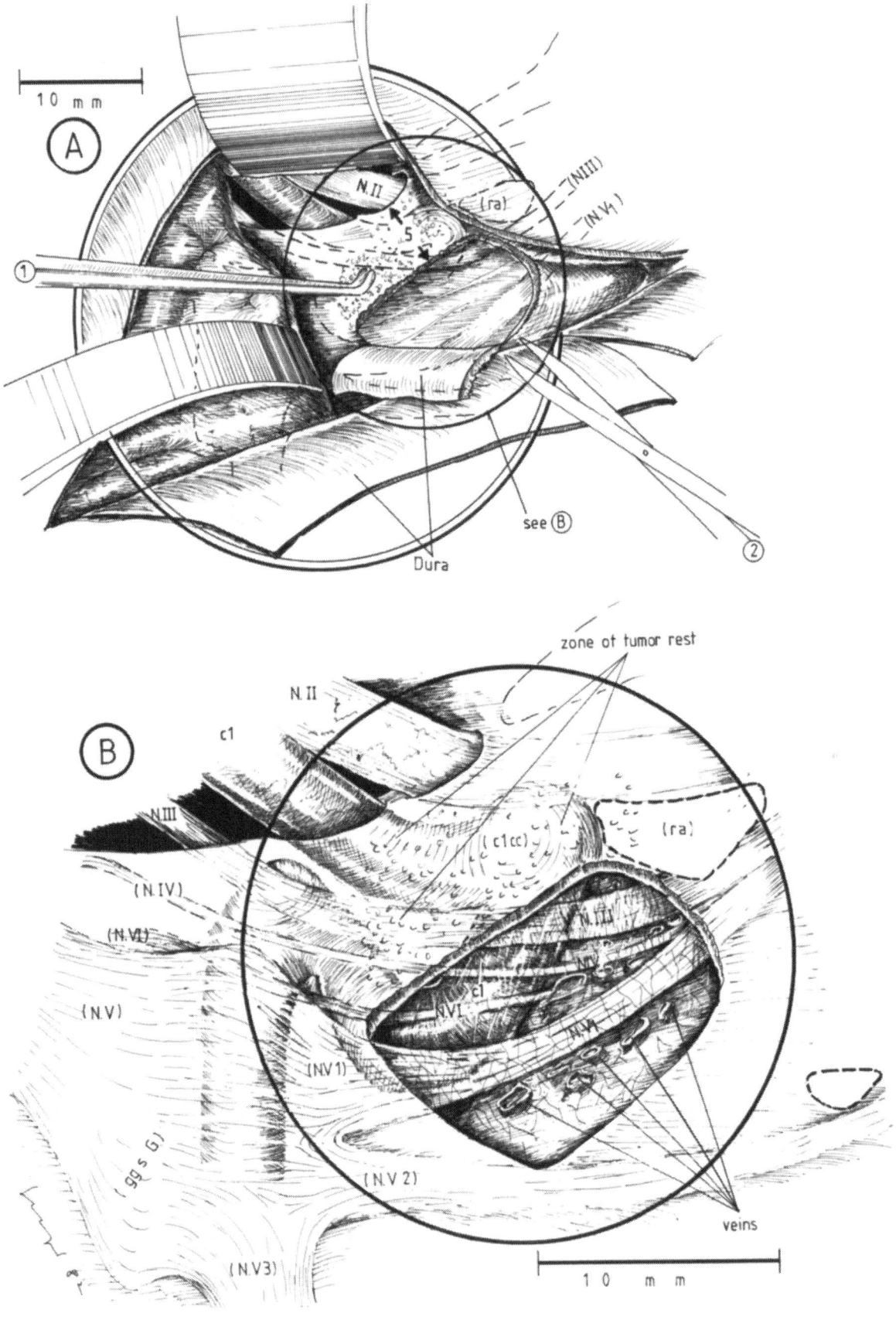
10 mm
A
N.II
5
(ra)
(N.III)
(N.V1)
1
see B
Dura
2
zone of tumor rest
B
N.II
c1
N.III
(c1cc)
(ra)
(N.IV)
(N.VI)
N.III
N.V
c1
N.VI
N.VI
(N.V)
(N.V1)
(gg s G)
(N.V 2)
veins
(N.V3)
10 mm

Fig. 80. Operations in the area surrounding Sinus cavernosus.
Tumors of Sinus cavernosus area.
Four tumor types with four operation examples shown. Anatomical transection sketches done according to operation site

A Sinus cavernosus region, section planes **B** to **E** drawn in. Broken lines = projection

B Lateral tumor lying outside nerves and vessels of the Sinus cavernosus area = radical operation possible (see clinical example Figs. 81 to 85)

C Tumor between superficial and deep nerve layer in lateral Sinus cavernosus area (s. clinical example Figs. 86 to 89, here with transition into posterior orbital region) = radical operation possible

D Tumor in all aeas of Sinus cavernosus except the Sella, but limited to one side (see clinical example Figs. 90 to 93). In most cases radical operation not possible. However, this example shows tumor radically operable, since intraorbital tumor portion caused blindness and led to enucleation of bulbus, whereby all the structures of Sinus cavernosus area could be resected except for A. carotis int.

E Tumor in all Sinus cavernosus areas extending contralaterally (see clinical example Figs. 99 to 95). Tumor inoperable, except for local nerve decompression, i. e. N.II and N.III

Abbreviations:

cl A. carotis int.

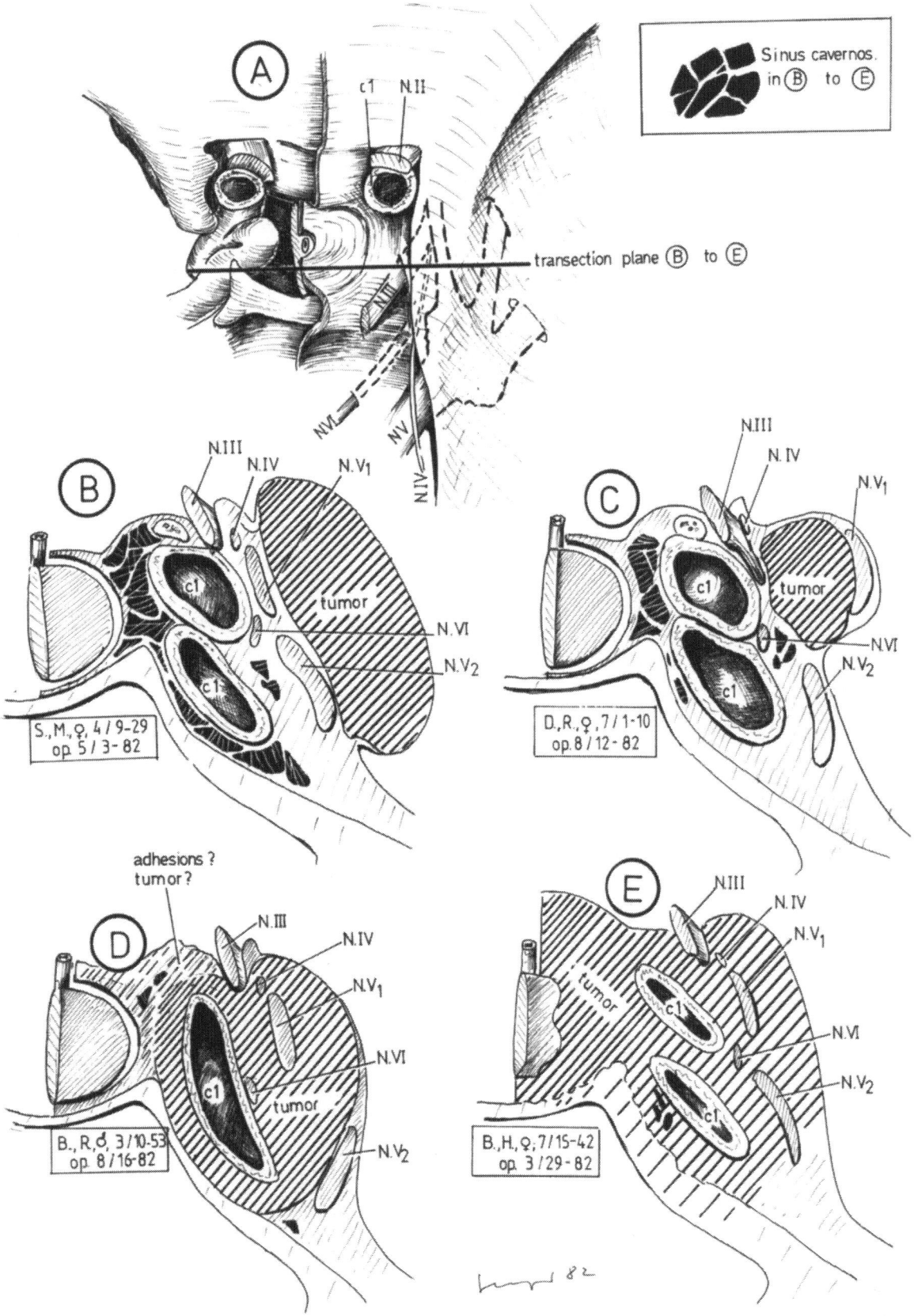
A
c1
N.II
Sinus cavernos. in B to E
transection plane B to E
N.VI
N.V
N.IV
B
N.III
N.IV
N.V1
c1
tumor
N.VI
N.V2
c1
S.,M.,♀, 4/9-29
op. 5/3-82
C
N.III
N.IV
N.V1
c1
tumor
N.VI
N.V2
c1
D.,R.,♀, 7/1-10
op. 8/12-82
adhesions ?
tumor ?
D
N.III
N.IV
N.V1
N.VI
c1
tumor
N.V2
B.,R.,♂, 3/10-53
op. 8/16-82
E
N.III
N.IV
N.V1
tumor
c1
N.VI
N.V2
c1
B.,H.,♀, 7/15-42
op. 3/29-82
82

Fig. 81. Operations in the area surrounding Sinus cavernosus.

Clinical example of **superficial lateral Sinus cavernosus tumor***. Histological finding: meningioma. Postoperative incomplete external N. oculomotorius paresis and diminished sensitivity of the three branches N. trigemini; complete postoperative recovery within few weeks. Postoperative improvement of organic psychosyndrome. Passing suspicions of seizure-activity in EEG

A + B Angiogram: displacement of cerebral arteries and tumor, uptake of contrast medium (histological: meningioma)

C – F CT: temporo-medial tumor arising from Sinus cavernosus area

G + H No tumor postoperatively demonstrable

---

* Operation performed by Dr. W. Hassler, author's coworker.

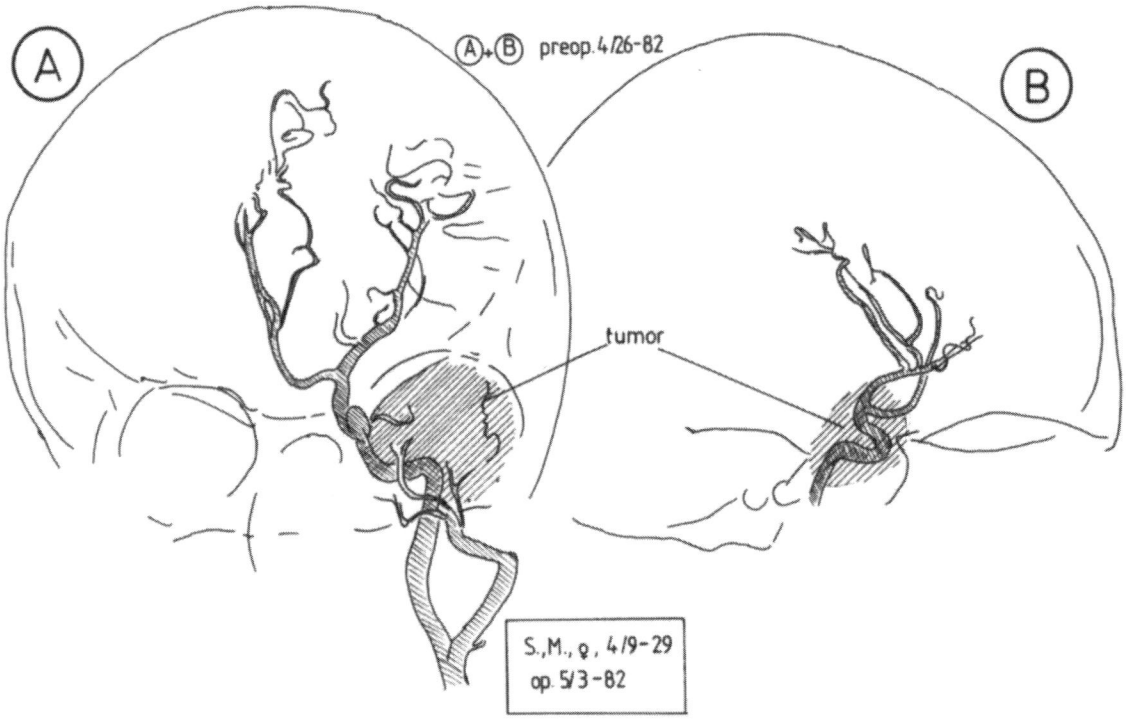
A
A+B preop. 4/26-82
B
tumor
S.,M., ♀, 4/9-29
op. 5/3-82

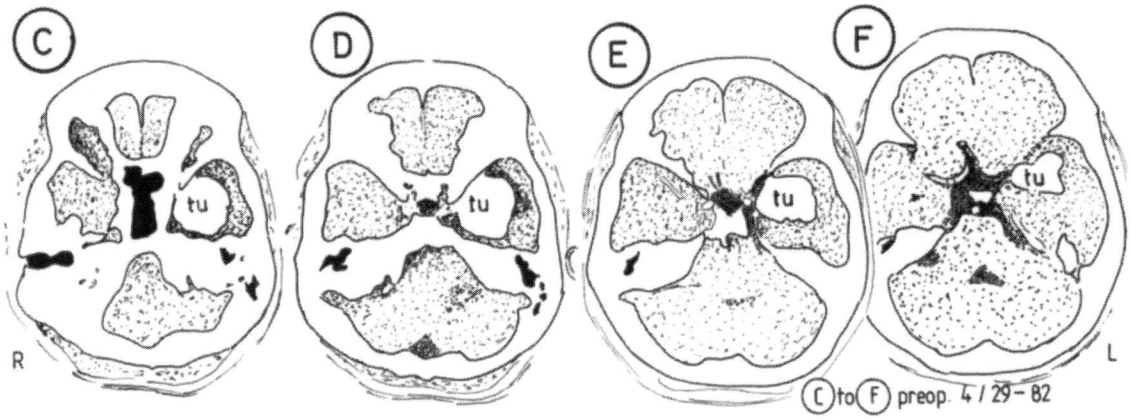
C
D
E
F
tu
tu
tu
tu
R
L
C to F preop. 4/29-82

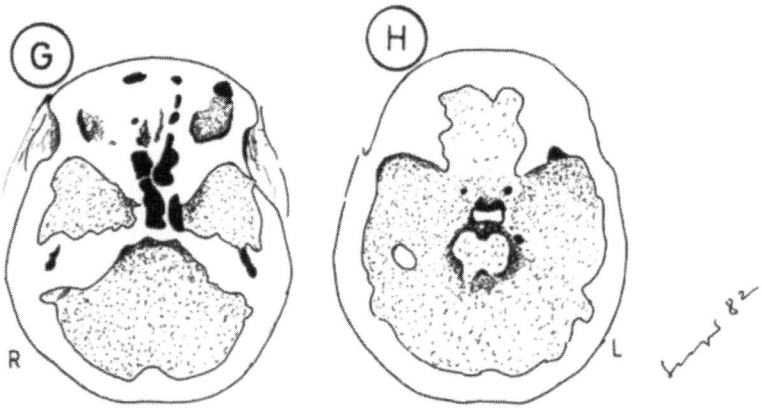
G
H
R
L
G+H immediate postop. 5/3-82

Fig. 82. Operations in the area surrounding Sinus cavernosus.
Operation site
A **Trepanation** sketched on skull
B Enlarged detail from **A**, microsurgical site of Fig. 83 sketched in

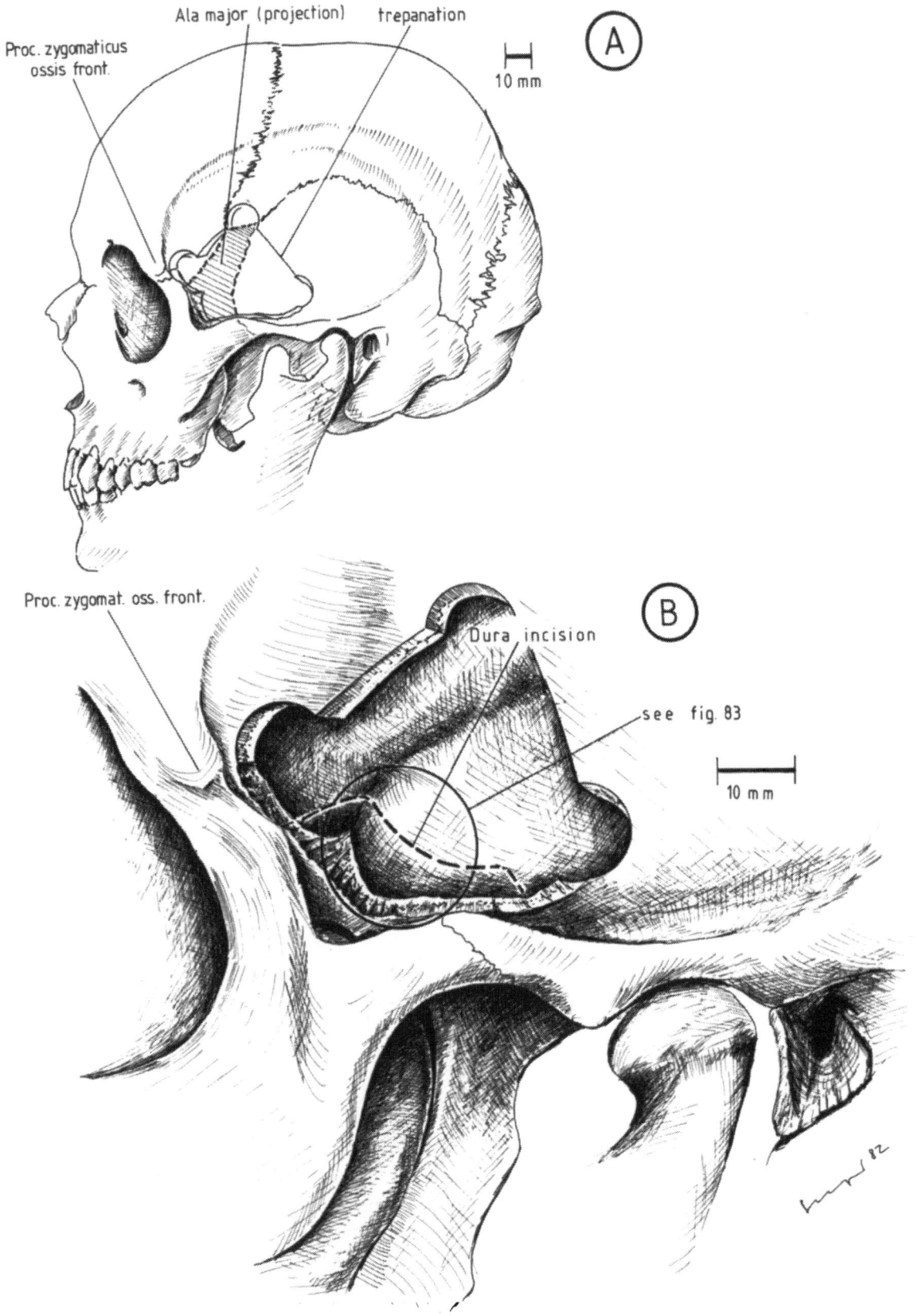
Ala major (projection)
trepanation
Proc. zygomaticus ossis front.
10 mm
A
Proc. zygomat. oss. front.
B
Dura incision
see fig. 83
10 mm

Fig. 83. Operations in the area surrounding Sinus cavernosus.
Operation site after Dura opening

A **1** Holding back **Arachnoidea** with small hook
2 Opening up Arachnoidea over Fissura lateralis Sylvii

B **1** Retraction of frontal lobe after splitting Arachnoidea of Fissura Sylvii
2 Slight pulling back of temporal lobe
3a Coagulation of tumor insertion in Dura
3b Thorough irrigation and suction

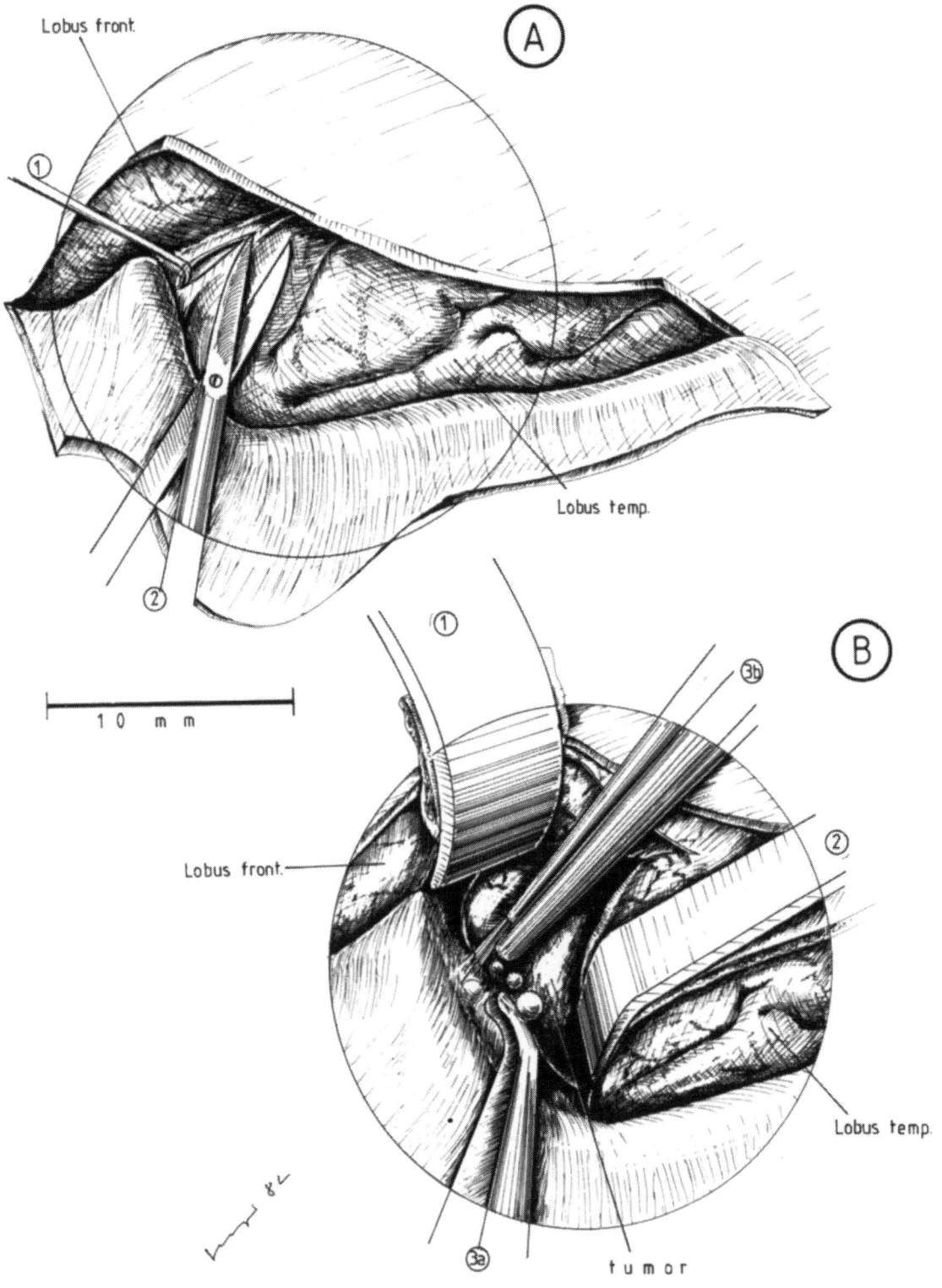
A
Lobus front.
1
2
Lobus temp.
10 mm
B
1
3b
2
Lobus front.
Lobus temp.
3a
tumor

Fig. 84. Operations in the area surrounding Sinus cavernosus.

Operation site

A **1** Incision of bipolarly coagulated tumor surface

2 Pushing back of tumor from Ala minor. Open arrow: change of microscopic view, see **B**

3 Squeezing of tumor by forceps, tumor coagulation and removal

B Site after **tumor removal.** Dura still infiltrated by tumor. Black arrow: new microscopic view as opposed to **A**

Abbreviations:

ap Ala minor

cl A. carotis int.

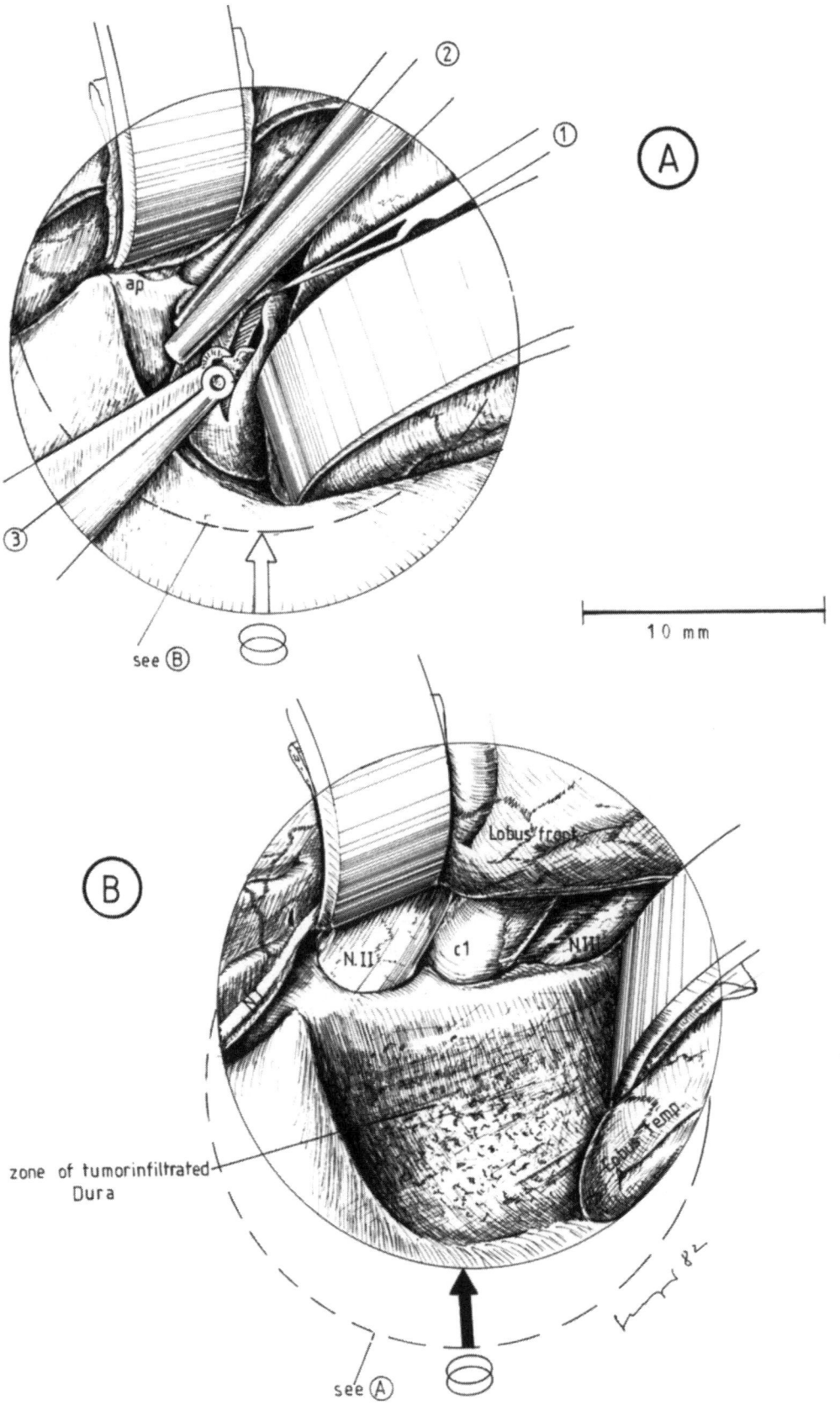
A
1
2
3
ap
see B
10 mm
B
Lobus front.
N. II
c1
N. III
Lobus temp.
zone of tumorinfiltrated
Dura
see A

Fig. 85. Operations in the area surrounding Sinus cavernosus.

Operation site

A **1** Retraction of incised superficial dura layer

2 Separation, by means of blunt preparation, of superficial dura layer from superficial nerve layer (N.V1 + N.V2)

Arrow: Change of microscopic view as opposed to Fig. 84 **B**

B **Excision of tumor-infiltrated Dura.** Superficial nerve layer (N.V1 + N.V2) is exposed nearly to Ganglion Gasseri. No tumor remnant can now be ascertained

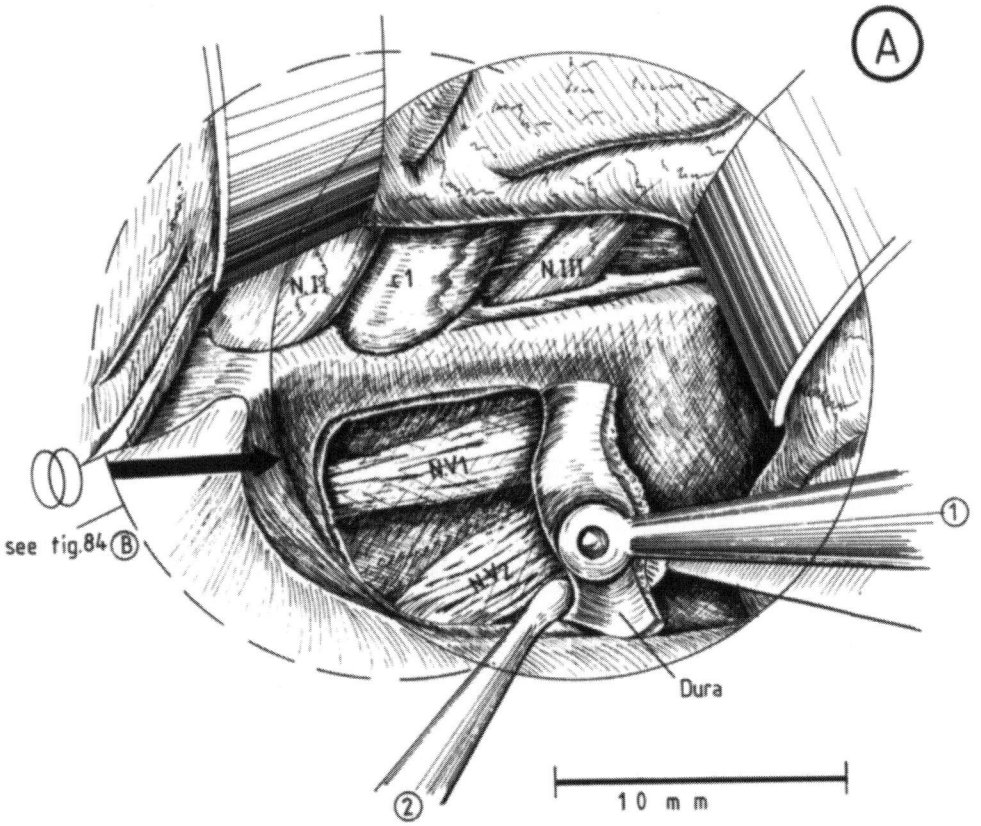
A
N.II
c1
N.III
N.V1
N.V2
see fig.84 B
1
2
Dura
10 mm

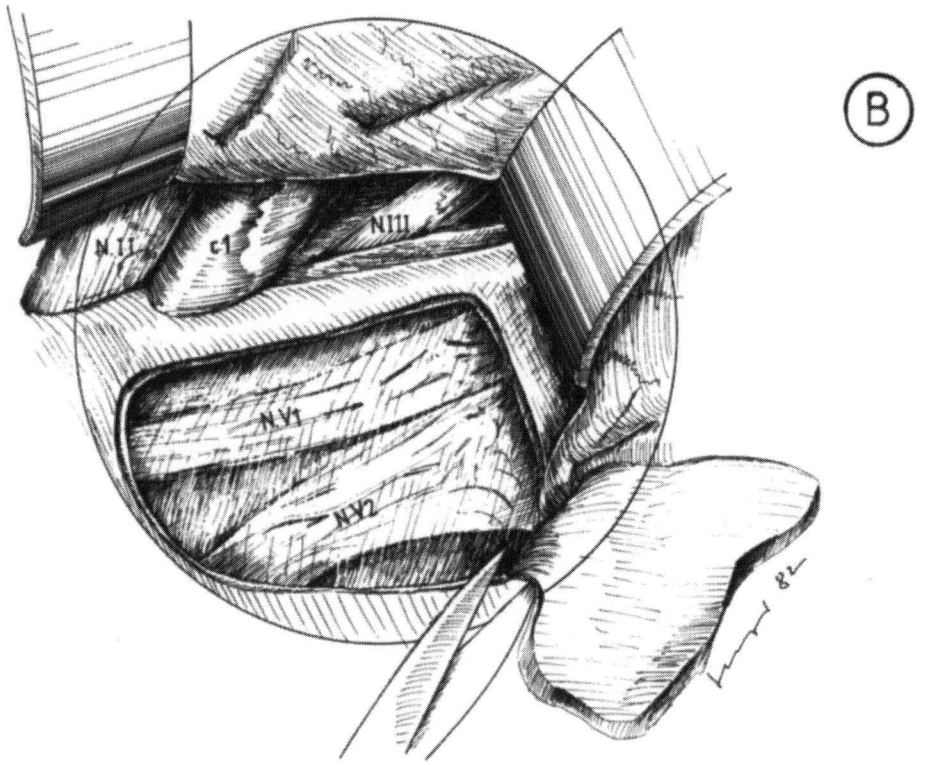
B
N.II
c1
N.III
N.V1
N.V2

Fig. 86. Operations in the area surrounding Sinus cavernosus.

Clinical example of **tumor located between Canalis opticus and Fissura orbitalis sup.*** (histologic: anaplastic meningioma). For 2 months leftsided trigeminal neuralgia, vertical diplopia; neurologica: leftsided ptosis. No additional postoperative deficits, trigeminal neuralgia disappeared

A	Lateral angiogram without tumor uptake of contrast medium
B	CT: Tumor of orbital cavity at orbito-cranial juncture in front of Processsus clinoideus ant. (with Pneumosinus dilatans, an accompanying finding in meningiomas located here)
C + D	CT-reconstructions showing tumor in posterior orbital area
C' + D'	Section planes of reconstructions **C + D**
E	Bone resection after complete tumor removal; posterior Processus clinoideus ant. portions remain

* Operation performed by Dr. W. Hassler, author's coworker.

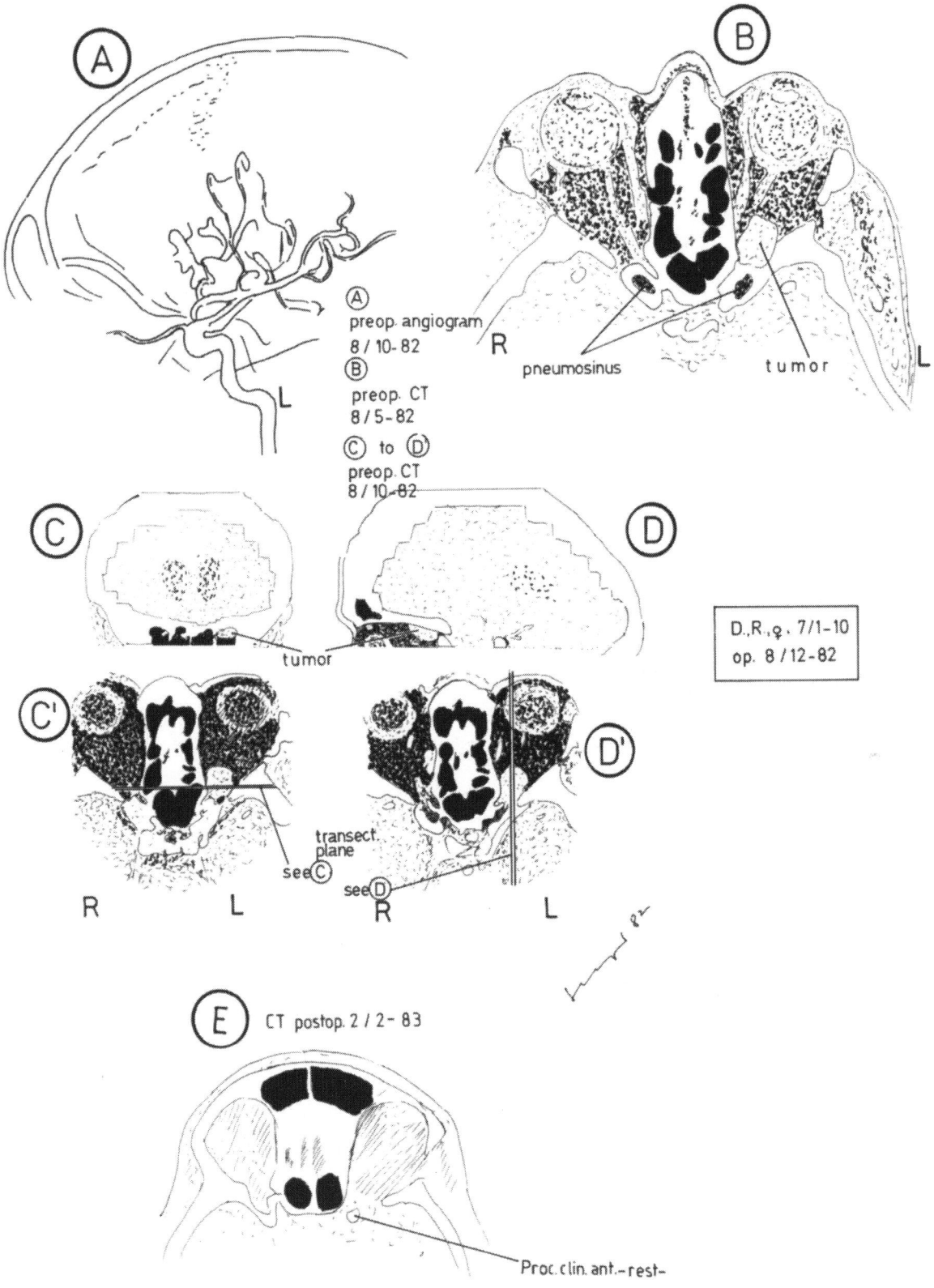
A
B
A
preop. angiogram
8 / 10-82
B
preop. CT
8 / 5-82
C to D
preop. CT
8 / 10-82
R
pneumosinus
tumor
L
L
C
D
tumor
D., R., ♀, 7/1-10
op. 8 / 12-82
C'
D'
transect. plane
see C
see D
R
L
R
L
E
CT postop. 2 / 2-83
Proc. clin. ant.-rest-

Fig. 87. Operations in the area surrounding Sinus cavernosus.

Operation site

A Skull sketch with various microsurgical view possibilities, pterional approach (arrows)

A' Skull sketch, **pterional trepanation** drawn in

B Microsurgical site after trepanation

1a Dura incision

1b Folding back of dura flaps

C Splitting of Fissura Sylvii

1 Opening up arachnoidea by small hook

2 Cutting of arachnoidal filaments with scissors

3 Gradual spreading apart of Fissura Sylvii

1 – 3 Fissura Sylvii is widely opened up

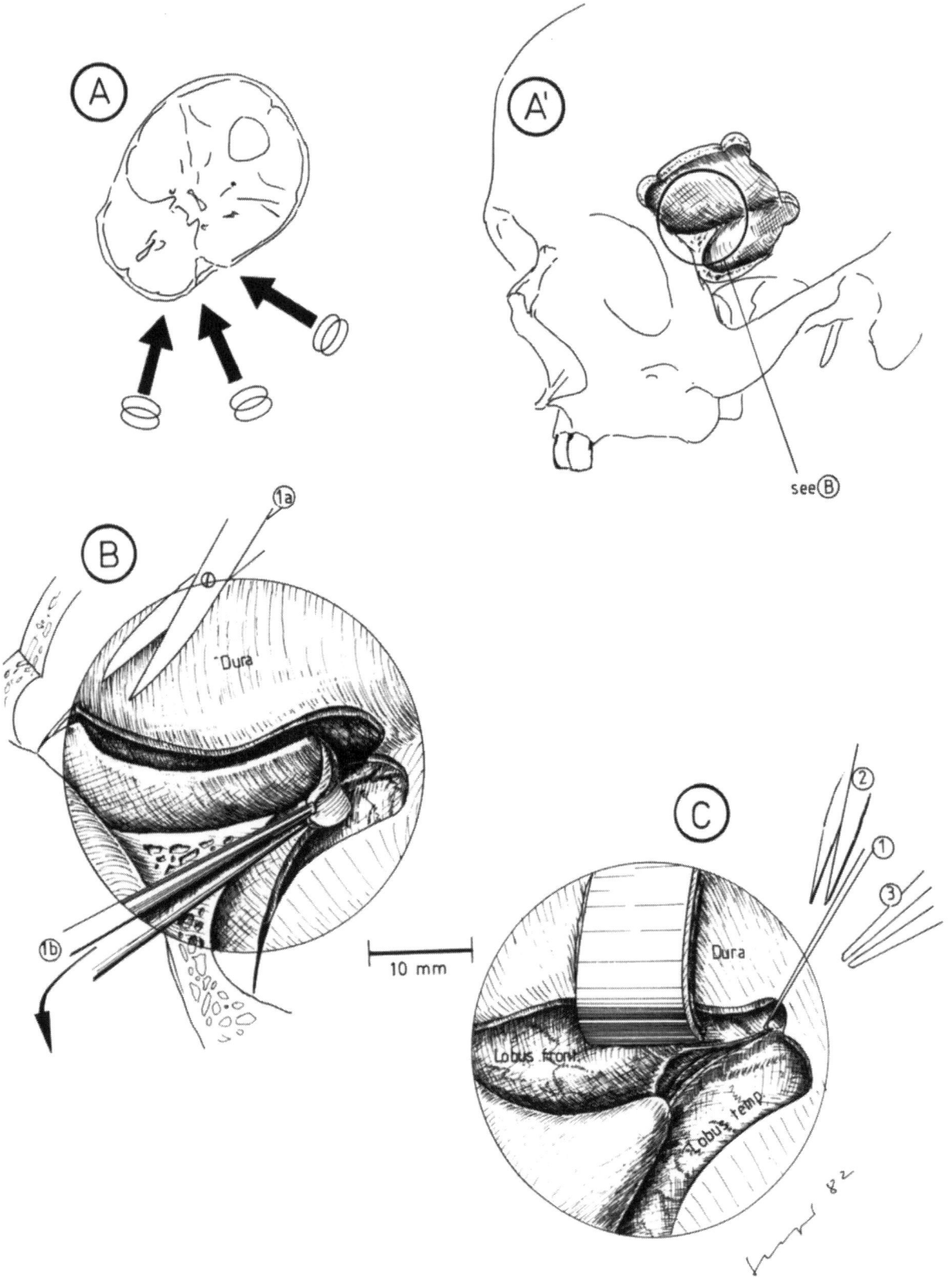
A
A'
see B
B
1a
1
Dura
1b
10 mm
C
2
1
3
Dura
Lobus front.
Lobus temp.

Fig. 88. Operations in the area surrounding Sinus cavernosus

A **1** **Reclination of Lobus frontalis** after opening of Fissura Sylvii arachnoidea

2 Slight retraction of Lobus temporalis

B Enlarged detail from **A. Opening of dura over Sinus cavernosus** area

1a Dura incision over N. oculomotorius path and over the palpable Processus clinoideus ant.

1b + 1c Wedening of incision until close to N.II and A. carotis int. *–c1–*

C **Resection of Processus clinoideus ant.,** a small residual of which is preserved lateral to A. carotis int. *–c1–*; N.III and N.V1 recognizable after dura resection

C' Topographical anatomical sketch for **C.** Thin-dotted line: dura resection. Heavy broken line: tumor localization

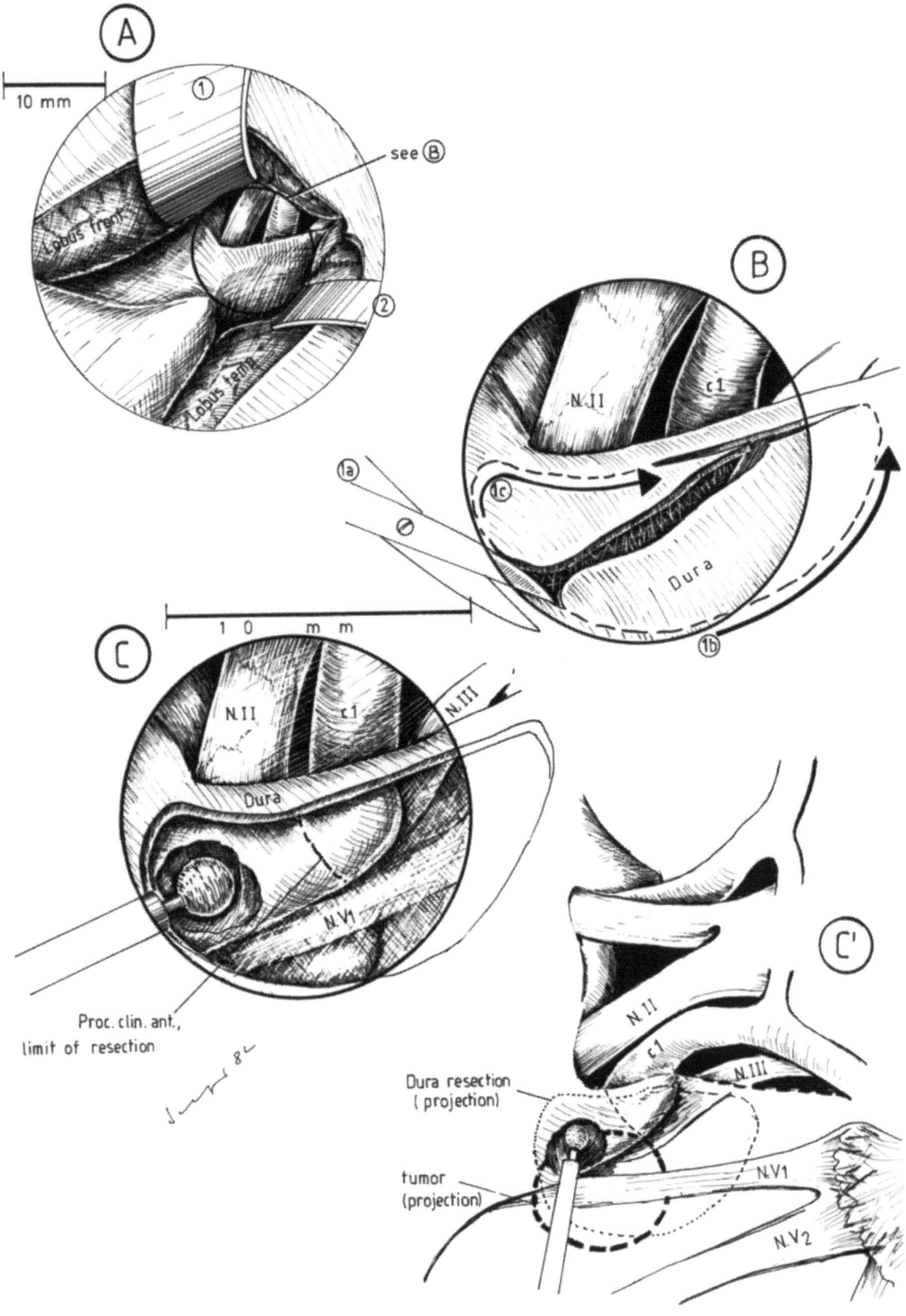
A
10 mm
1
see B
Lobus front.
2
Lobus temp.
B
N.II
c1
1a
1c
Dura
1b
10 mm
C
N.II
c1
N.III
Dura
N.V1
Proc. clin. ant.,
limit of resection
C'
N.II
c1
N.III
Dura resection
(projection)
tumor
(projection)
N.V1
N.V2

Fig. 89. Operations in the area surrounding Sinus cavernosus

A **1a + 1b** Incision of tumor surface above and below N.V1

2 Hollowing of tumor with curette

3 Removal of loosened tumor tissue

B **1a + 1b** Removal of loosened tumor bulk from tumor bed

C Site after **tumor removal**

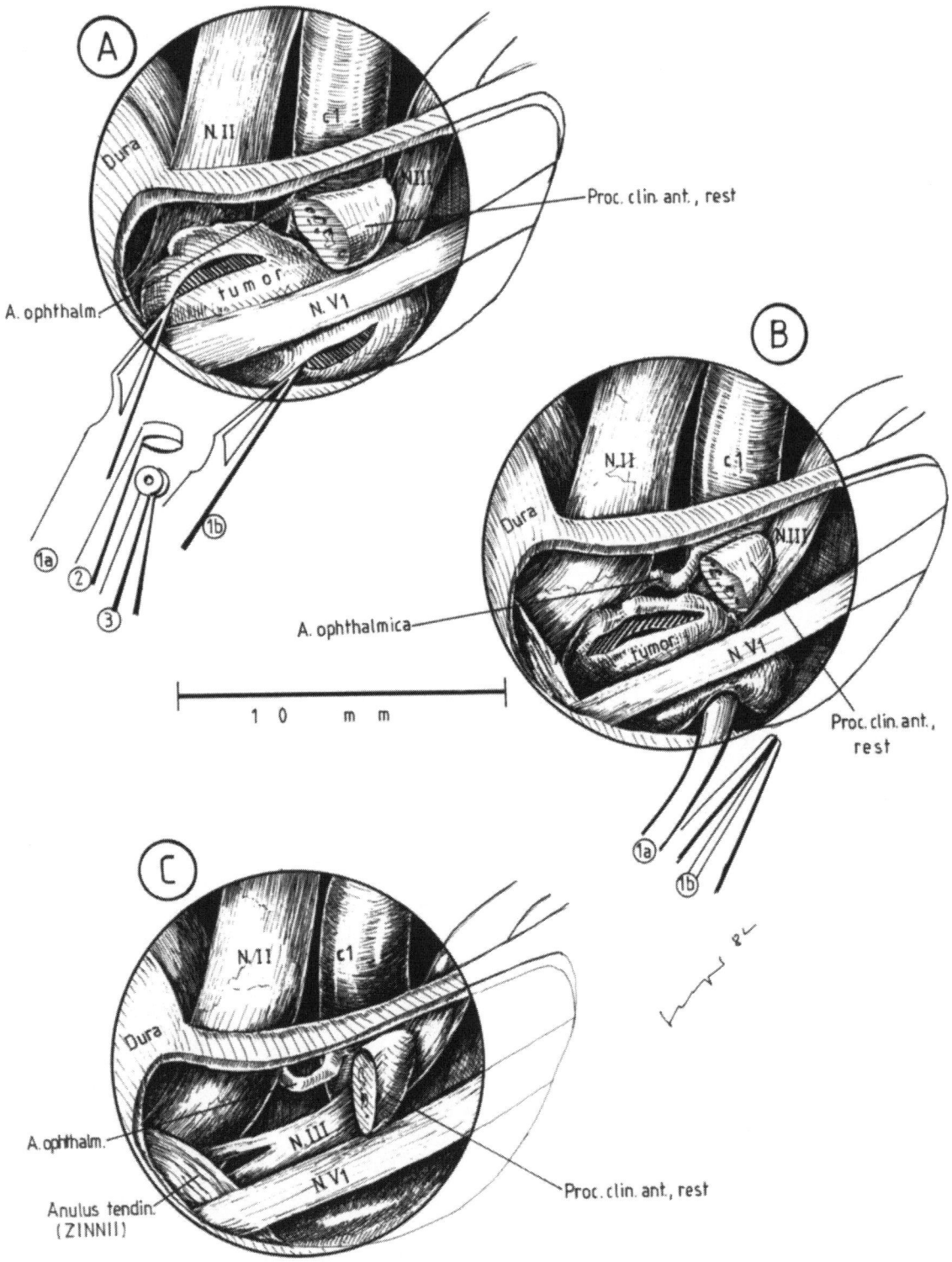
A
Dura
N.II
c1
N.III
Proc. clin. ant., rest
tumor
A. ophthalm.
N.V1
1a
2
3
1b
B
N.II
c1
Dura
N.III
A. ophthalmica
tumor
N.V1
Proc. clin. ant., rest
1a
1b
1 0 m m
C
N.II
c1
Dura
A. ophthalm.
N.III
N.V1
Anulus tendin. (ZINNII)
Proc. clin. ant., rest

Fig. 90. Operations in the area surrounding Sinus cavernosus.

Clinical example of **meningioma recidivation occupying total left Sinus cavernosus** area*. Normally, this type tumor inoperable. In this case, as patient was already blind, the intraorbital portion of tumor, together with bulbus, was enucleated. Since here it was unnecessary to save the already destroyed nerves of the Sinus cavernosus area, radical tumor removal was possible

A + B In angiogram: contrast medium uptake by tumor

C CT, preoperative: basal tumor with exophthalmus (histological: meningioma)

D Reconstruction, coronal section. Narrowing of basal cisterns by tumor

D' Section planes of reconstruction **D**

E Situation after eye enucleation and tumor removal. Extensive bone resection with defect of Processus clinoideus ant. and close-by portions of Ala minor and Ala major

* Operation performed by Dr. W. Hassler, author's coworker.

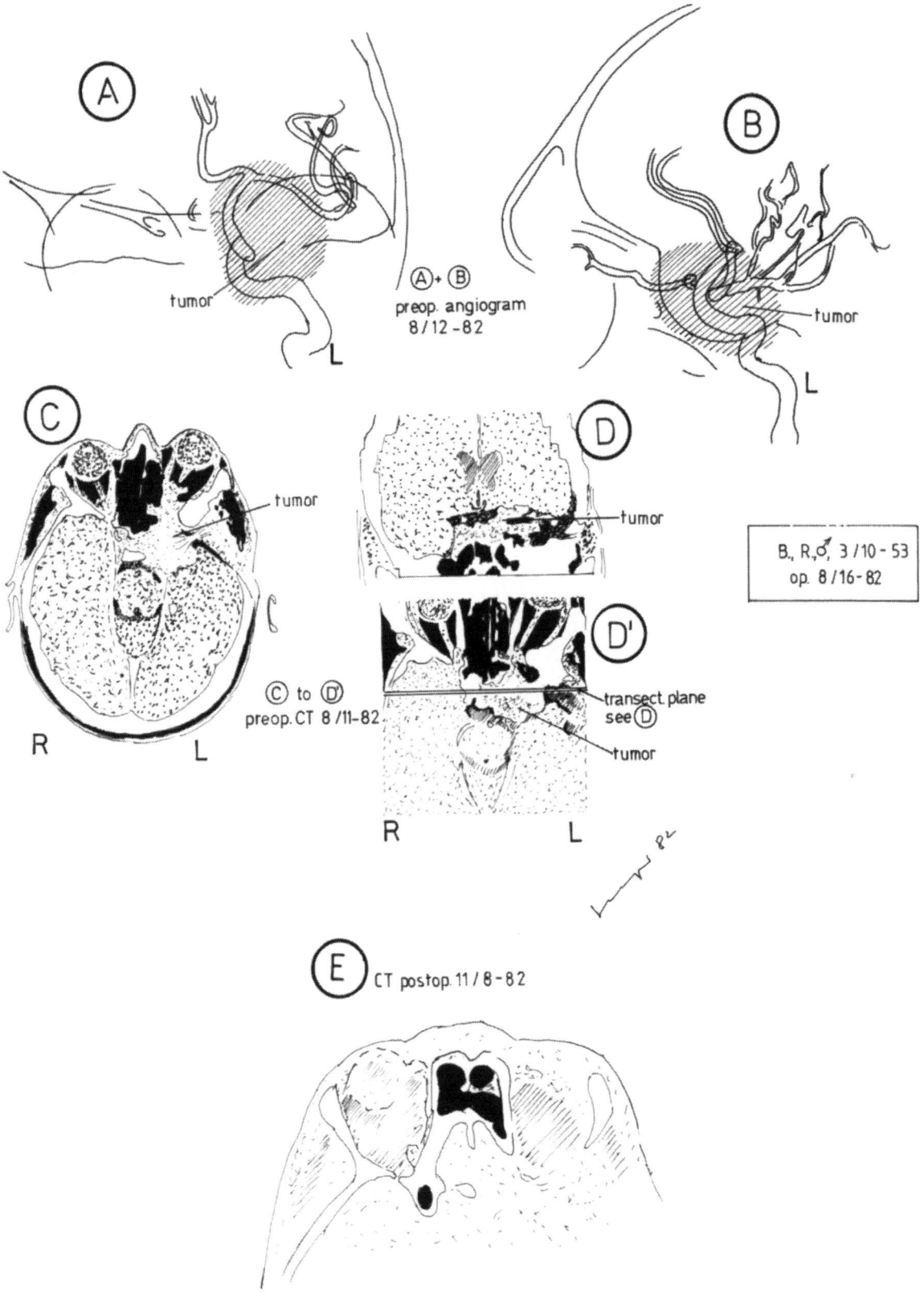
A
tumor
L
A + B
preop. angiogram
8/12-82
B
tumor
L
C
tumor
R
L
C to D'
preop. CT 8/11-82
D
tumor
D'
transect. plane
see D
tumor
R
L
B., R., ♂, 3/10-53
op. 8/16-82
E
CT postop. 11/8-82

Fig. 91. Operations in the area surrounding Sinus cavernosus

A Skull sketch, various microsurgical view positions shown

B Skull sketch with **pterional trepanation** drawn in. Recognizable previous trepanations were more extensive than present ones, corresponding to previous tumor size. In the approach to Sinus cavernosus and to orbital cavity a small pterional approach is sufficient

C Microsurgical site, corresponding to sketch **B. Drilling** of greatly thickened Ala minor and adjoining portions of orbita roof

D After drilling of Ala minor and major, juncture of Fossa cranii, media dura and perorbita dura is exposed medially, Foramen rotundum was not opened

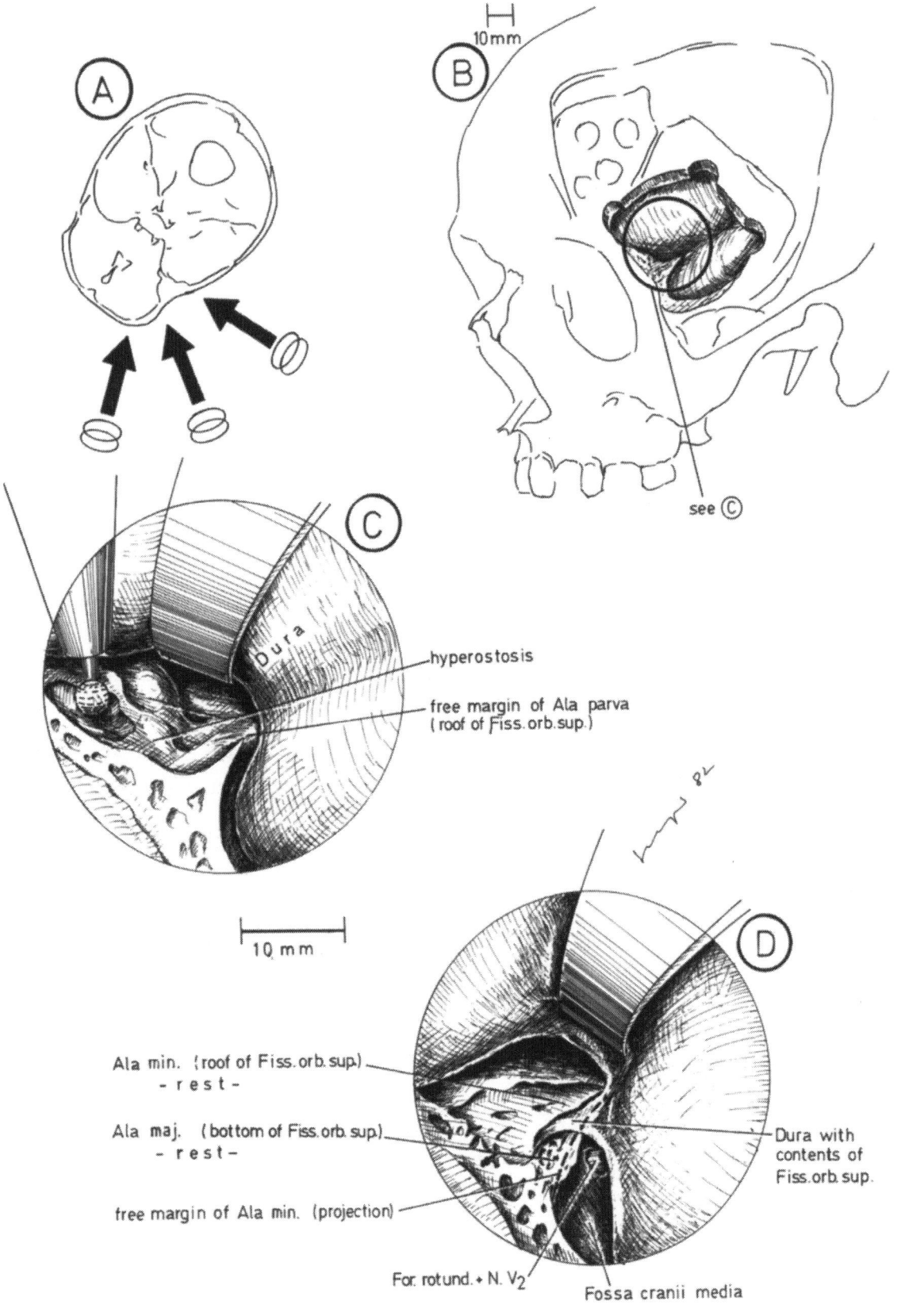
A
B
10 mm
see C
C
Dura
hyperostosis
free margin of Ala parva
(roof of Fiss. orb. sup.)
10 mm
D
Ala min. (roof of Fiss. orb. sup.)
- rest -
Ala maj. (bottom of Fiss. orb. sup.)
- rest -
free margin of Ala min. (projection)
Dura with
contents of
Fiss. orb. sup.
For. rotund. + N. V2
Fossa cranii media

Fig. 92. Operations in the area surrounding Sinus cavernosus

A **1** **Opening of dura**
- **2** Separation of adhesions from previous operations, between brain surface and dura
- **3** Snaring and pulling out of small basal dura flap

B **1a** Stretching of arachnoidal filaments over Fissura lateralis Sylvii by means of small hook
- **1b** Separation of these adhesions
- **2** After **opening of Fissura Sylvii,** insertion of spatula and reclination of frontal lobe
- **3** Dura incision over tumor near N.II and A. carotis int. *–c1–*
- **4a + 4b** Hollowing of tumor

C **1** Further insertion of spatula and **reclination of frontal brain** after opening of arachnoidea over N.II and A. carotis int.
- **2** Slight retraction of temporal pole
- **3** Coagulation of dura over tumor
- **4** **Incision of tumor** along A. carotis int. path
- **5** Stretching of tumor during incision

Abbreviations:

c1 A. carotis int.

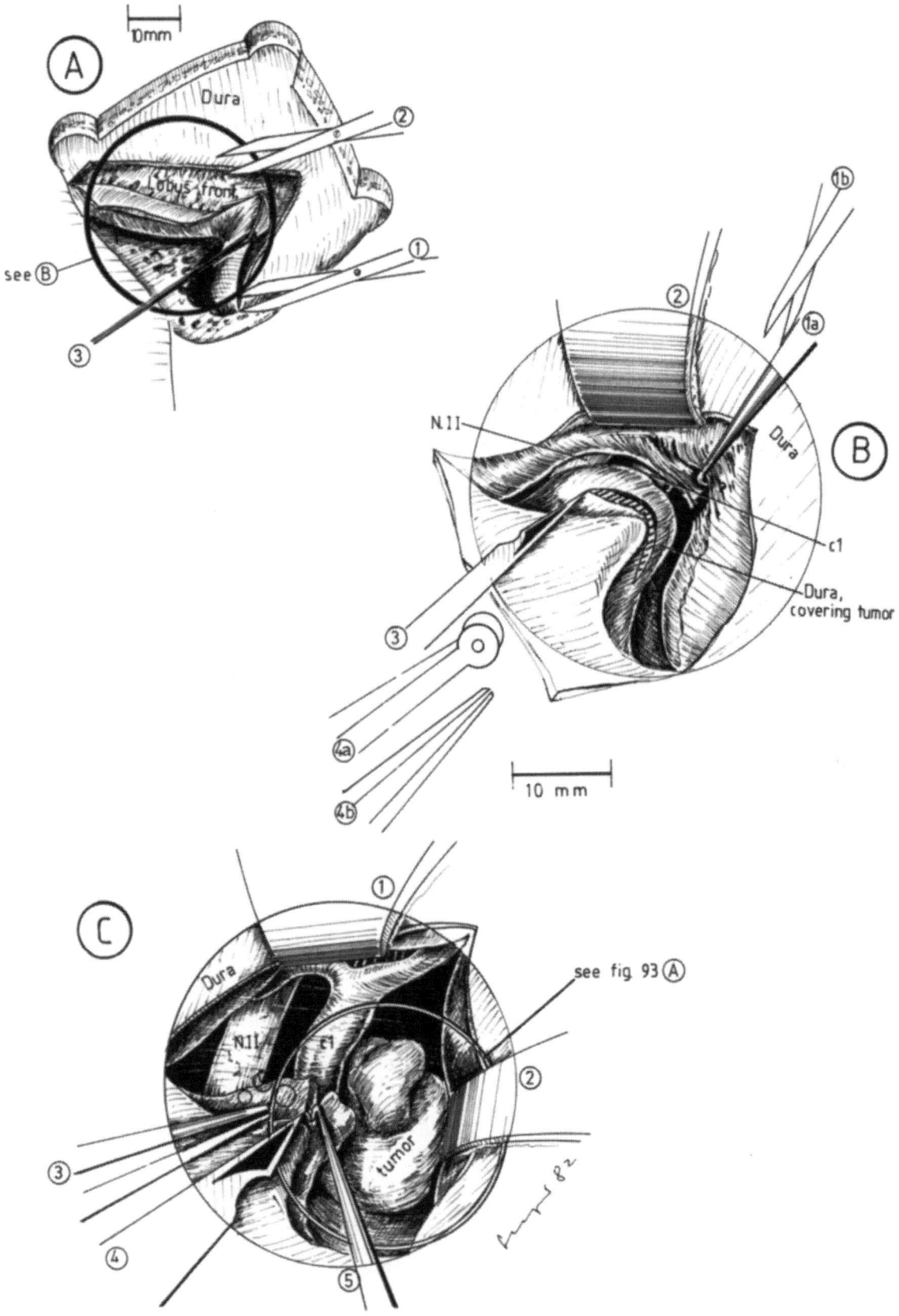
10mm
A
Dura
Lobus front
see B
1
2
3
1b
1a
N.II
Dura
B
c1
Dura, covering tumor
4a
4b
10 mm
C
Dura
N.II
c1
tumor
see fig. 93 A
1
2
3
4
5

Fig. 93. Operations in the area surrounding Sinus cavernosus

A Nerves running through Sinus cavernosus area can no longer be identified within tumor. For the already mentioned reasons, care need not be taken to save these nerves

1 Slight reclination of Lobus temporalis to posterior tumor edge

2 Incision of tumor along A. carotis int. path

B **1** Loosening of tumor from **A. ophthalmica,** which is afterward ligated

2 + 3 Loosening of tumor remnant from deep dura layer and bone.

broken lines: cranial nerves N.III, N.IV, N.V1 were not identifiable

B' Topographical anatomical sketch of **B,** left anterior view

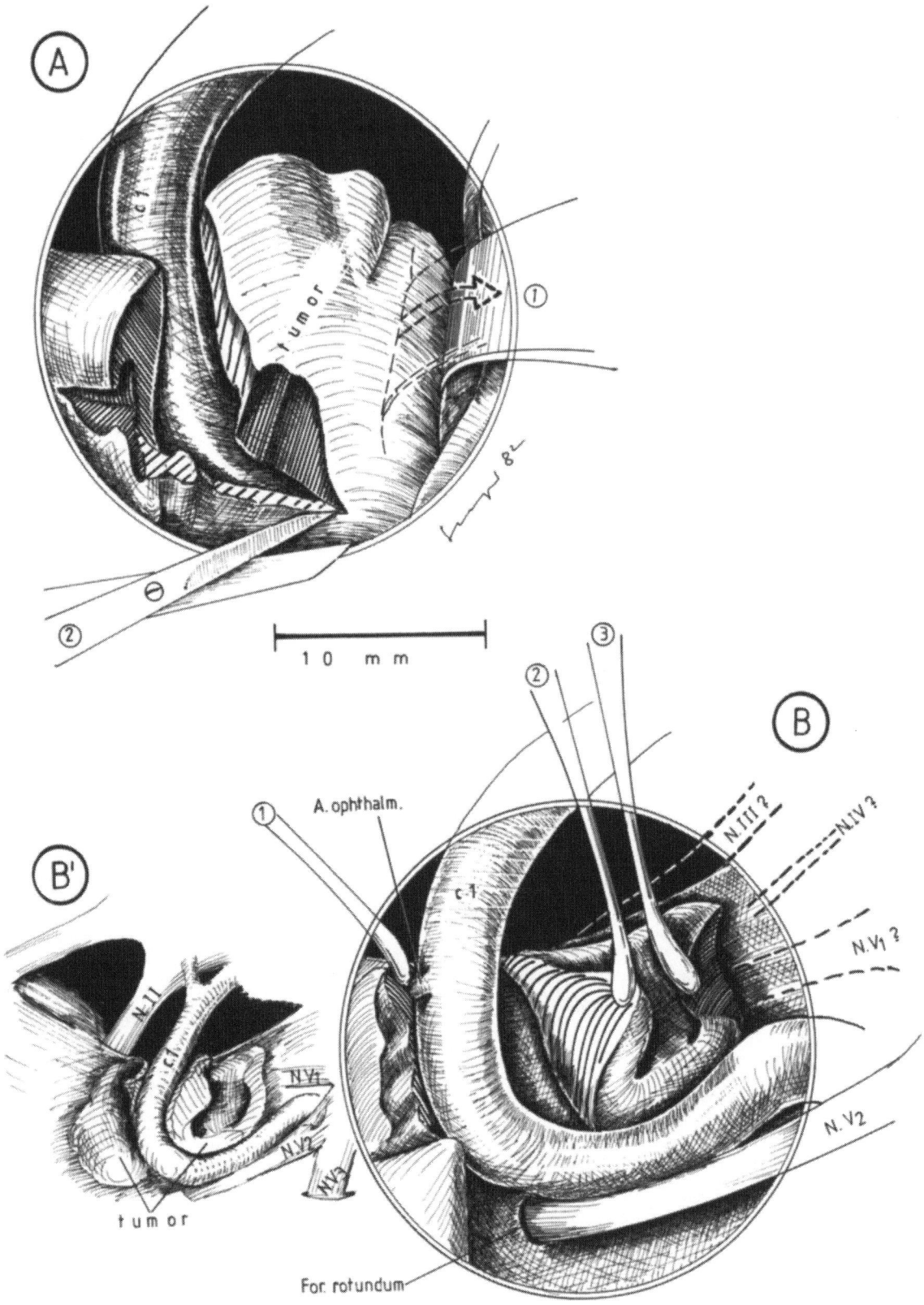
A
tumor
c.1
1
2
8°
10 mm
B
B'
1
2
3
A. ophthalm.
c.1
N.III ?
N.IV ?
N.V1 ?
N.V2
For. rotundum
N.II
c.1
N.V1
N.V2
N.V3
tumor

Fig. 94. Operations in the area surrounding Sinus cavernosus.

Clinical example of **inoperable tumor** (histological: meningioma) with contralateral extension*. In this case only a decompression of N. opticus and A. carotis int. is possible

A + B No contrast-medium uptake by tumor. Arrow: stenosis of A. carotis int. as it passes through Sinus cavernosus. The tumor being inoperable, even a decompression of A. carotis int. is out of the question because of danger to the nerves of Sinus cavernosus area. Carotis externa-interna bypass would be indicated if signs of an imminent cerebrovascular decompensation were present

C Section planes of reconstruction **C'** and **C''** sketched in, showing tumor infiltrating as a thin sheet towards the base

D + E Tumor is limited to Sinus cavernosus area. No sure indication of intradural growth. We have not presented postoperative CT because it was identical to preoperative CT: major portion of tumor was not removed

---

* Operation performed by Dr. H. R. Eggert, author's coworker.

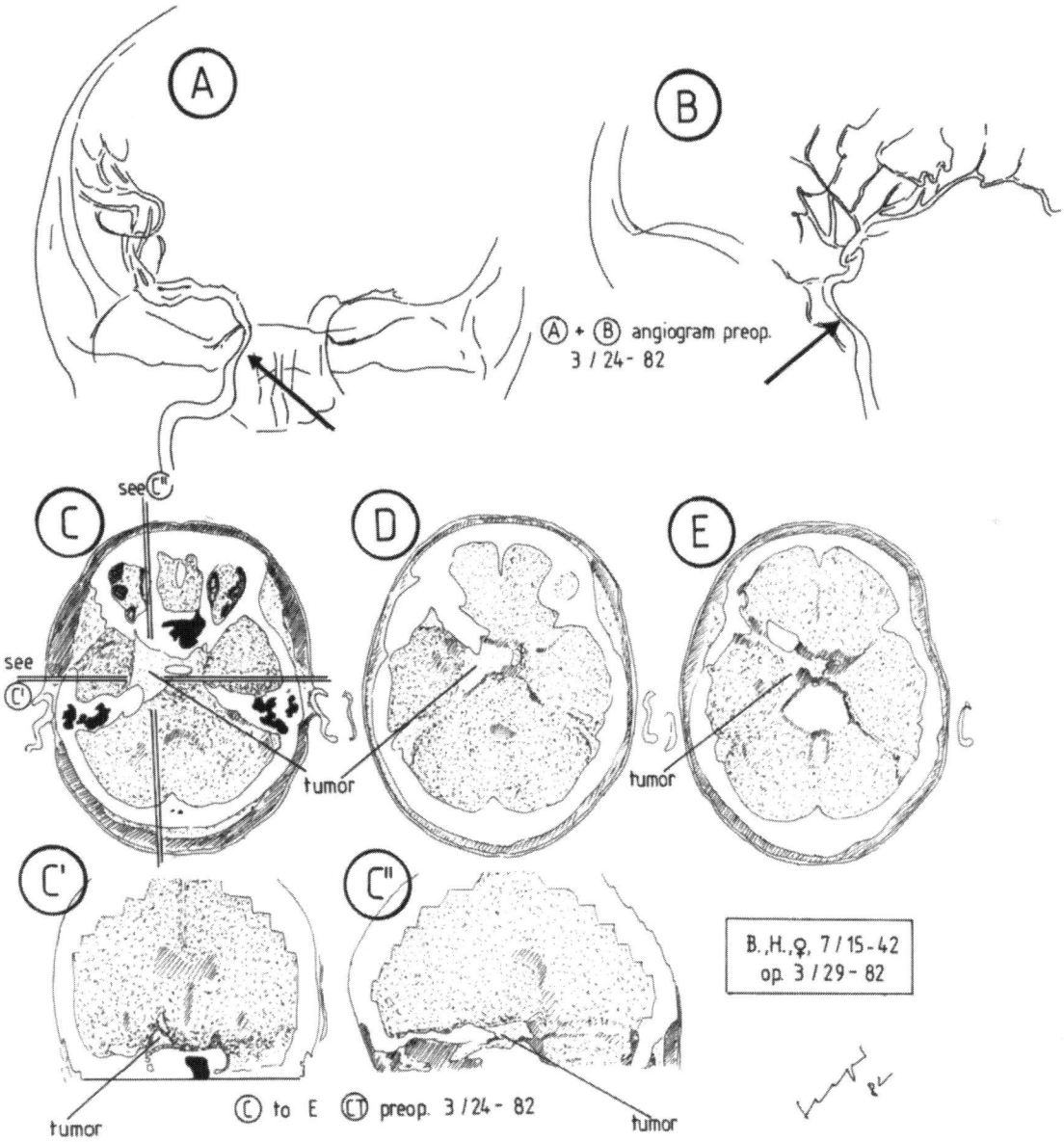
A
B
Ⓐ + Ⓑ angiogram preop.
3 / 24 - 82
see C''
C
see C'
tumor
D
E
tumor
C'
C''
B.,H.,♀, 7 / 15 - 42
op. 3 / 29 - 82
tumor
Ⓒ to E CT preop. 3 / 24 - 82
tumor

Fig. 95. Operations in the area surrounding Sinus cavernosus.
Microsurgical site

A Spreading of Fissura Sylvii exposes topographical relation of tumor, N. oculomotorius, A. carotis int. *–cl–*, N. opticus on both sides, as well as Chiasma

B Coagulation of tumors's dura cover accompanied by extensive irrigation

C **Tumor slightly shrunken, N.II and N.III are decompressed** at dura penetration points.
Effect of decompression is unsatisfactory, because tumor portions still impinge upon these two nerves at the skull base

B' Anatomical sketch for **B**

C' Anatomical sketch for **C**
Open arrows: Shrinking of tumor by bipolar electrocoagulation

Abbreviations:

ap Ala minor
cl A. carotis int.

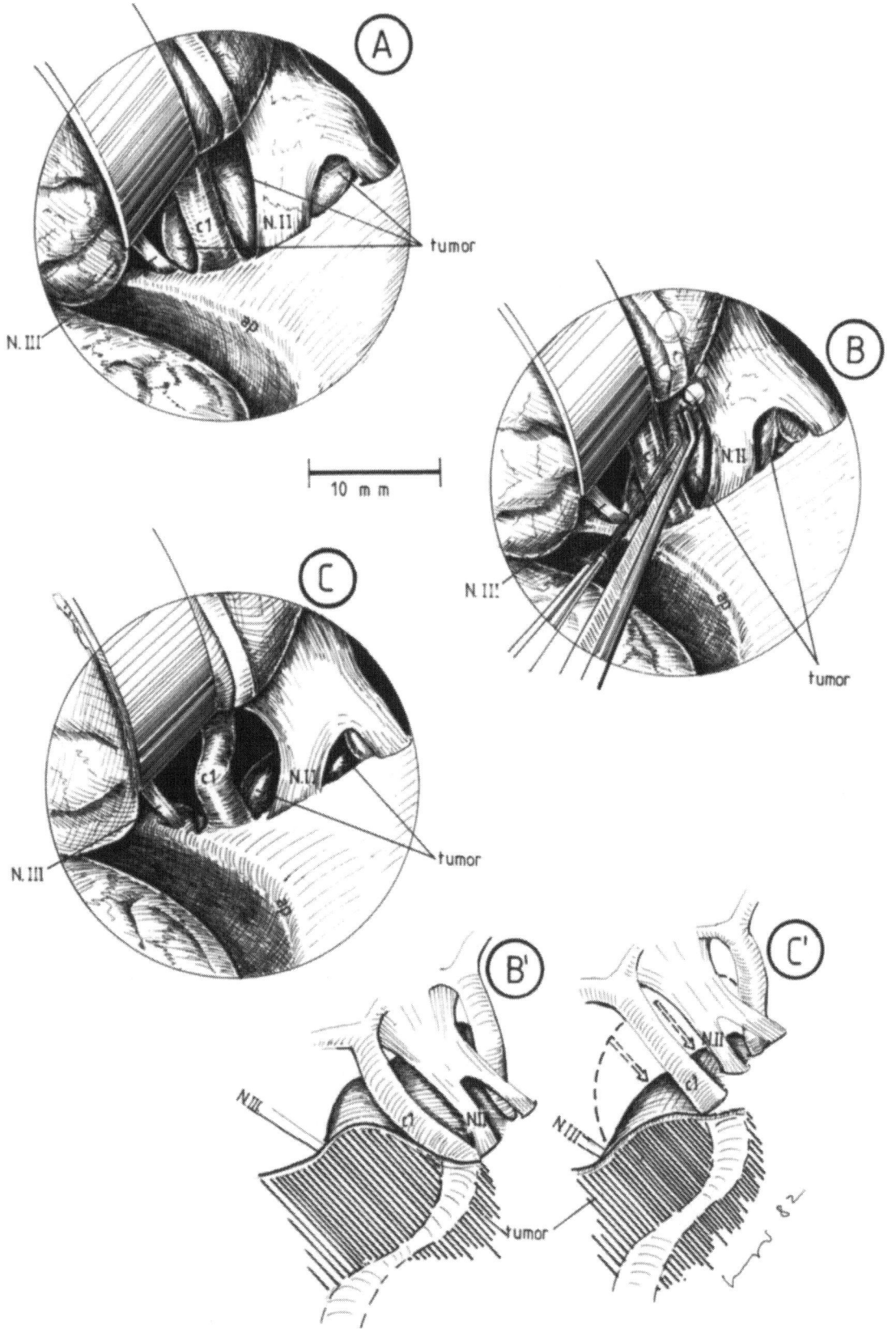
A
c1
N. II
tumor
N. III
ap
B
N. II
N. III
ap
tumor
10 mm
C
c1
N. II
tumor
N. III
ap
B'
N. III
c1
N. II
tumor
C'
N. II
c1
N. III

Fig. 96. Operations in the area surrounding Sinus cavernosus.
Clinical example of **Cavum Meckeli-meningioma** *

A + A' Angiogram shows contrast medium uptake by tumor

B + B' CT (level see **D**) shows: tumor caused atrophy of Os petrosum tip and Dorsum sellae on the right side

E CT one day after operation: air marks the site of radically removed tumor

* Operation performed by Dr. H. R. Eggert, author's coworker.

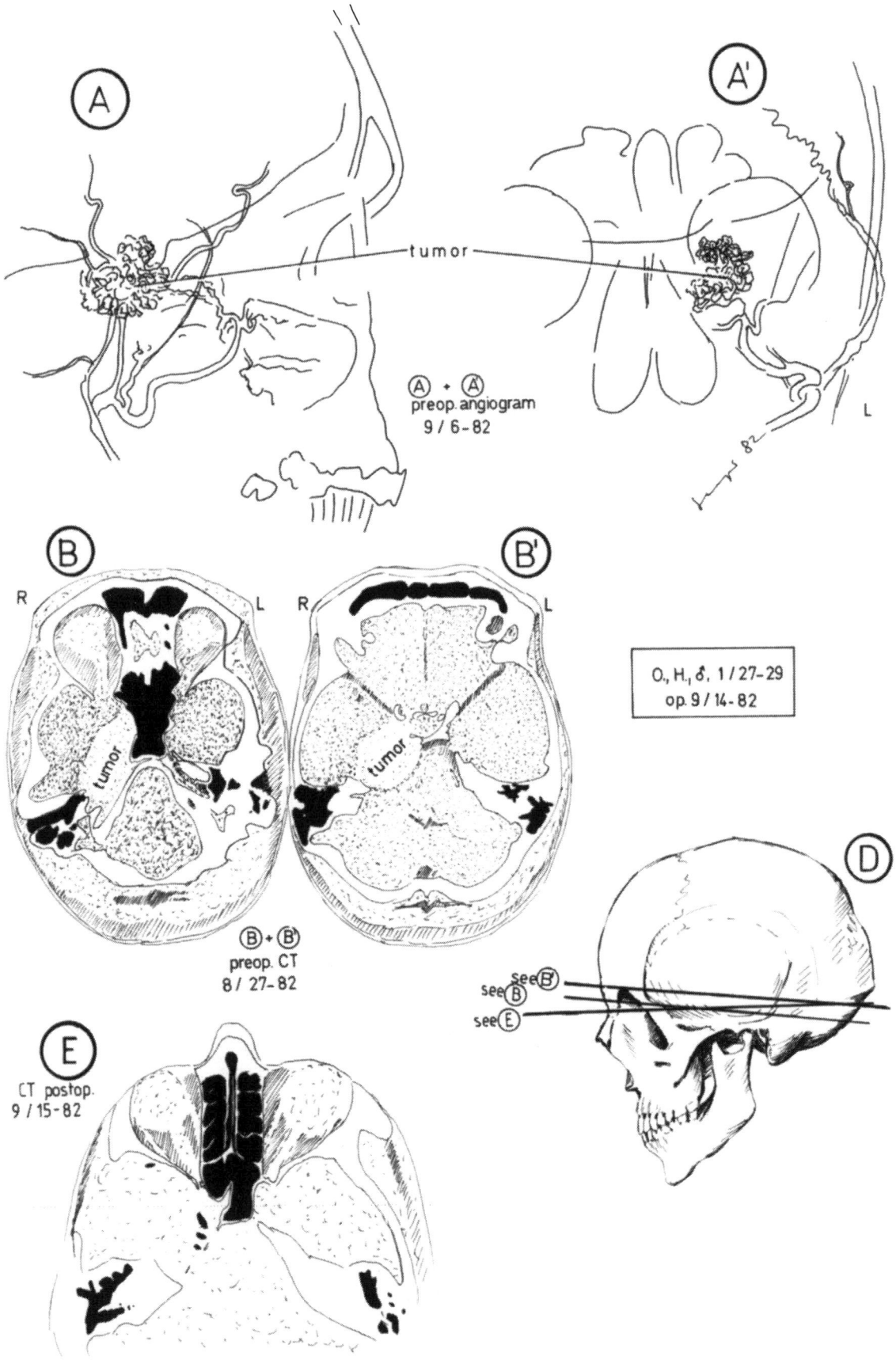
A
A'
tumor
Ⓐ + Ⓐ'
preop. angiogram
9 / 6-82
L
B
B'
R
L
R
L
tumor
tumor
O., H., ♂, 1 / 27-29
op. 9 / 14-82
Ⓑ + Ⓑ'
preop. CT
8 / 27-82
D
see Ⓑ'
see Ⓑ
see Ⓔ
E
CT postop.
9 / 15-82

Fig. 97. Operations in the area surrounding Sinus cavernosus.

Topographical anatomical sketch

A Skull sketch, overview for **A' + A''**

A' Detail of skull base with senile bone atrophy. One sees the close topographical relation of Impressio n. trigemini *–imp–*, Foramen lacerum *–lc–* (which surrounds A. carotis int. in the unmacerated skull) and Foramen ovale *–ov–*. Impressio n. trigemini corresponds to position of N.V, Foramen lacerum lies below Cavum Meckeli

A'' Sketch for **A'** with dura, Ganglion Gasseri and several adjoining structures drawn in; broken line indicates site of tumor which, in hourglass form, has distended Cavum Meckeli *–x–* and has penetrated into posterior fossa, with a second tumor lump along path of N. trigeminus *–y–*

B – B'' Another projection, corresponding to **A – A''**. This skull preparation shows two Impressiones trigemini: the smaller one, lying higher *–impn–* caused by N. trigeminus; the larger one, farther lateral, *–impg–* caused by Ganglion Gasseri

C There are two possible ways for tumor to spread into posterior fossa:

a dura distension dorsal to N. trigeminus (as operatively verified in this presented case) – the better possibility

b spreading of tumor along N. trigeminus through its penetration point in tentorium, and growing around N. trigeminus – less advantageous for operation

Abbreviations:

ac Porus acusticus int.
ca Processus clinoideus ant.
cv Cavum Meckeli (transection)
cl A. carotis int.
ds Diaphragma sellae
Ggl.G. Ganglion semilunare (Gasseri)
imp Impressio trigemini, normal finding
impg Impression by Ganglion Gasseri
impn Impression by N. trigeminus
lc Foramen lacerum
ov Foramen ovale
ps Sinus petrosus sup.
te Tentorium
x, y Tumor limit, projection

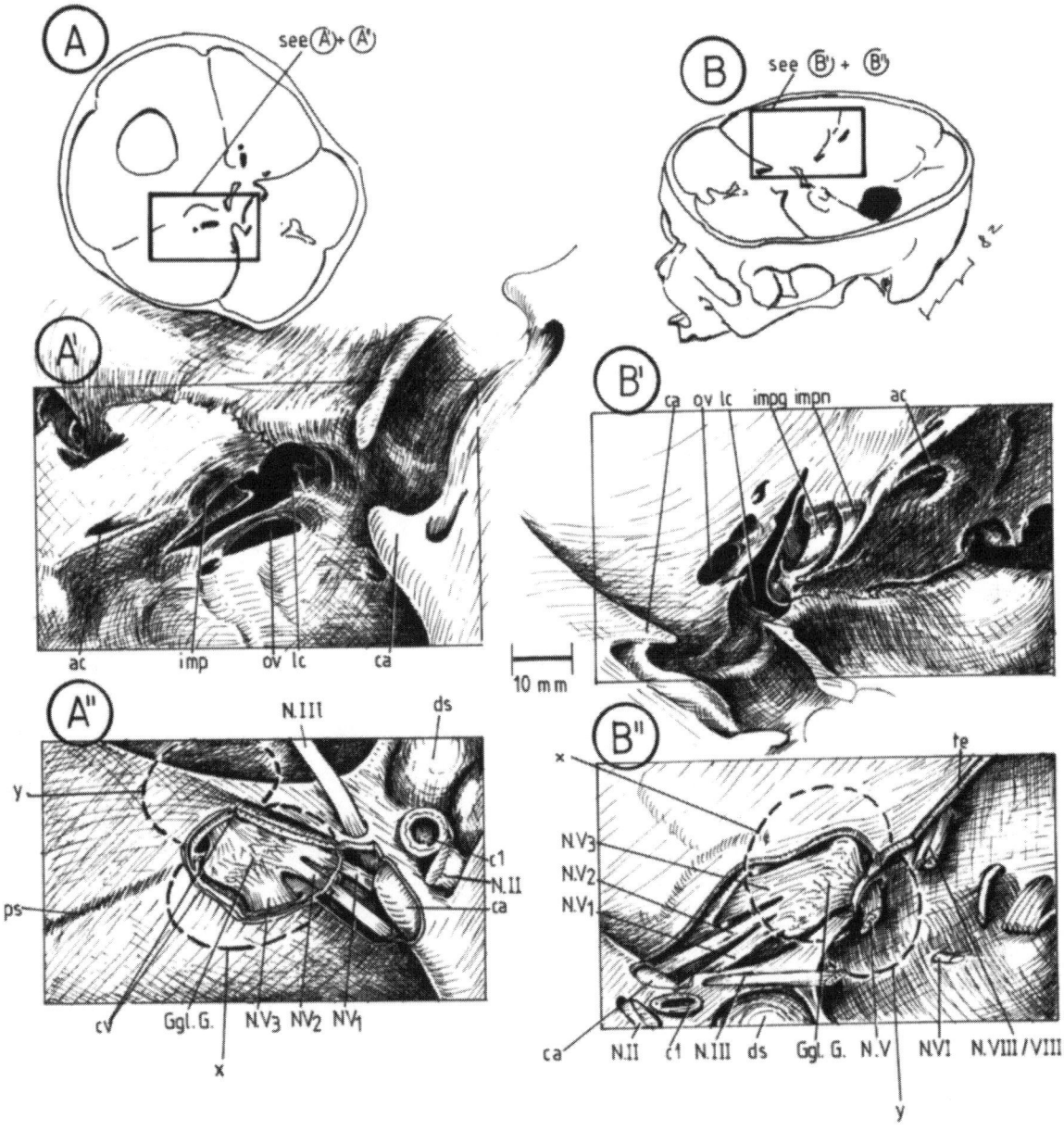
A
see A' + A''
B
see B' + B''
A'
ac
imp
ov
lc
ca
B'
ca
ov
lc
impg
impn
ac
10 mm
A''
N.III
ds
y
c1
N.II
ps
ca
cv
Ggl. G.
N.V3
N.V2
N.V1
x
B''
te
x
N.V3
N.V2
N.V1
ca
N.II
c1
N.III
ds
Ggl. G.
N.V
N.VI
N.VIII/VIII
y

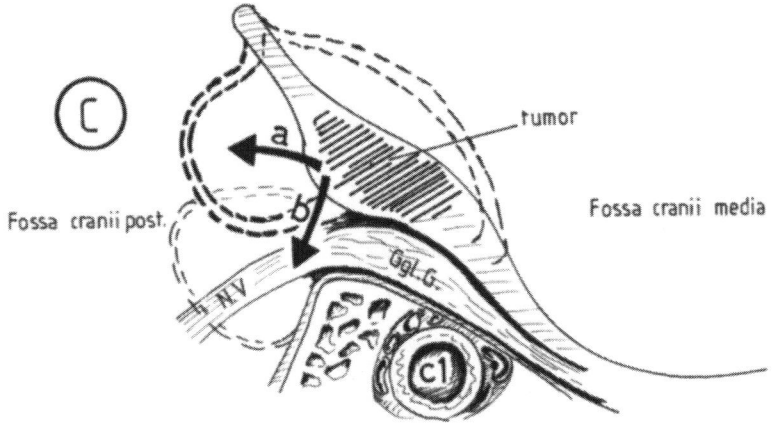
C
tumor
a
b
Fossa cranii post.
Fossa cranii media
Ggl. G.
N.V
c1

Fig. 98. Operations in the area surrounding Sinus cavernosus.
Microsurgical site
Lateral-anterior view

A Lifting of temporal pole after spreading Fissura Sylvii. Richly vascularized tumor has penetrated dura at one small spot

B Enlarged detail from **A**

1 Tumor coagulation

2 **Dura incision around tumor** as far as Sinus petrosus sup. *–sp–*

3a + 3b After incision of dura, its edges are pushed away from tumor (open arrows)

C **1** Coagulation of tumor surface, outer edges of tumor are pulled from its bed

2 Only after thorough tumor coagulation, is richly vascularized tumor hollowed out, and then its interior is coagulated, using extensive irrigation

Abbreviations:

(ac) Processus clinoideus ant. (projection)
sp Sinus petrosus sup.

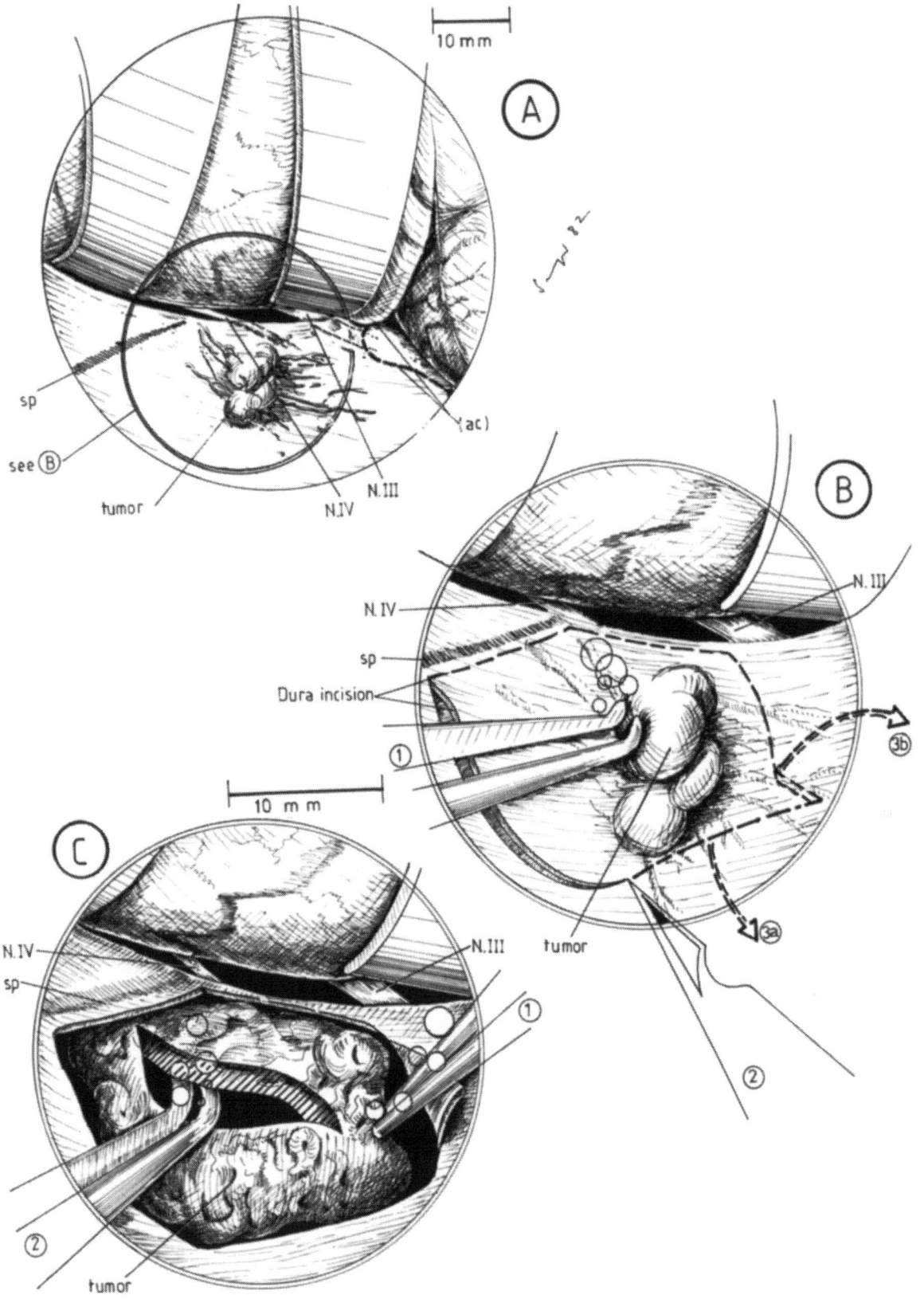
10 mm
A
sp
see B
tumor
N.IV
N.III
(ac)
B
N.IV
sp
Dura incision
N.III
1
3b
3a
tumor
2
10 mm
C
N.IV
sp
N.III
1
2
tumor

Fig. 99. Operations in the area surrounding Sinus cavernosus.

Operation site and anatomical model presentations

A Microsurgical site. In front of Sinus petrosus sup. –*sp*–, tumor is severed transversely, and anterior portion, located in Fossa cranii media, is removed

B Anatomical skull sketch, overview for **C** + **D**, *s* corresponding to section plane **C'**

C Detail of skull preparation, N. trigeminus and its branches drawn in

D As **C**, showing deeply excavated Impressio trigemini. Scalpel and broken line mark site of tumor incision in **A**

C' Section sketch of bone, dura, A. carotis int. and N. trigeminus. Sketch corresponding to section plane –*s*– in **C**

D' As **C**, tumor and tumor incision as in **A** sketched in. Section plane corresponding to *s* in **D**

E Microsurgical site after tumor removal. Ganglion Gasseri and N. trigeminus branches lie in base of tumor bed, covered by translucent dura layer.
(N.V **C'**): Sketch shows original normal path of N. trigeminus preceding tumor development
(N.V **D'**): Path of N. trigeminus, when rotated operation microscope views posterior fossa

Abbreviations:

cl A. carotis int.
sp Sinus petrosus sup.
te Tentorium

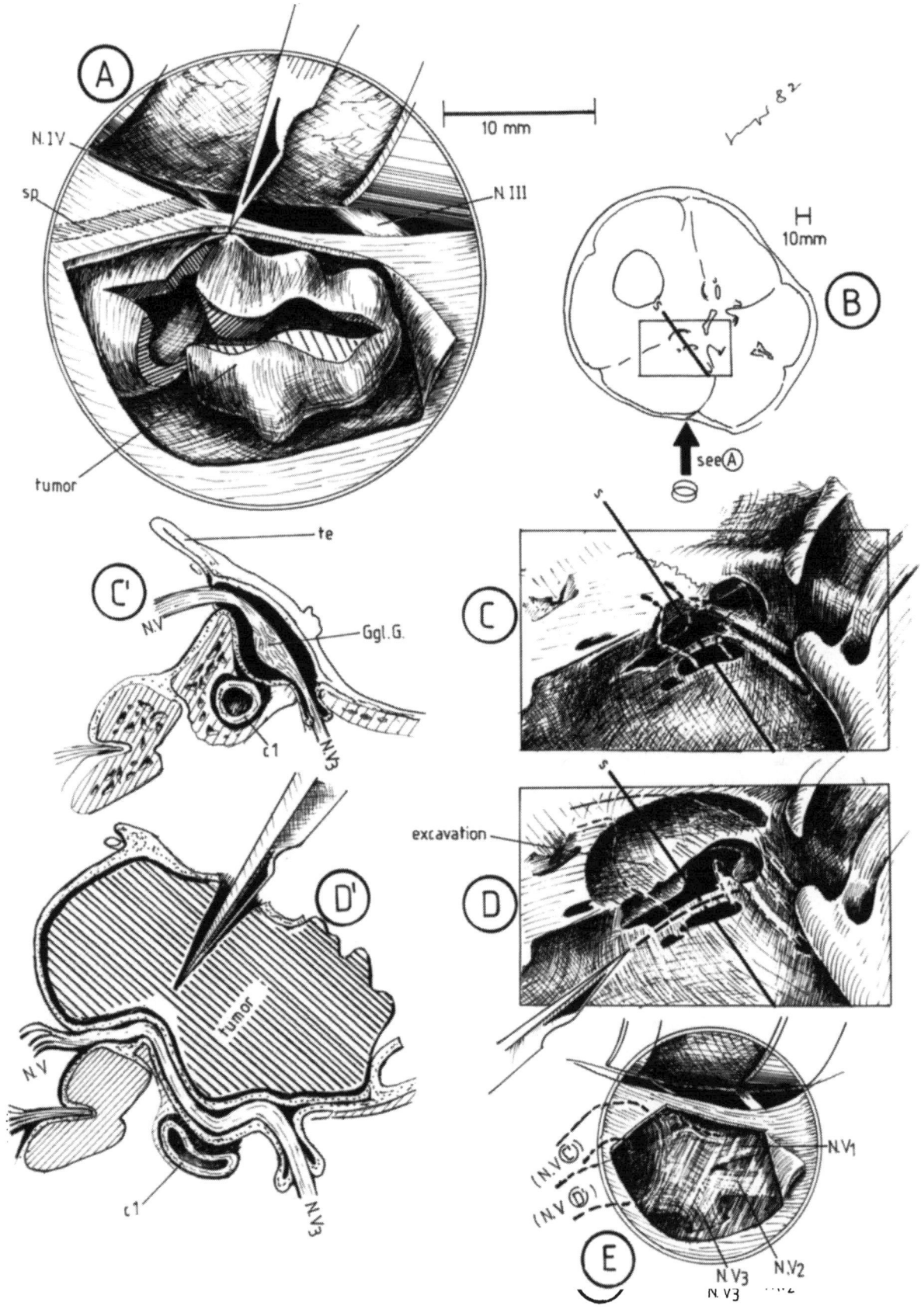
A
N. IV
sp
N. III
tumor
10 mm
B
10mm
see A
C'
te
N.V
Ggl. G.
c1
N.V3
C
s
D'
tumor
N.V
c1
N.V3
D
s
excavation
E
N.V1
(N.V C)
(N.V D)
N.V3
N.V2

Chapter 3
Frontobasal Operations
(Figs. 100 to 134)

Tumor (olfactory groove meningioma) (Figs. 100 to 115)

Fig. 100. Frontobasal operations.
Clinical example of Olfactorius meningioma. For half a year diminishing performance, 2 weeks ago grand mal, bilateral but predominantly left hyposmia. Postoperative bilateral anosmia, no additional deficits, no more seizures; performance improved.
Diagnostic procedures

A – B' Preoperative angiograms show the typical displacement syndrome (arrows). Tumor vascularization mainly from A. ophthalmica through ethmoidal branches. Vessels entry into tumor within a hyperostosis (= enostosis) (see also CT **D – E'**)

C – E' Preoperative CT-findings showing tumor with basal-central hyperostosis. Angiogram shows extensive tumor vascularization. Hyperostosis encloses a **recesse of Sinus sphenoidalis.**
Danger of postoperative liquor fistula!

F Postoperatively, a cavity filled with CS-fluid is seen, instead of tumor

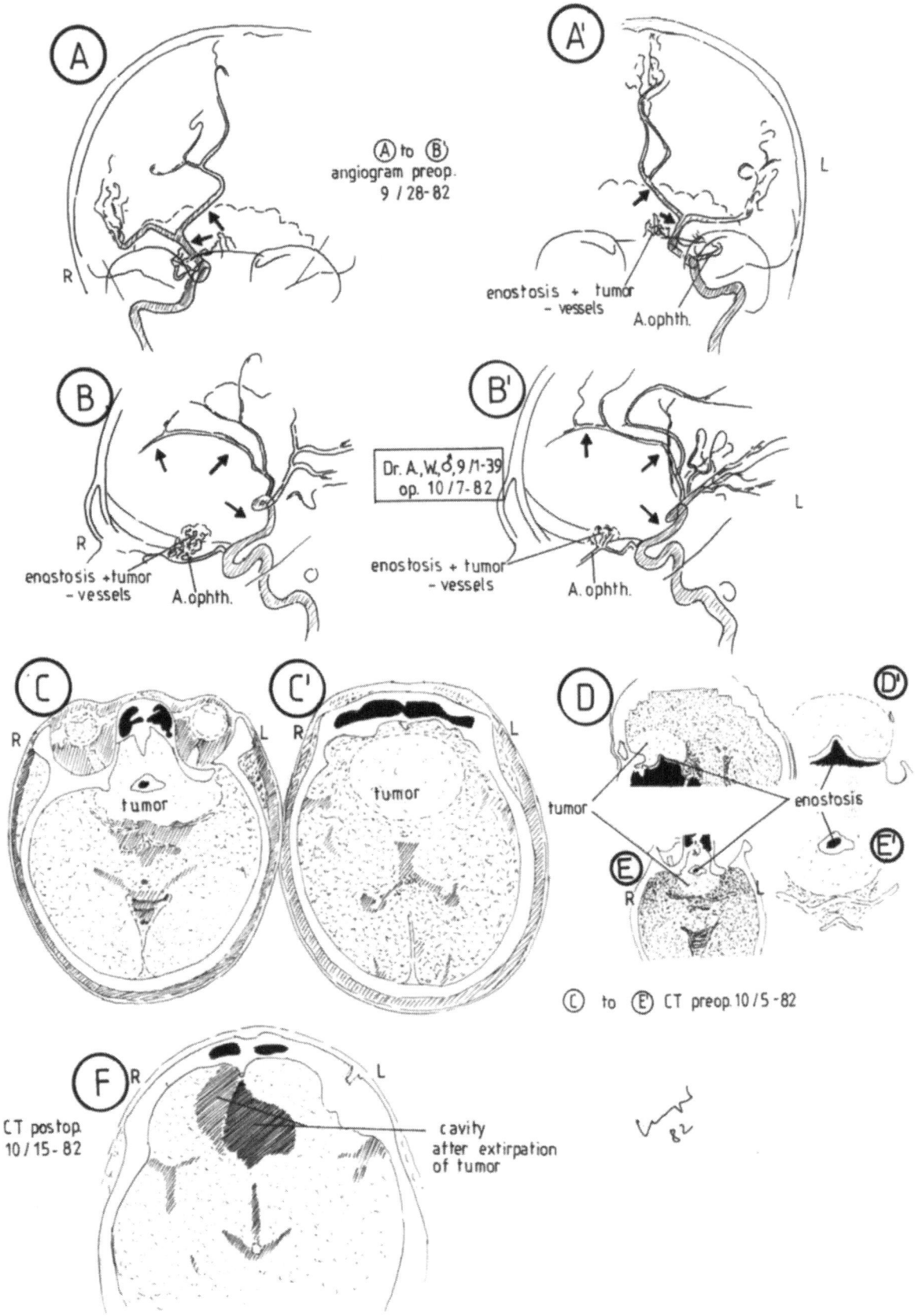
A
A'
Ⓐ to Ⓑ'
angiogram preop.
9 / 28-82
R
L
enostosis + tumor
- vessels
A.ophth.
B
B'
Dr. A., W., ♂, 9/1-39
op. 10/7-82
R
L
enostosis + tumor
- vessels
A.ophth.
C
C'
R
L
tumor
D
D'
tumor
enostosis
E
E'
R
L
Ⓒ to Ⓔ' CT preop. 10/5-82
F
R
L
CT postop.
10/15-82
cavity
after extirpation
of tumor
82

Fig. 101. Frontobasal operations.
Olfactorius meningioma, steps from skin incision to trepanation. Broken lines: projection of trepanation and skull structures

A **1** Skin incision. At first periosteum is left on skull surface

A' As **A,** schematic anatomical transection

B Preparation of skin and galea, as well as periosteum

- **1** Pushing of skin from periosteum medially as far as nasion, lateraly as far as orbital edge
- **2** Periosteum incision
- **3** Pushing of periosteum also as far as orbita and nasion *

C Preparation of periosteum and M. temporalis prior to trepanation

- **1a, 1b, 1c** Galea-skin flap is pulled back by retractors until orbital edges become clearly visible
- **2** Only then can periosteum be pushed back as far as orbital edge and nasion
- **3** Incision of Fascia and Aponeurosis temporalis at anterior sector of linea temporalis sup.
- **4** Pushing away of M. temporalis in the area of incision **3,** in order to place lateral burr hole there (cosmetic result better than burr hole medial of linea temporalis sup.)
- **5a** Retention of periosteum
- **5b** Drilling of burr holes

C' As **C,** lateral view

- **1** see **C 3**
- **2** see **C 4**
- **x** see **C**

D **1** Loosening dura from inner skull surface in the area of all burr holes, using curved dissector

- **2** Drilling of bone

Abbreviations:

cu Cutis
ga Galea aponeurotica (Aponeurosis of M. epicranius)
mf Musculus frontalis (present nomenclature: M. epicranius, Venter frontalis)
p Periost
sk Skull
x Marking of burr hole trepanation in the most anterior area of Fossa temporalis

---

* Difficult and in some cases incorrect. Better method: Cutis, Galea and periosteum detached from skull in one piece (see Fig. 119).

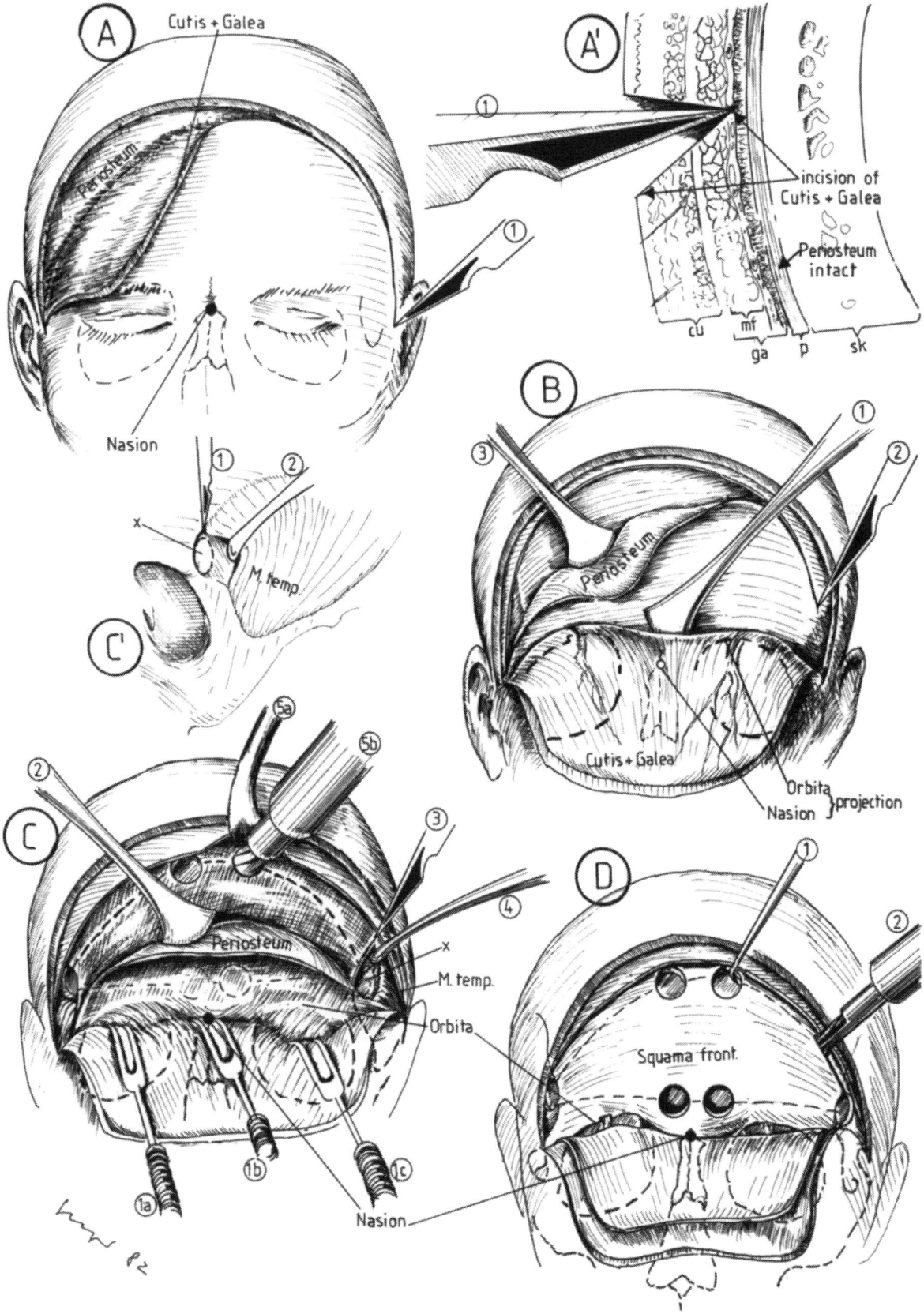
A
Cutis + Galea
Periosteum
Nasion
A'
incision of
Cutis + Galea
Periosteum
intact
cu
mf
ga
p
sk
B
Periosteum
Cutis + Galea
Orbita
Nasion
projection
C'
M. temp.
C
Periosteum
M. temp.
Orbita
Nasion
D
Squama front.

Fig. 102. Frontobasal operations.
Olfactorius meningioma. Basal enlargement of trepanation as far as nasion

A Medio-basal burr holes lie in the Sinus frontalis area above nasion

B Simplified anatomical sagittal section
- **1** Removal of Sinus frontalis mucosa, as far as possible (if mucosa fragments remain, they can be removed after trepanation)
- **2** Drilling posterior wall of Sinus frontalis

C Enlargement of burr hole, on the side of major tumor spread, towards skull base as far as nasion (see **C'** also)

D Posterior wall of Sinus frontalis is also removed as far as skull base

B' – D' Corresponding to **B – D,** but anterior view

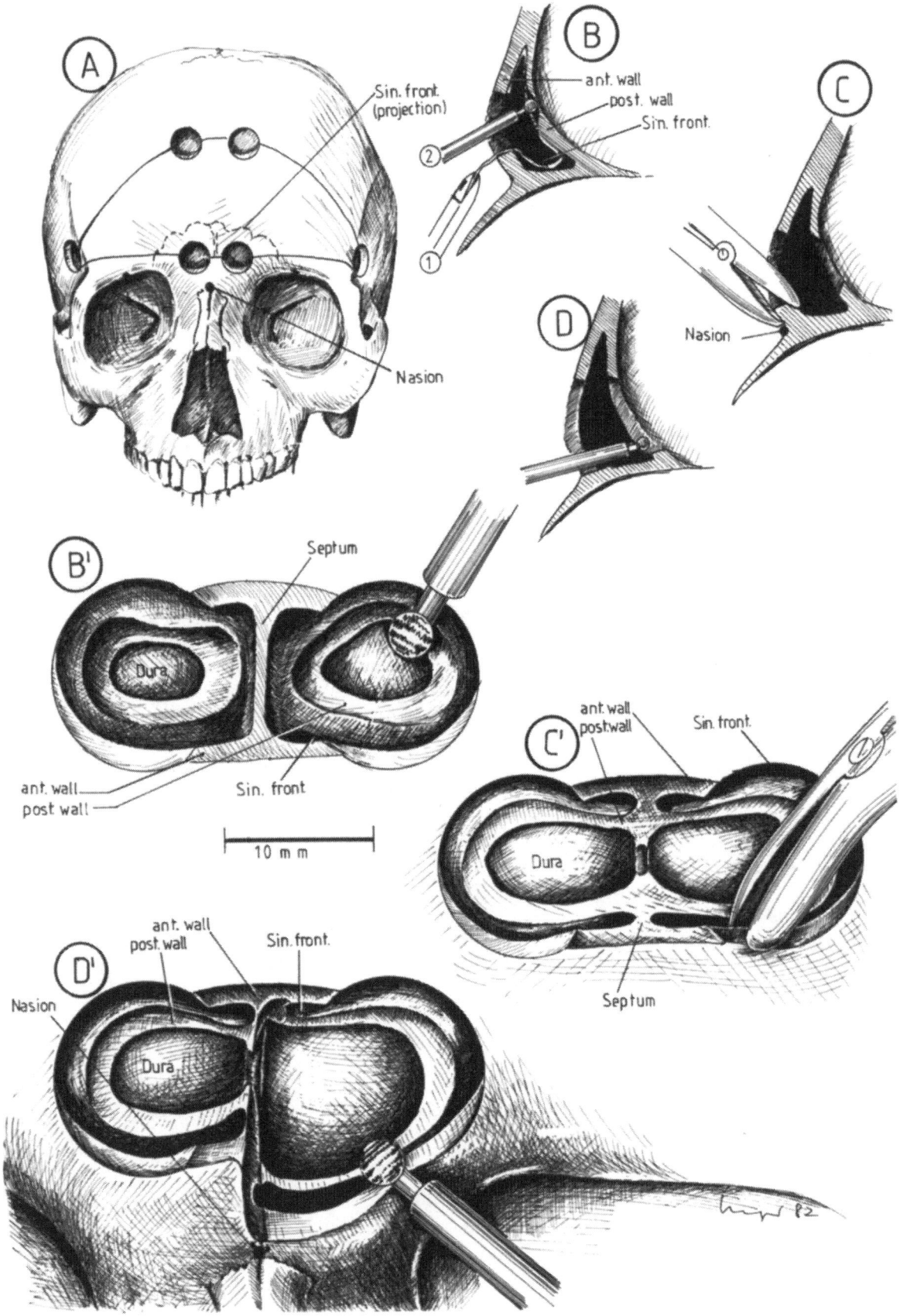
A
Sin. front.
(projection)
Nasion
B
ant. wall
post. wall
Sin. front.
2
1
C
1
Nasion
D
B'
Septum
Dura
ant. wall
post. wall
Sin. front
10 m m
C'
ant. wall
post. wall
Sin. front.
Dura
Septum
D'
ant. wall
post. wall
Sin. front.
Nasion
Dura

Fig. 103. Frontobasal operations.
Olfactorius meningioma. Tumor extirpation

A Microsurgical site of the following figures, sketched on skull

B Enlarged detail from **A.** Position of dura incision (broken lines)

C Small dura flaps folded outwards

- **1a + 1b** Cotton wool packing of Sinus frontalis after clearing it carefully of mucosa remnants
- **2a** Covering Sinus frontalis with cotton wool
- **2b** Folding out dura
- **3** Coagulation of leptomeninges
- **4** Incision of leptomeninges and fibrous remnants of brain tissue lying between tumor surface and leptomeninges

C' Schematic section for **C**

D

- **1a** Coagulation of tumor surface (with leptomeninges and thin fibrous brain tissue)
- **1b** Thorough irrigation; surrounding dura – especially Sinus sagittalis sup. – and brain tissue is covered with cotton wool as protection against heat (sketch omits cotton wool to show anatomical topography)
- **2** Incision of tumor surface
- **3a** Spreading movements of forceps within tumor to loosen tumor parenchyma
- **3b** Removal of loosened tumor tissue and holding tumor vessels, using sucker

D' Schematic section for **D**

Abbreviations:

a Arachnoidea, outer layer
a' Arachnoidea cover of tumor
c Remnants of fibrous brain tissue
cow Cotton wool
d Dura
sf Sin. front.
ss Sin. sagitt. sup.

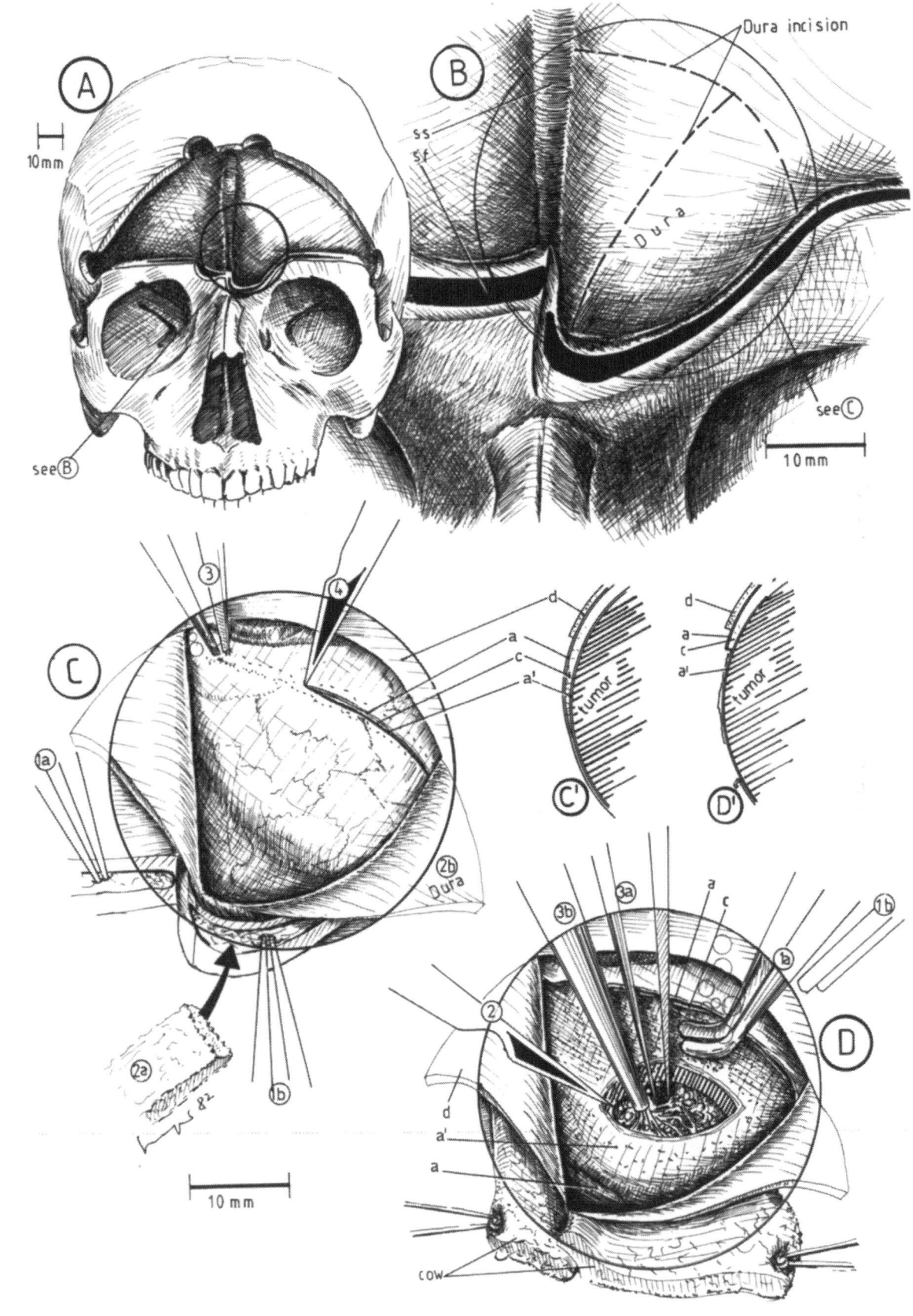
A
10mm
see B
B
Dura incision
ss
sf
Dura
see C
10 mm
C
3
4
1a
2b
Dura
2a
1b
10 mm
d
a
c
a'
tumor
C'
d
a
c
a'
tumor
D'
D
3b
3a
a
c
1b
b
2
d
a'
a
cow

Fig. 104. Frontobasal operations.
Olfactorius meningioma. Anatomical appendix to microsurgical operation

A Schematic anatomical median section (tumor sectioned somewhat lateral of median plane). *x:* start of tumor hollowing

A' Enlarged detail from **A.** Note topographical relation of excavation to enostosis *–en–*, to projection of Crista galli *–(cg)–* and to projection of posterior falx edge *–(fx)–*.

B Schematic oblique skull transection, sketched-in section planes of tumor *S1, S2* and *S3* parallel to median plane

A'' Corresponding to **B** after skull opening and removal of basal tumor portions *–x–*, as in **A + A'**

Abbreviations:

(cg)	Crista galli (projection)
ct	Cutis
d	Dura
en	Enostosis
(fx)	Falx (projection)
mt	M. temporalis
sf	Sinus frontalis
sk	Skull bone
S1, S2, S3	Corner points of transection planes
x	Start of tumor hollowing

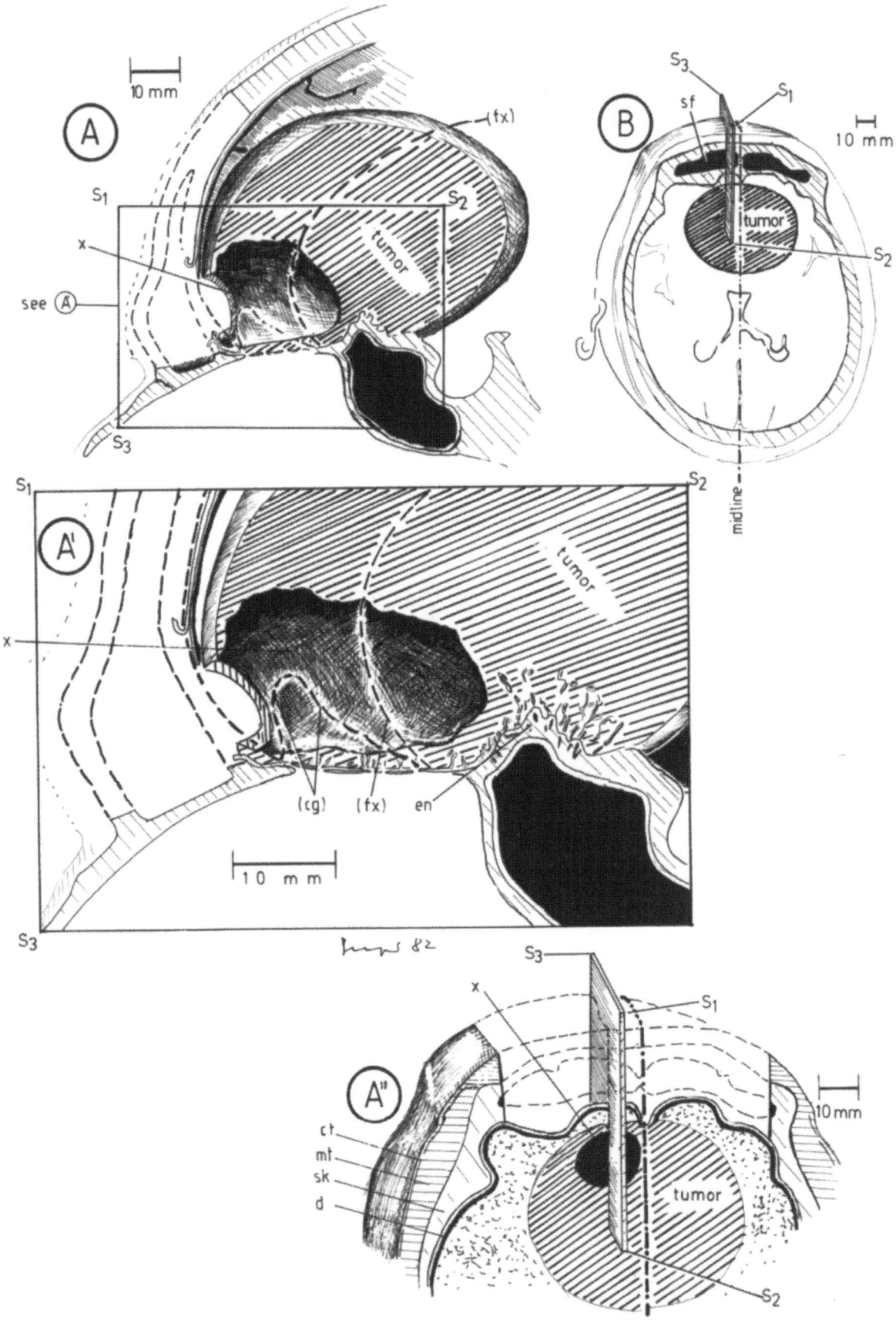
A
10 mm
(fx)
S1
S2
S3
x
see A
tumor
B
S3
S1
sf
10 mm
tumor
S2
midline
A'
S1
S2
S3
x
tumor
(cg)
(fx)
en
10 mm
A''
S3
x
S1
10 mm
ct
mt
sk
d
tumor
S2

Fig. 105. Frontobasal operations.
Olfactorius meningioma. Basal tumor hollowing with early elimination of tumor vessels

A **1** Holding tumor vessels by sucker after siphoning off loosened tumor parenchyma

2 Electrocoagulation of tumor vessels held by suction

3 Separation of coagulated vessels in enostosis area

Close behind enostosis one can already expect N.II and A. carotis int., on both sides lateral of midline

A' Schematic horizontal section through tumor. Anatomical topographical relation of enostosis, N.II and A. carotis int. *–c1–* sketched in

B After cessation of tumor bleeding tendency, hollowing of tumor may proceed on a larger scale

C After thorough hollowing of tumor, its outer surface can be loosened from surrounding brain tissue. Preparation has to be carried out exactly between arachnoideal cover of the brain *–a–* and arachnoidal tumor cover *–a'–*, to prevent unnecessary traumatization of brain tissue or less than radical tumor removal.

Arrows: tumor and brain tissue may spread apart spontaneously. In this case one must ascertain that this separation has taken place correctly between the arachnoidal layers*

D Microsurgical site for **B + C**

1 Blunt squeezing of tumor using forceps

2 Siphoning off tumor tissue and holding fast of vessels

3 Coagulation of vessels stretched by suction

Principally, when loosening extracerebral tumors from surrounding brain tissue, the preparation must take place between arachnoidal cover of brain and arachnoidal tumor cover. If this is not possible, because one of these arachnoidal covers was ruptured by tumor, then one must seek another site from which correct preparation can proceed. Following this method will result in unprotected brain zones remaining small. This is essential to prevent postoperative epilepsy.

Abbreviations:

a External arachnoidal layer of brain
a' Arachnoidal tumor cover
en Enostosis (main tumor vascularization occurs in this area)
fx Falx

---

* The author thanks Prof. Dr. G. Yaşargil, Zürich, for his reference to this principle of arachnoidal preparation in cases of acoustic meningioma, which can be applied to all operations of extracerebral tumors.

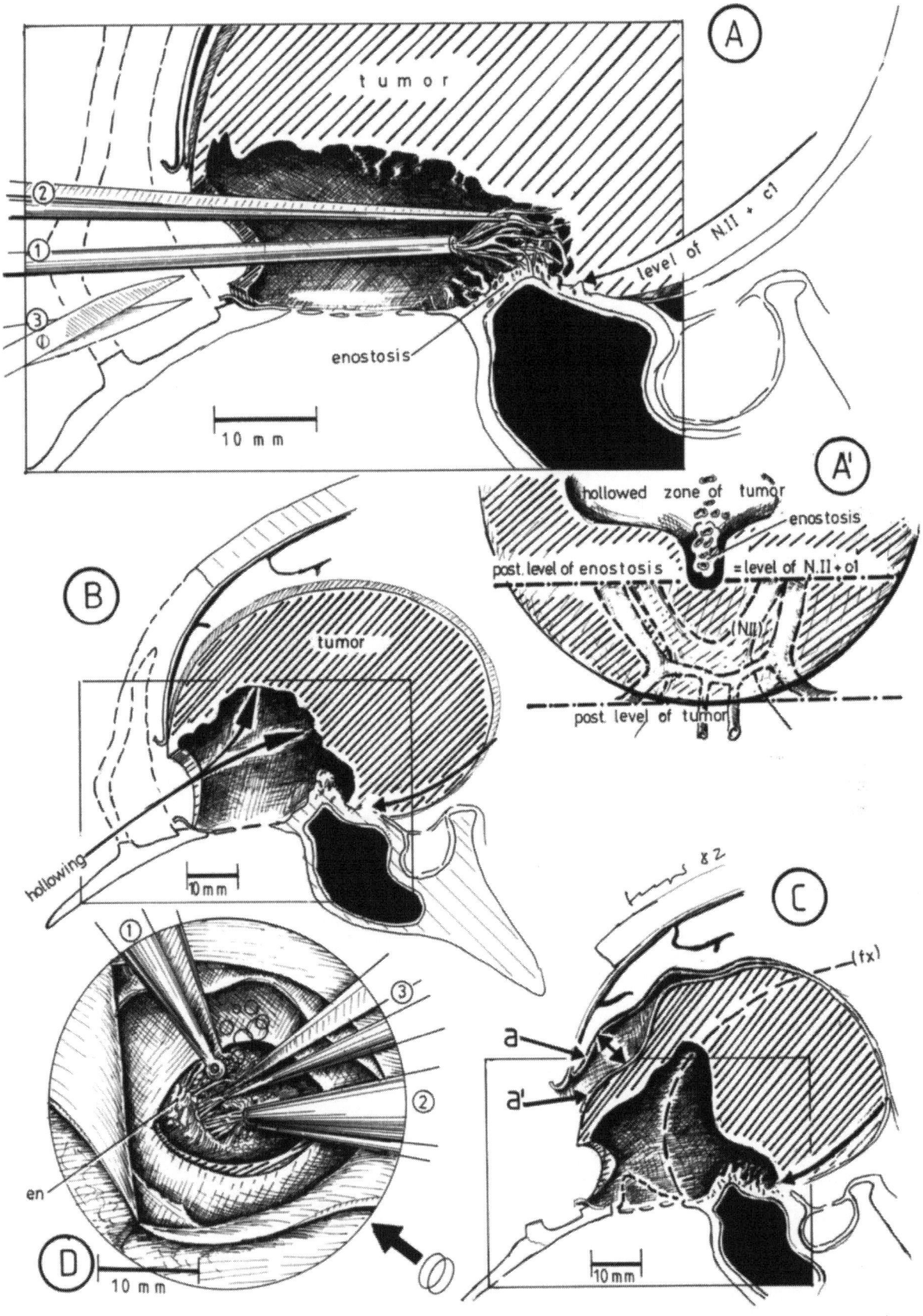
A
tumor
level of N.II + c1
enostosis
10 mm
A'
hollowed zone of tumor
enostosis
post. level of enostosis
= level of N.II + o1
(N.II)
post. level of tumor
B
tumor
hollowing
10 mm
C
&z
(fx)
a
a'
10 mm
D
en
10 mm

Fig. 106. Frontobasal operations.
Olfactorius meningioma. Tumor extirpation

A Anatomical longitudinal transection sketch similar to preceding fig. Arrows: tumor collapse
- **1** Collapsing tumor portions are removed by cutting around original tumor incision

B After further hollowing, collapsing tumor portions are circularly sliced away (*s1 – s4*), see microsurgical sites **E – G**

C After further tumor hollowing, falx *–fx–* becomes visible medially. Basal hollowing must not be done yet because of the danger of injury to N. opticus and/or A. carotis int.

D If tumor shows tendency to collapse, spatula can be positioned into tumor cavity

E – G Microsurgical sites

E
- **1** Pulling back arachnoidal layer of brain from tumor surface
- **2** As **1**
- **3** Circular tumor resection around previous incision

F
- **1, 2, 3** Hollowing of tumor and coagulation of tumor vessels as before
- **4** Preparation again of outer arachnoidal layer away from tumor surface (tumor arachnoidea)
- **5** Further tumor incision with removal of tumor portions

G
- **1** Insertion of spatula to prevent sinking of tumor and of Lobus frontalis lying above tumor. Falx *–fx–* exposed
- **2** Tumor hollowing extends into the opposite side, however not quite as far as skull-base

Abbreviations:

(cg) Crista galli (projection)
en Enostosis
(en) Enostosis (projection)
fx Falx
lc Lamina cribrosa

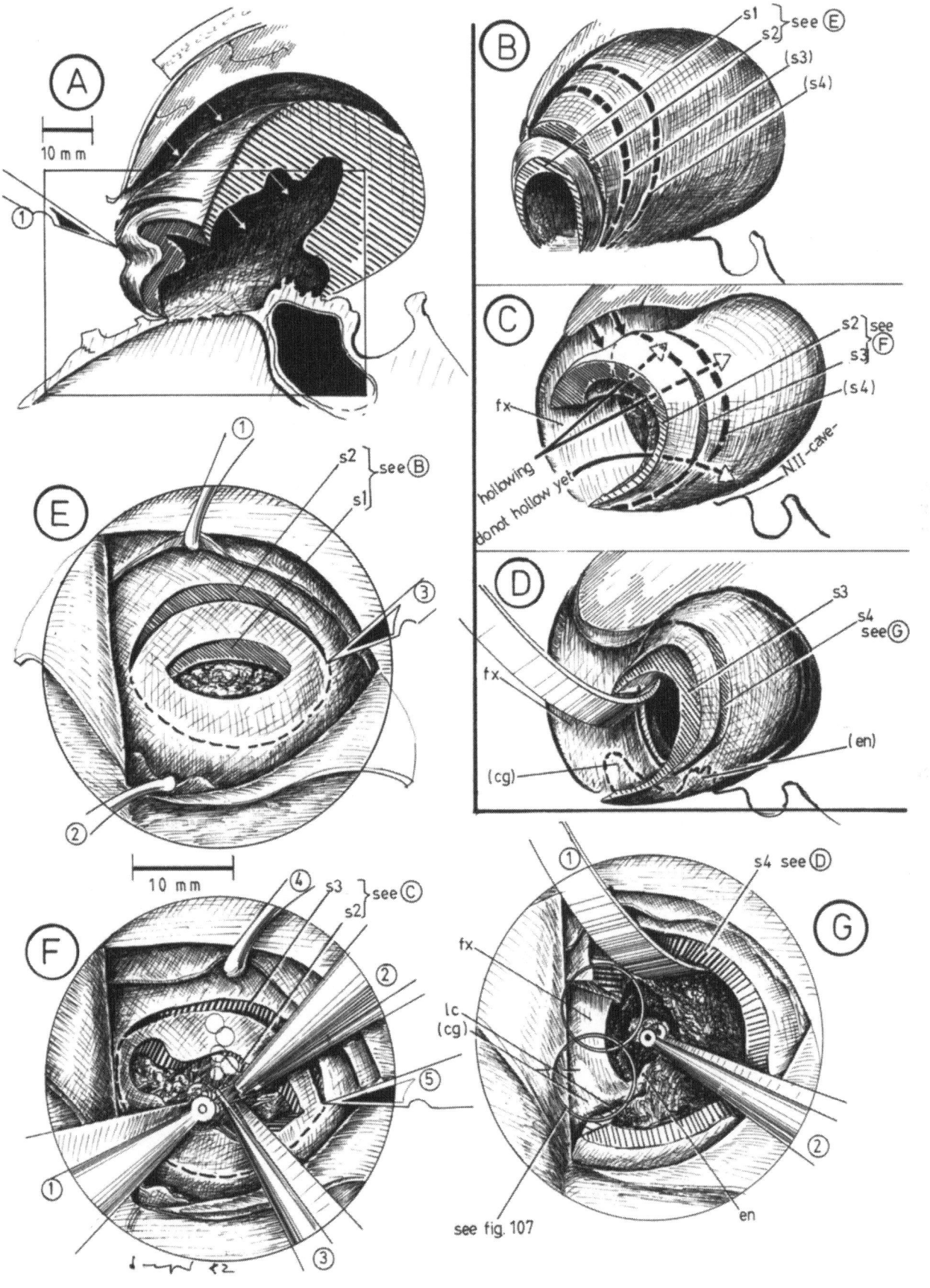
A
10 mm
1
B
s1
s2
see E
(s3)
(s4)
C
s2
see F
s3
(s4)
fx
hollowing
donot hollow yet
NIII-cave-
D
s3
s4
see G
fx
(en)
(cg)
E
1
s2
see B
s1
3
2
10 mm
F
4
s3
s2
see C
2
5
1
3
G
1
s4 see D
fx
lc
(cg)
2
see fig. 107
en

Fig. 107. Frontobasal operations.
Olfactorius meningioma. Tumor extirpation

A Enlarged detail from Fig. 106 **G**
- **1** Incision of falx leaf around Crista galli on tumor side along Sinus sagittalis sup. *–ss–*
- **2** Resection of Crista galli
- **3** Transcision of falx nearly as far as Sinus sagittalis sup. *–ss–*

A' Schematic horizontal section through tumor and neighboring structures. Arrow: direction of microscopic view. *p:* due to oblique microscopic view projection, falx appears foreshortened

A'' Anatomical section sketch of **B,** to show topographical relation of incised falx leaf *–i–*, Crista galli and Sinus sagittalis sup. *–ss–*

B **1a** Loosening of contralateral tumor from incised falx portion
- **1b** Stretching of falx (both leafs)
- **2** Incision of contralateral falx leaf after Crista galli removal. White arrows: excision of incised falx portion

C Bleeding from incised falx portion is controlled by suture (not by clip) *

Abbreviations:

en Enostosis
p Seemingly foreshortened falx
ss Sinus sagittalis sup.

---

* For this suggestion I thank PD Dr. A. M. Landolt, Neurosurgical Clinic, University of Zürich, Switzerland.

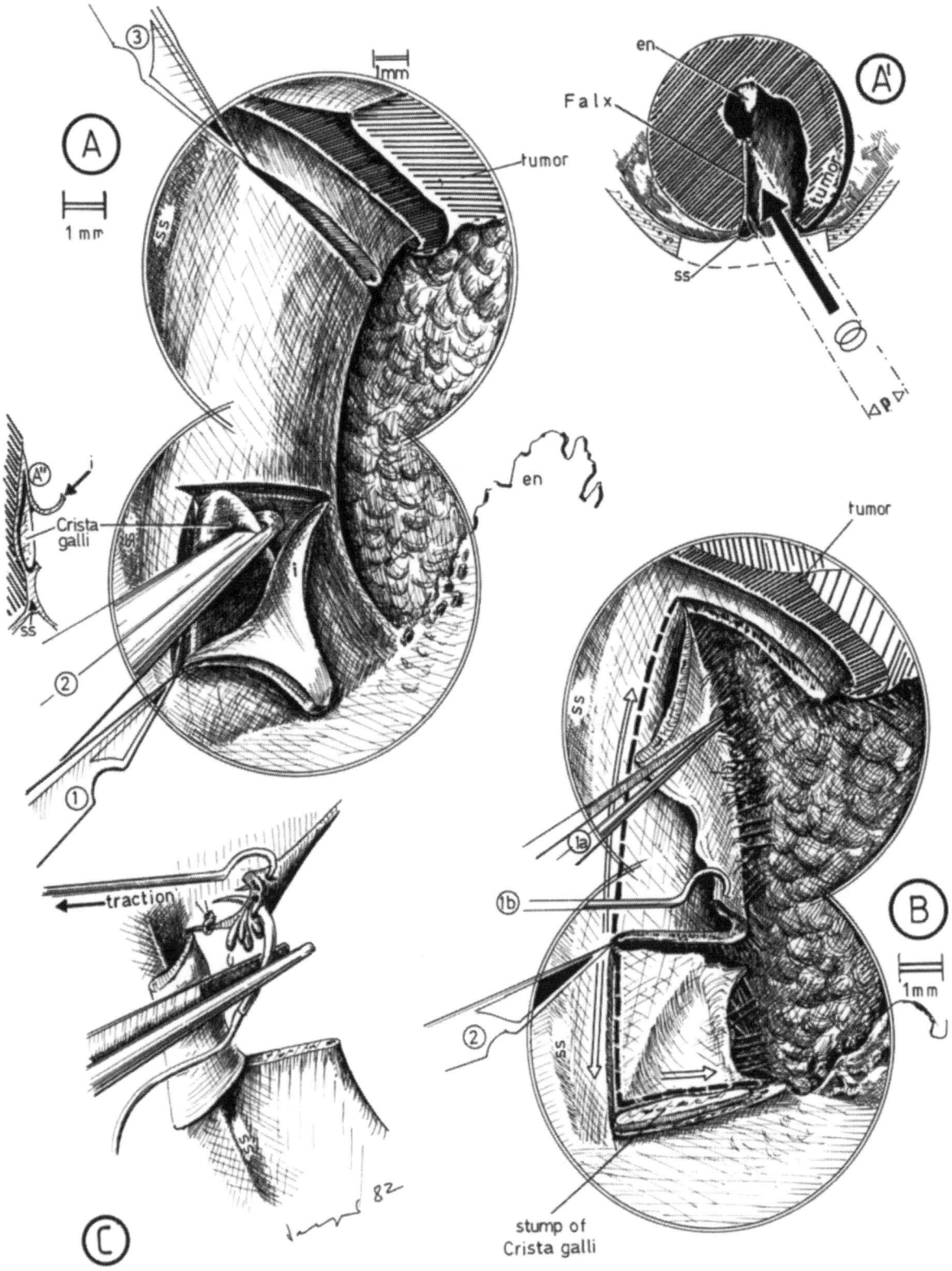
A
1 mm
3
1mm
tumor
ss
en
A'
Falx
tumor
ss
p
A''
i
Crista galli
ss
i
en
2
1
tumor
ss
1a
1b
2
ss
B
1mm
stump of Crista galli
traction
C

Fig. 108. Frontobasal operations.
Olfactorius meningioma. Tumor extirpation

A Microsurgical site
- **1** Spatula repositioned, then slight pulling
- **2** Further falxincisions and falx-resections (broken line) until contralateral tumor surface is reached

A' Schematic horizontal anatomical section. Arrow: direction of microscope view

A'' Schematic sagittal anatomical section, corresponding to microsurgical site **A**

B **1a + 1b** Further tumor hollowing as before
- **2** Pulling arachnoidal layer of brain from tumor arachnoidal layer
- **3** Resection line (broken line) of superficial tumor portions

B' Schematic anatomical horizontal section for situation **B.** Arrow: direction of microsurgical view in **B**

C Microsurgical site. Tumor greatly diminished. Its surface can also be seen contralaterally dorsally. Spatula no longer lies in tumor lumen, but rather underneath brain (protected by layer of cotton wool *–cow–*)

C' Schematic anatomical horizontal section, situation corresponds to **C.** Arrow: direction of microsurgical view, corresponding to **C**

Abbreviation:

cow Cotton wool

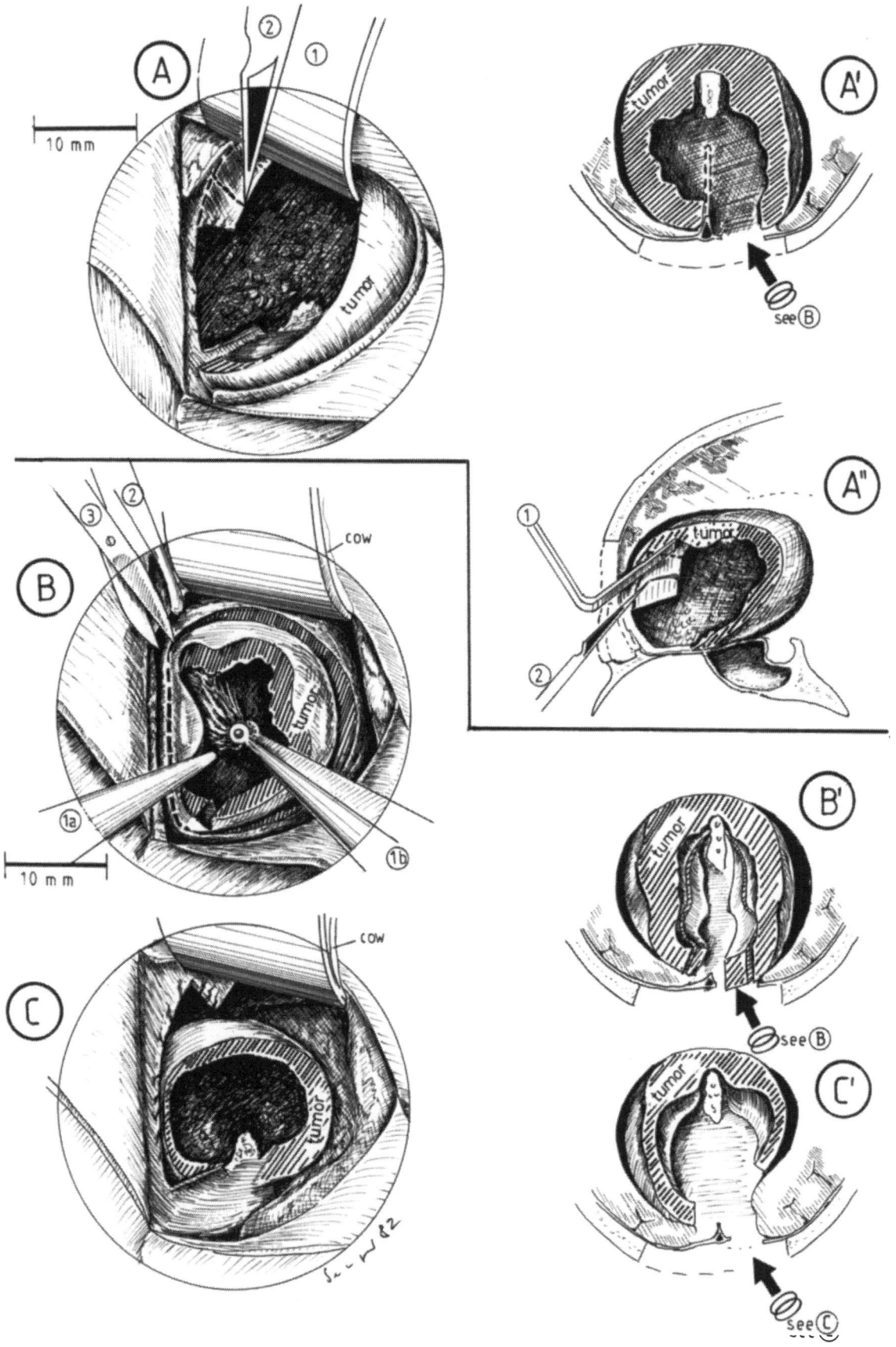
A
2
1
10 mm
tumor
A'
tumor
see B
A"
1
tumor
2
B
3
2
cow
tumor
1a
1b
10 mm
B'
tumor
see B
C
cow
tumor
C'
tumor
see C

Fig. 109. Frontobasal operations.
Olfactorius meningioma. Tumor extirpation

A Microsurgical site. Tumor removed exept for a bowl-shaped remnant deep basally. Until now, Aa. carotis intt. and Nn. optici were not yet visible. Over tumor one can see, in the depth of Fissura mediana, Aa. cerebri antt. and left A. frontopolaris

A' Anatomical horizontal section sketch for **A**

A'' Anatomical sagittal section sketch for **A.** Midline defined first by falx remnant and enostosis, later by A. cerebri ant.

B Sectional enlargement from **A**

1a Drilling of enostosis *–en–*

1b Pressing of wax *–wx–* using cotton wool *–cow–* onto resection surface of enostosis

2a + 2b Pushing tumor away from arachnoidea of Cisterna optica *–co–*, from N.II and from Chiasma *–ch–*

C **1a + 1b** Scraping off tumor remnants in the area of Tuberculum sellae and Planum sphenoidale

2 Cautions coagulation of bleeding points in the area of Planum sphenoidale und Tuberculum sellae

3 Blind coagulation at posterior edge of Tuberculum sellae. Hypophyseal stalk may lie close by; danger of unnoticed opening of Sinus sphenoidalis exists if anterior Sella wall is thin

4 In case of dura defects, control of bone bleeding using wax and cotton wool

D + E Anatomical model of preparation in Nn. optici area

D Marking of midline (see also **A'**)

E Pushing off tumor first from midline area, and only then, from Nn. optici

Abbreviations:

ch Chiasma
co Cisterna optica (arachnoidea)
cow Cotton wool
en enostosis
fx Falx remnant
wx Wax

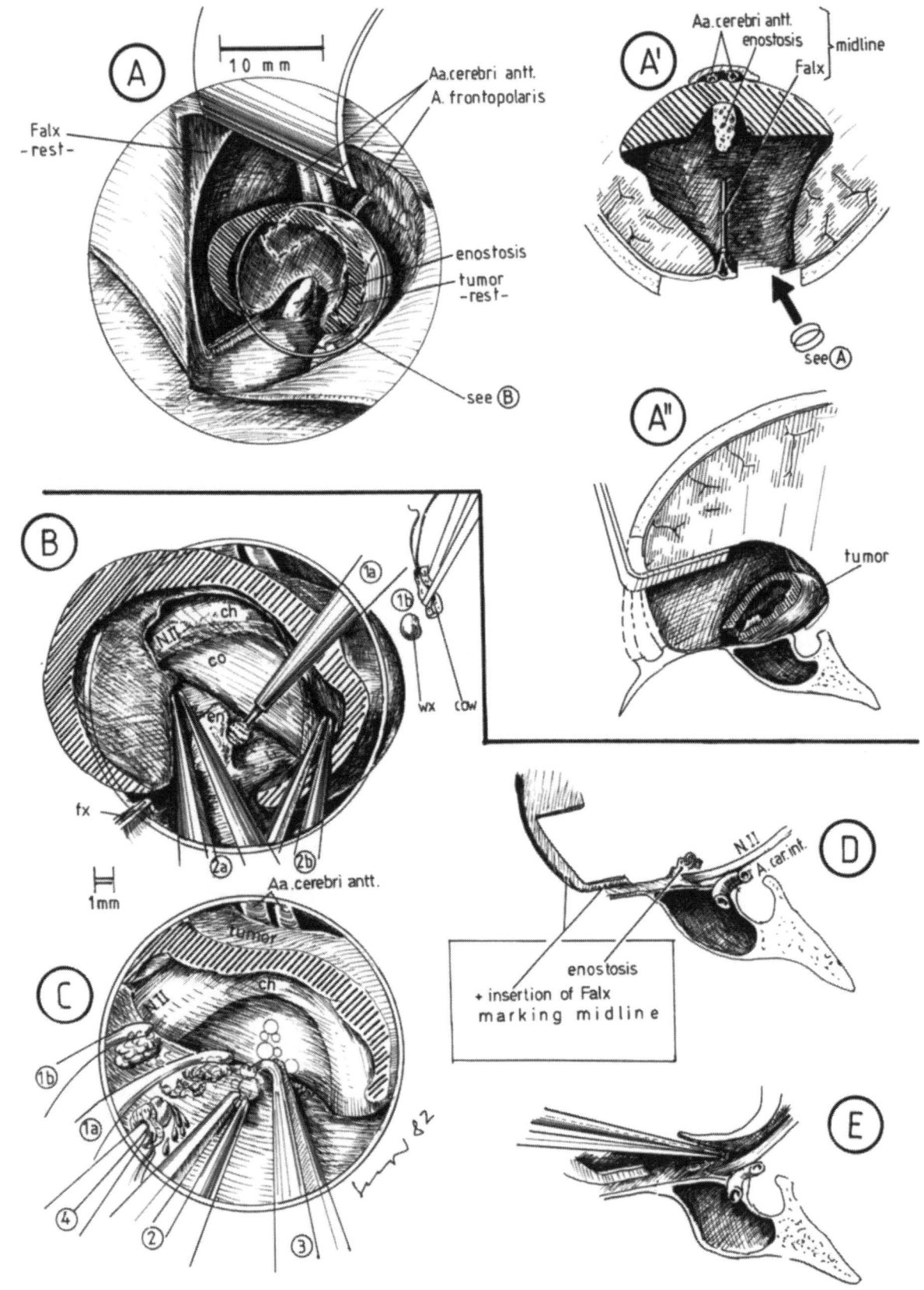
A
10 mm
Falx
-rest-
Aa.cerebri antt.
A. frontopolaris
enostosis
tumor
-rest-
see B
A'
Aa.cerebri antt.
enostosis
Falx
midline
see A
A''
tumor
B
1a
1b
ch
NII
co
en
wx
cow
fx
2a
2b
1mm
Aa.cerebri antt.
C
tumor
ch
NII
1b
1a
4
2
3
D
NII
A. car. int.
enostosis
+ insertion of Falx
marking midline
E

Fig. 110. Frontobasal operations.
Olfactorius meningioma. Grafting procedures

A Microsurgical site after tumor removal
1 After enostosis, drilling defect of dura and Planum sphenoidale exists. Injury to Sinus sphenoidalis mucosa cannot be seen

A' Anatomical topographical sketch (view from above), of microsurgical site **A**

A'' As **A,** sagittal section

B Microsurgical site after tumor removal. Closure of dura and bone gap in Planum sphenoidale (roof of Sinus sphenoidalis closed by stitching on periosteum)

B' + B'' Enlarged detail from **A''** before and after application of graft

Abbreviations:

co Cisterna optica, covered by arachnoidea
(en) Enostosis (projection)

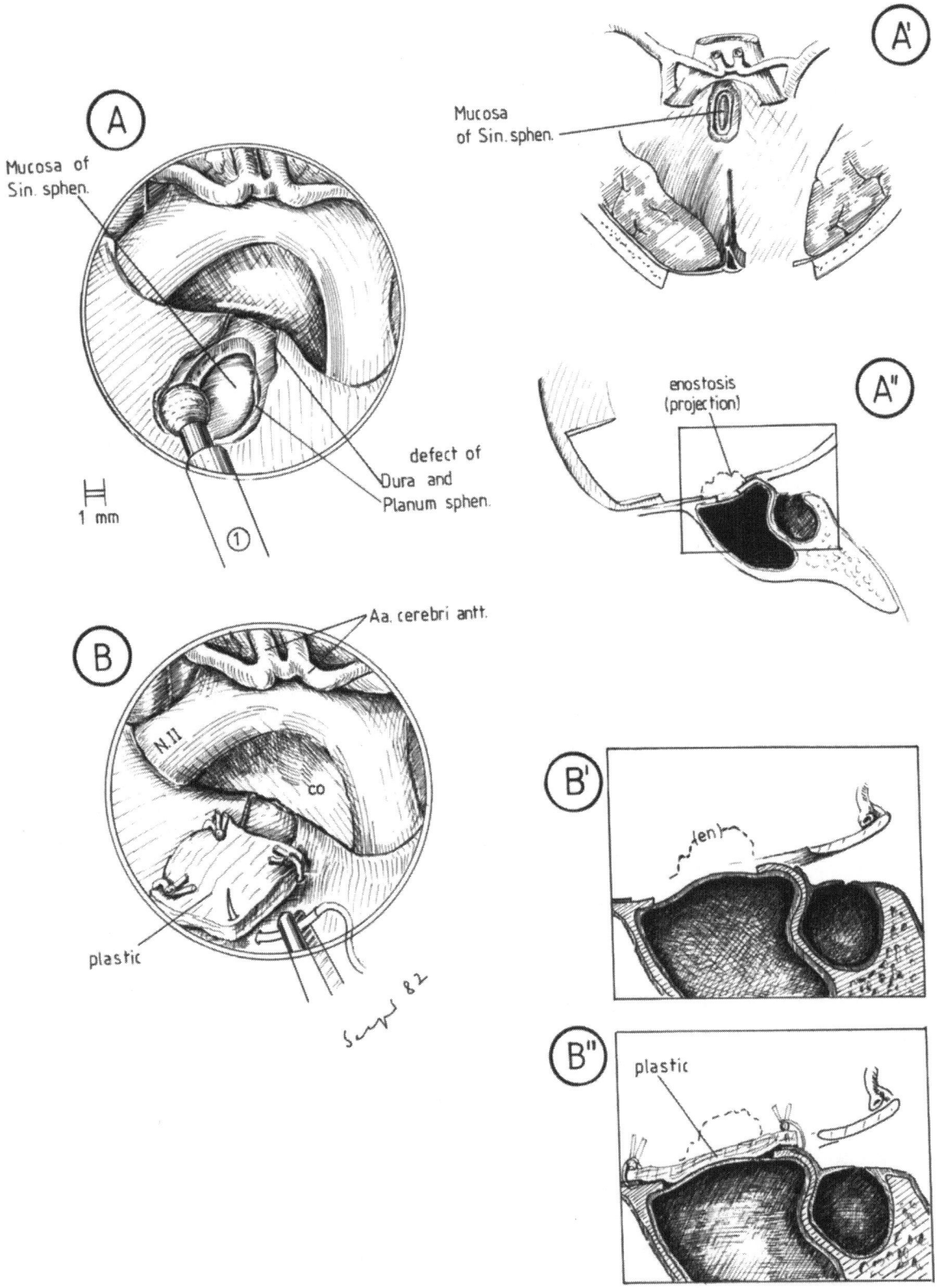
A
Mucosa of
Sin. sphen.
defect of
Dura and
Planum sphen.
1 mm
1
A'
Mucosa
of Sin. sphen.
A"
enostosis
(projection)
B
Aa. cerebri antt.
N.II
co
plastic
B'
B"
plastic

Fig. 111. Frontobasal operations.
Olfactorius meningioma. Grafting procedures

A Graft closure of dura
A' Anatomical section sketch for **A**
B Dura closed
B' Anatomical horizontal section sketch for **B**
B'' Anatomical sagittal section sketch for **B**

Abbreviations:

a Dura graft (galea or periosteum)
b Medial dura flap
c Latero-basal dura flap
d Dura of convexity

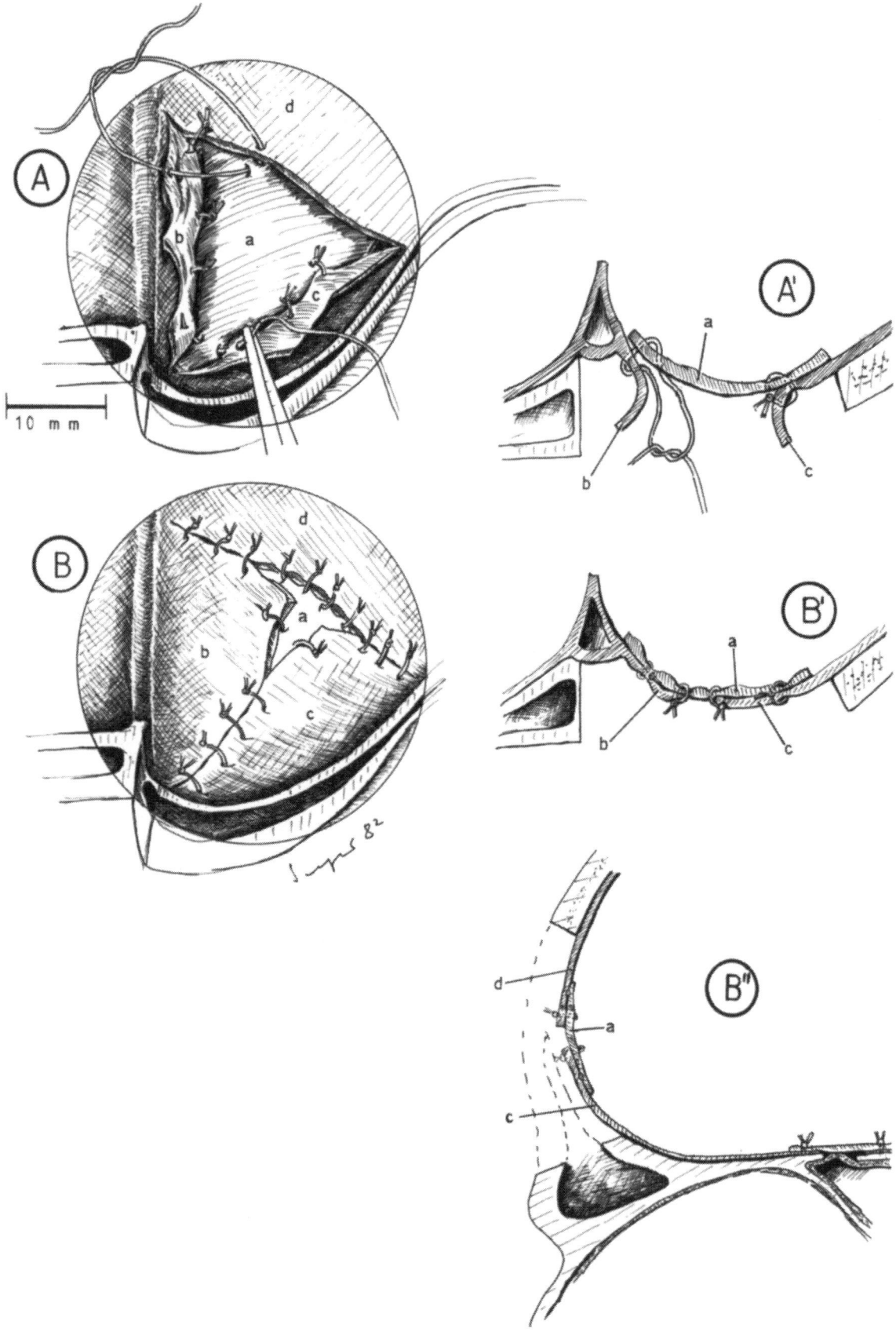
A
d
a
b
c
10 mm
A'
a
b
c
B
d
a
b
c
B'
a
b
c
B''
d
a
c

Fig. 112. Frontobasal operations.
Olfactorius meningioma. Grafting procedures

A Operation site after dura closure

B Anatomical topographical sketch, view from above, mucosa portions of Sinus frontalis still preserved. Light arrows: epidural cleft, in which periosteum graft is placed later on, on both sides

C Anatomical topographical sketch. **1, 2, 3** removing mucosa remnants from Sinus frontalis

C' Anatomical topographical sketch. Mucosa remnants carefully removed from all niches of Sinus frontalis. One looks into Ductus fronto-nasalis on both sides

D Operation site. Median incision of periosteum flap
1 Splitting of periosteum flap.
Light arrow: tucking periosteal flap into epidural cleft *

E – E'' Schematic anatomical sagittal sketches

E A piece of M. temporalis is placed into Sinus frontalis. Light arrow: tucking of periosteum into epidural cleft

E' Periosteum is fastened to dura by suture

E'' Tissue glue ** injected from beneath into periosteum layer and musculature
1 Injection of tissue glue from lateral direction
2 Pressing of periosteum flap and muscles into Sinus frontalis

---

* This method is not applicable in frontalbasal fractures (see appropriate chapter).
** Fibrinogen concentrate, Immuno.

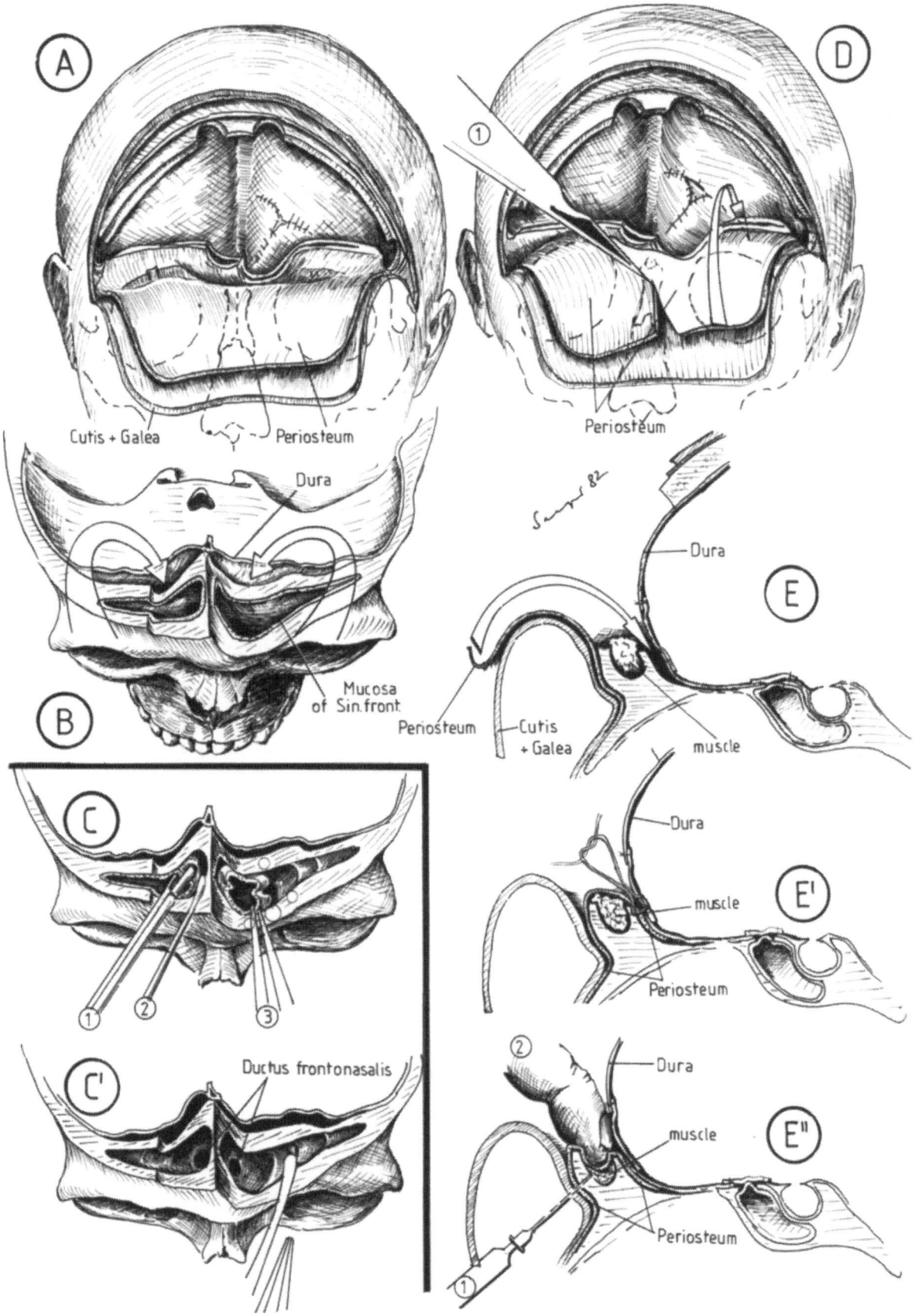
A
Cutis + Galea
Periosteum
D
1
Periosteum
Dura
B
Mucosa
of Sin.front
Dura
E
Periosteum
Cutis
+ Galea
muscle
C
1
2
3
Dura
E'
muscle
Periosteum
C'
Ductus frontonasalis
2
Dura
muscle
E''
Periosteum
1

Fig. 113. Frontobasal operations.
Olfactorius meningioma. Grafting procedures

A
- **1a** (Arrow): left periosteal flap positioned epidurally and fastened (see preceding figure)
- **1b** (Arrow): right periosteal flap is positioned in the same way

A'
- **2** Fastening periosteal flap to dura
- **3a** + **3b** Periosteum flap, as well as muscle, positioned into Sinus frontalis, are injected from beneath with fibrin glue

A'' Immediately after injection of tissue glue, periosteum graft, and muscle positioned in Sinus frontalis, are firmly compressed. Graft forms a depression in Sinus frontalis.

B – B'' Periosteum graft can be fastened to lateral bone edge at base with nails*

C Wound closure
- **1** Reinsertion of bone flap, then attached by sutures
- **2a** Burr holes, especially above nasion, are filled with bone shavings
- **2b** Gluing of bone shavings with fibrin glue
- **3** (arrow) placing of drain, suture of Galea and skin

---

* Method of Prof. T. Riechert, author's predecessor.

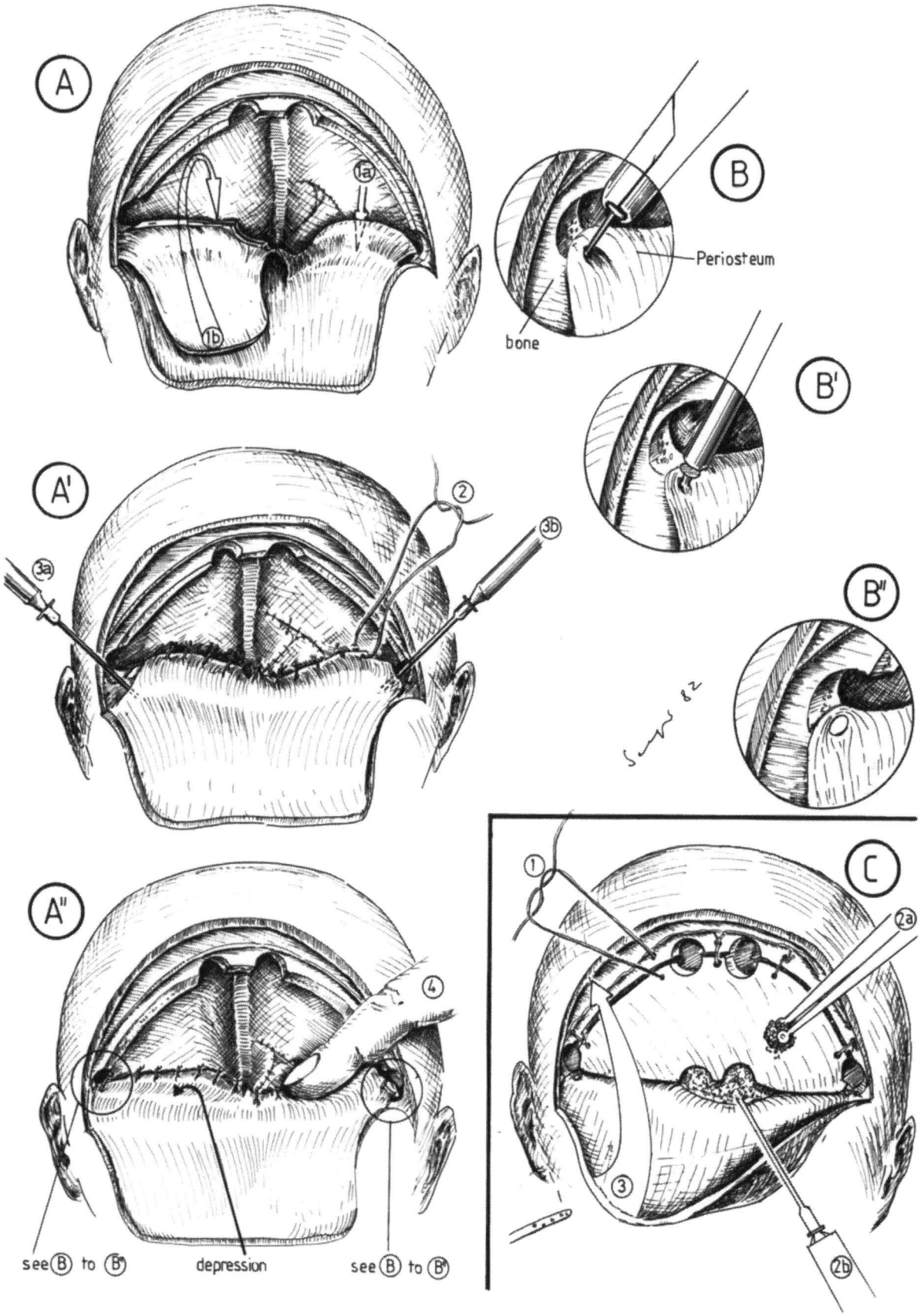
A
1a
1b
B
Periosteum
bone
B'
A'
2
3a
3b
B''
A''
4
see B to B'
depression
see B to B''
C
1
2a
3
2b

Fig. 114. Frontobasal operations.
Olfactorius meningioma. Grafting procedures
Appendix to Fig. 113: Riechert's technique of bone nailing

A Nail holder, overview, with hammer
A' Nail holder with nail, greatly enlarged
Arrows: grooves for holding nailhead
A'' Nail
B Hammer
C Instrument for deeper nailing. Nail is partly hammered in using holder **A,** then holder is changed for instrument **C** to enable firm nailing
C' Enlarged detail of **C**
D Thick-walled corticalis cannot be nailed
D' Thin-walled corticalis should not be nailed too forcefully
E Nailing is possible in strong spongiosa, whether or not thin compacta is present

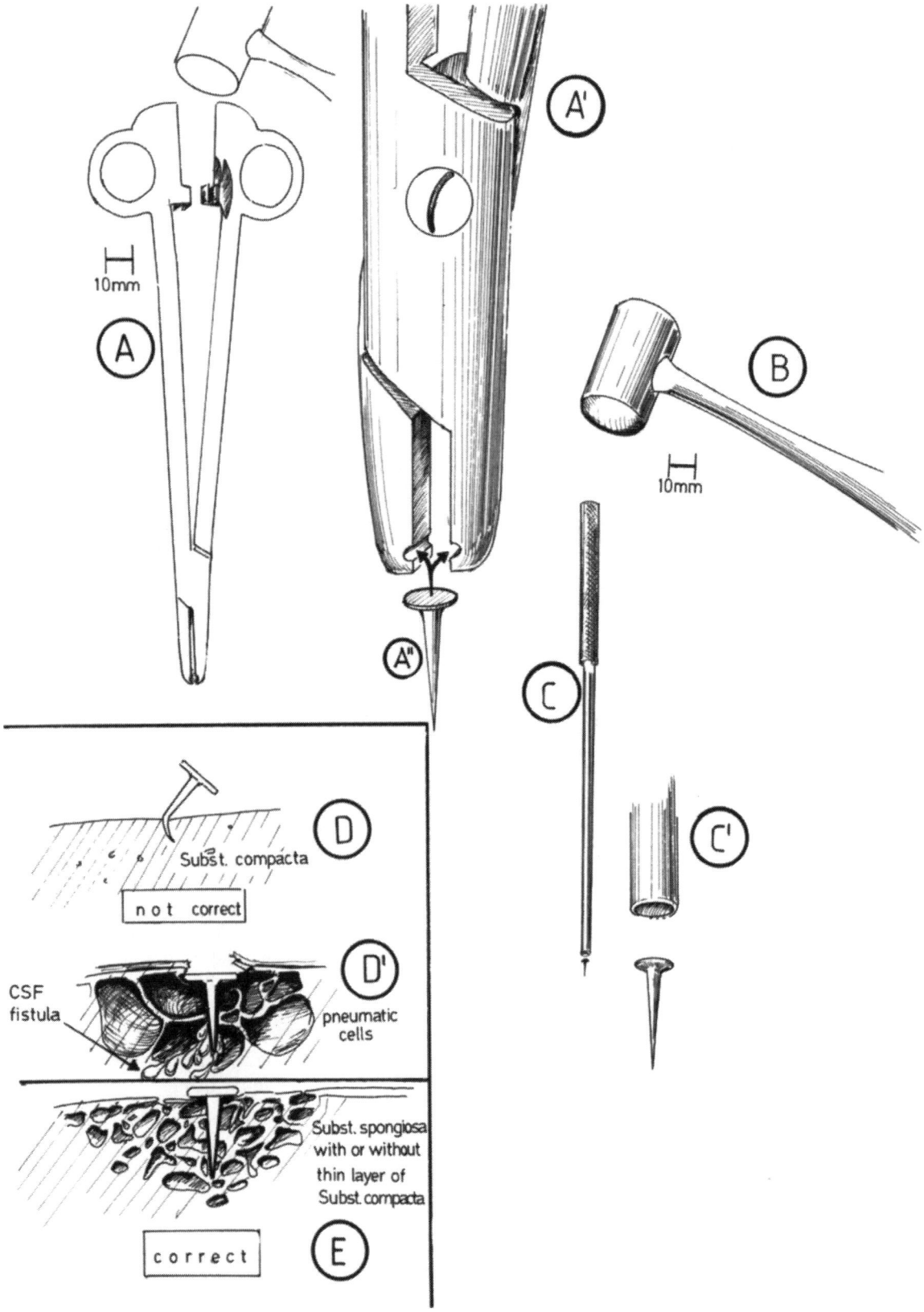
A'
10mm
A
B
10mm
A"
C
C'
D
Subst. compacta
not correct
D'
CSF
fistula
pneumatic
cells
Subst. spongiosa
with or without
thin layer of
Subst. compacta
correct
E

Fig. 115. Frontobasal operations.
Frontobasal fracture with liquor fistula. Anatomy of Lamina cribrosa, four enlargements, details from skull preparations*, frequently occurring normal findings

A Lamina cribrosa with varying excavations, Foramen coecum not exactly in mid-line, but lying to the side of Sulcus sagittalis

B Similar asymmetry –*x*– of Lamina cribrosa as in **A.** Foramen coecum unusually voluminous with marked bony edges –*y*– circling Foramen coecum, contrary to **A** where foramen edges diverge frontwards in two bony branches from Crista galli

C Crista frontalis without Sulcus sagittalis sup.. Probably corresponding to lack of anterior Sinus sagittalis sup. portion (according to Kaplan, atresia of anterior Sinus sagittalis sup. portion occurs in 7% of normal individuals). In skulls with senile atrophy larger gaps are found especially in anterior Lamina cribrosa area –*z*–

D Small Foramen coecum, bone edge structures –*y*– neither ring-like as in **B,** nor surrounded by two diverging bony branches as in **A** and **C.** Behind foramen, most anterior Lamina cribrosa portion lies quite deep. During preparation of Bulbus olfactorius one must expect these structural irregularities. Normally, large gaps in Lamina cribrosa (*z* in **A + C**) are covered only by a thin dura layer (and in the area of Meatus nasi superior by a thin mucosa layer).
Contact here with instruments creates especially great danger of liquor fistula

Abbreviations:

x Lateral excavation of Lamina cribrosa
y Bone bulging in Foramen coecum area
z Larger gaps in Lamina cribrosa

---

* Schematic presentations of variants can be found in J. Lang (in: Lanz – Wachsmuth, 1979).

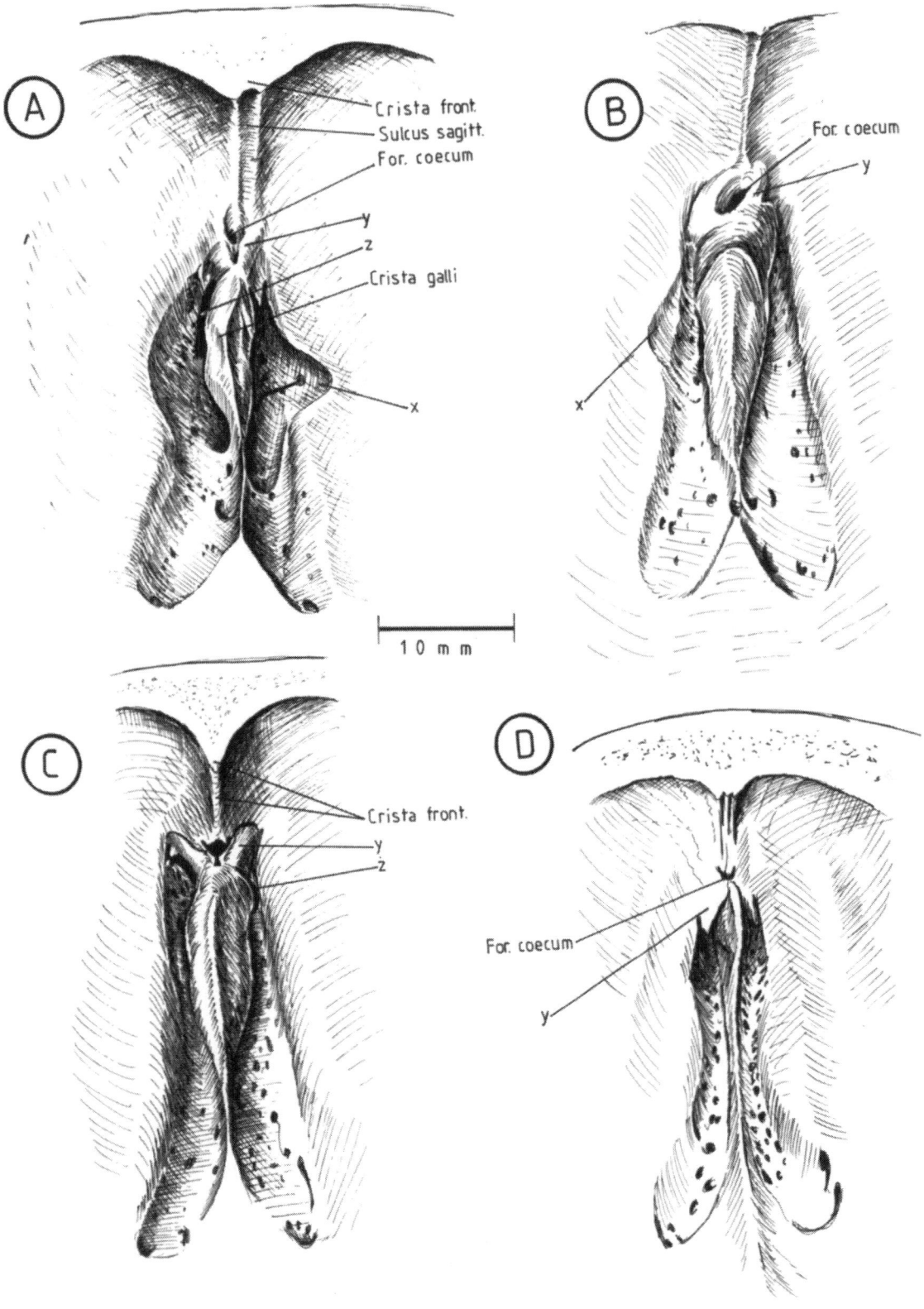
A
Crista front.
Sulcus sagitt.
For. coecum
y
z
Crista galli
x
B
For. coecum
y
x
10 mm
C
Crista front.
y
z
D
For. coecum
y

Frontobasal fracture with liquorhea (Figs. 116 to 134)

Fig. 116. Frontobasal operations.
Frontobasal fracture with liquor fistula. Anatomy. Schematic projection of sinuses onto skull base. Localization possibilities of liquor fistulas

A Projection of nasal sinuses onto skull base in cases of extensive pneumatization. Location of Cellulae ethmoidales remains nearly constant, Sinus frontales vary greatly. Anatomical topographical relation between Sinus sphenoidalis and skull base can be quite complicated. In rare cases, Sinus sphenoidalis is missing. Most often it is located beneath Planum sphenoidale and Sella; it may incorporate Dorsum sellae and Clivus. Frequently Processus clinoidei antt. are also pneumatized (see also Pneumosinus dilatans). Foramen rotundum may lie in Sinus sphenoidalis wall. Then the medial wall of Foramen rotundum protrudes into Sinus sphenoidalis (see chapter on Hypophysis)

A' Enlarged detail from **A'**, bone relief drawn in. Localization of liquor fistula

- **a** Lamina cribrosa, most frequent localization for liquor fistula
- **a'** Planum sphenoidale
- **b** Tuberculum sellae, liquor fistula difficult to identify (see **B**)
- **c** Drilling roof and medial wall of Canalis opticus may easily lead to opening of Sinus sphenoidalis (i. e. as in operations for A. ophthalmica aneurysms or N. opticus tumors)
- **d** When pneumatization of Processus clinoideus ant. is present, operations for Os sphenoidale meningiomas, A. ophthalmica aneurysms, and N. opticus processes may lead to liquor fistulae
- **e** Operations for Dorsum sellae meningiomas, radical transcranial hypophysectomy, with dura extirpation as far as sella entrance, may lead to liquor fistulas, since the typical vascularization may also require extensive electrocoagulation on the Dorsum sellae
- **a + b** Are common localizations of liquor fistulas following skullbrain trauma
- **c** to **e** Are less frequent and easily accessible through surgery

B Traumatic liquor fistula, schematic sagittal section

- **a** Lamina cribrosa
- **a'** Planum sphenoidale
- **b** Anterior sella wall below Tuberculum sellae
- **f** Posterior wall of Sinus frontalis

Traumatic liquor fistulae occur predominantly near midline; they are easily recognized in the area of **a + a'**. By a direct view of areas **b + f** these fistulae are difficult to see (but they can be seen by using a warmed dental mirror or curved bulb-headed probe)

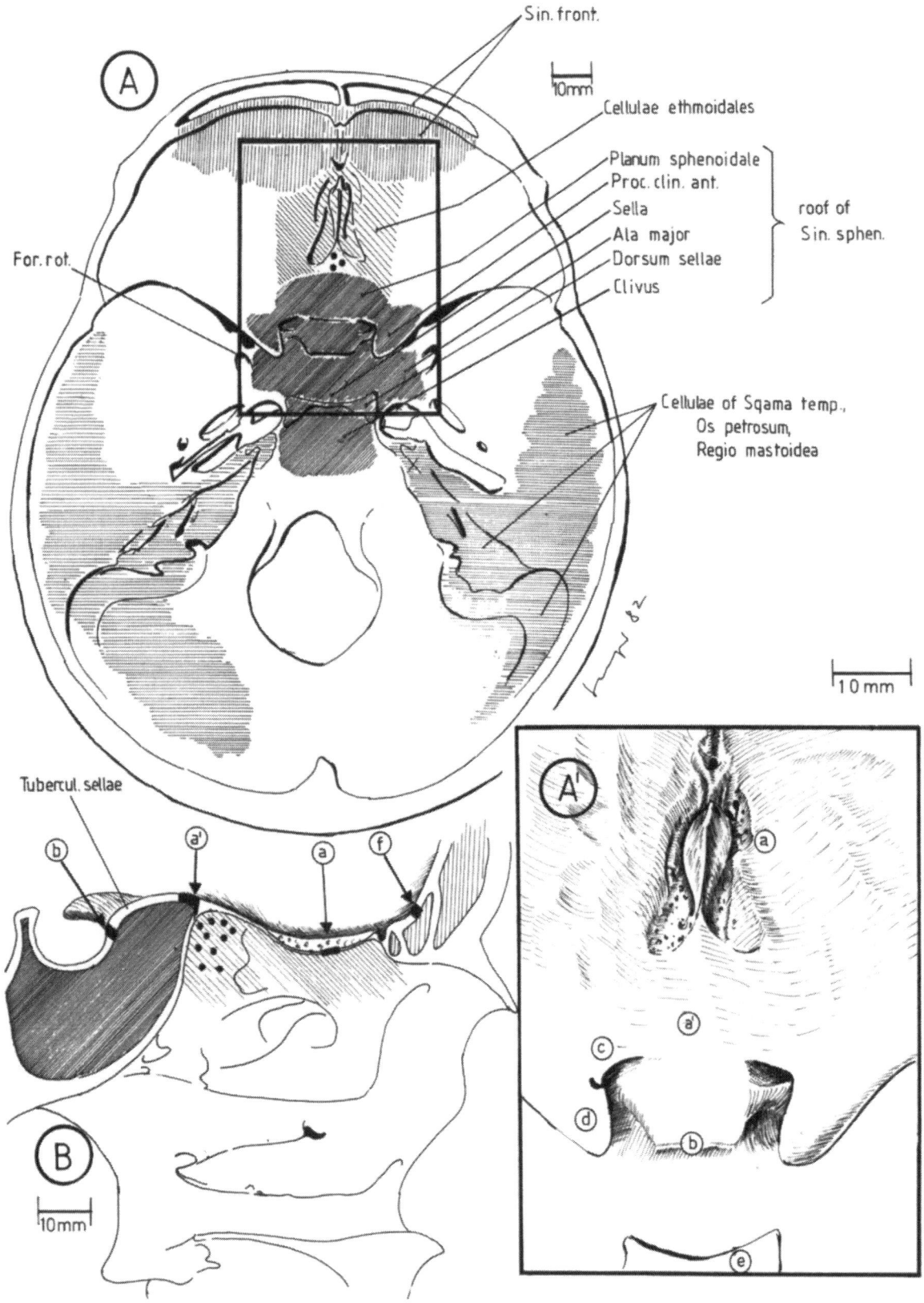
A
Sin. front.
10mm
Cellulae ethmoidales
Planum sphenoidale
Proc. clin. ant.
Sella
Ala major
Dorsum sellae
Clivus
roof of
Sin. sphen.
For. rot.
Cellulae of Sqama temp.,
Os petrosum,
Regio mastoidea
10 mm
Tubercul. sellae
b
a'
a
f
B
10mm
A'
a
a'
c
d
b
e

Fig. 117. Frontobasal operations.
Frontobasal fracture with liquor fistula
Clinical example of a patient with multiple frontobasal fractures. Full consciousness for four weeks prior to operation. Then 2 days comatose; after tracheotomy quick regaining of consciousness in outside hospital. Referred to us completely oriented. Bilateral anosmia, decreasing visual acuity on right side, otherwise no neurological findings. Craniotomy, immediately thereafter enucleation of injured right eye ball*. No additional postoperative findings. Quick recuperation. Preoperative psychosyndrome disappeared within few weeks
Clinical findings

A – C	X-ray-studies show multiple fracture zones *–x–*
D – E	CT findings: multiple fracture zones *–x–*
A' – B'	Postoperative x-ray: bone fragments removed
D'	Postoperative CT: fracture fragment removed; intracranial air accumulation *–y–* typical finding immediately after operation

Abbreviations:

x Multiple fracture zone
y Air accumulation

---

* Enucleation performed by Prof. Dr. H. Wietschel, Universitäts-Augenklinik Freiburg (Director: Prof. Dr. G. Mackensen).

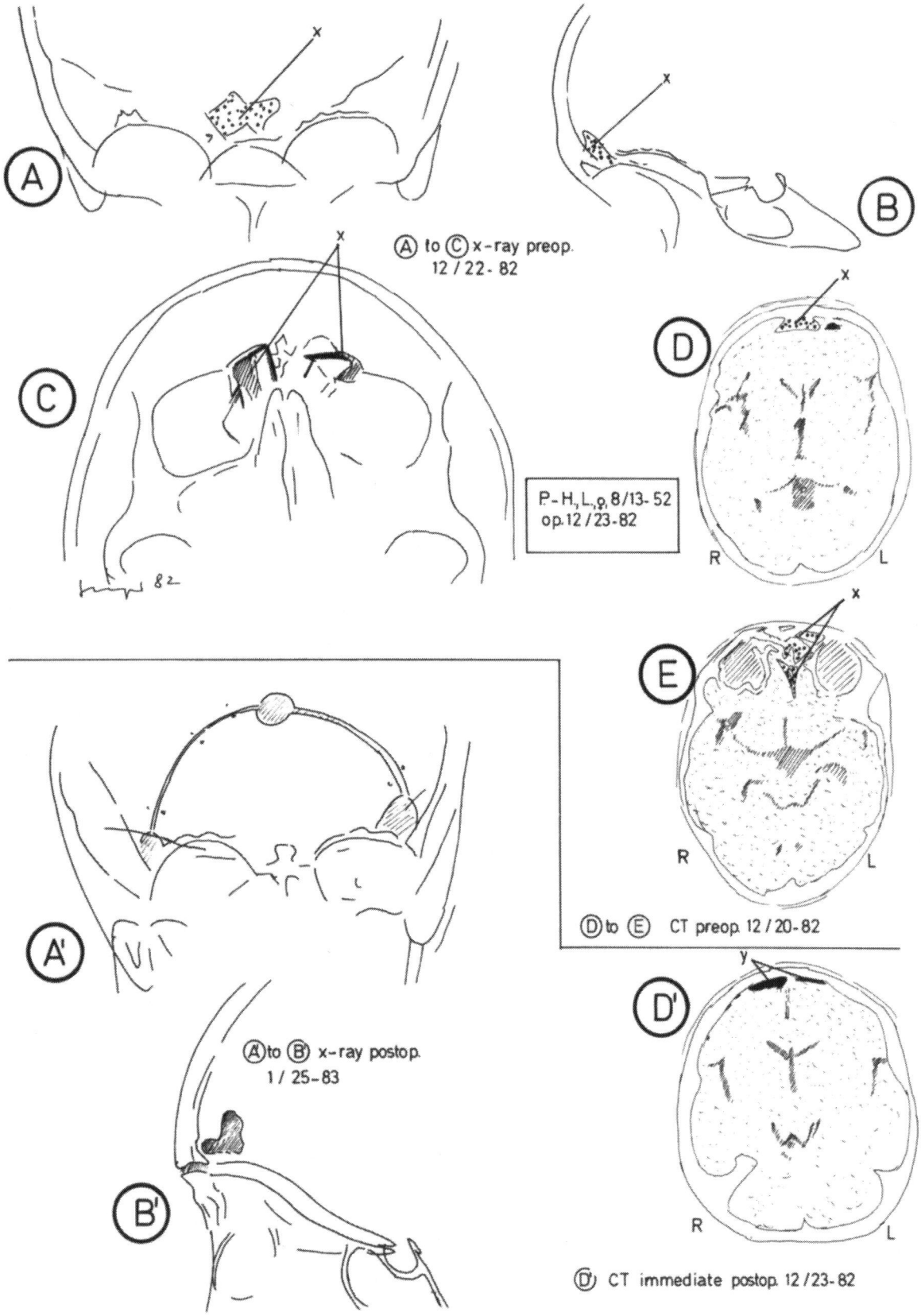
A
B
C
D
E
A'
B'
D'
x
y
R
L
Ⓐ to Ⓒ x-ray preop.
12 / 22 - 82
P-H, L, ♀, 8/13-52
op. 12 / 23-82
Ⓓ to Ⓔ CT preop. 12 / 20-82
Ⓐ to Ⓑ x-ray postop.
1 / 25-83
Ⓓ CT immediate postop. 12 / 23-82

Fig. 118. Frontobasal operations.
Frontobasal fracture with liquor fistula
Anatomical model presentation of clinical case

A Arrow *1:* Impression fracture of medial portions of Squama frontalis and Sinus frontalis
Arrow *2:* Impression fracture of Os sphenoidale with dislocation into skull

B Arrows as in **A.** Note compression of Falx and of anterior portion of Sinus sagittalis sup.

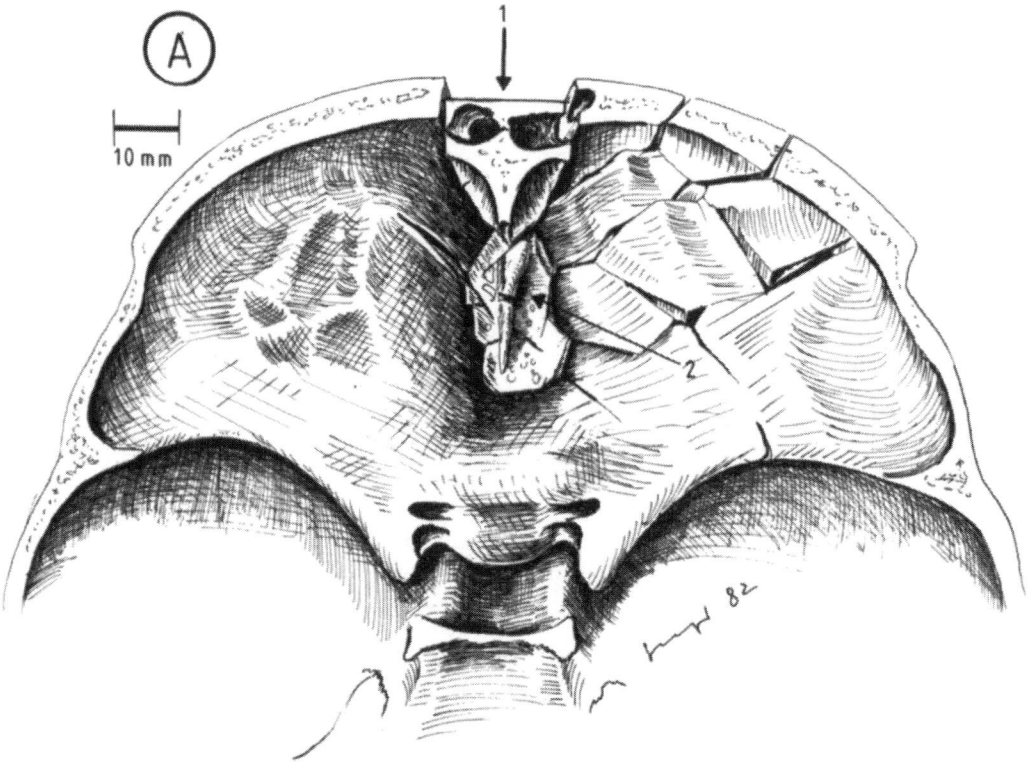
A
10 mm
1
2

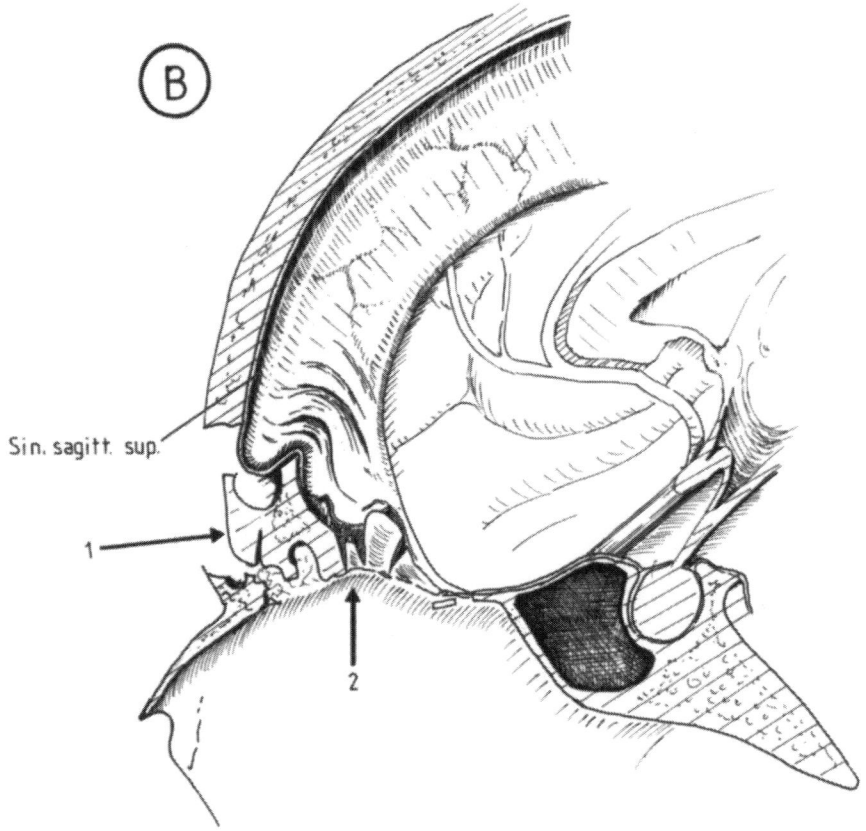
B
Sin. sagitt. sup.
1
2

Fig. 119. Frontobasal operations.
Frontobasal fracture with liquor fistula
Incision and preparation of skin and periosteum. Possible mistakes

A Incorrect incision: frontal branch of N.VII is severed, causing paralysis of anterior portions of M. epicranius –*m*– (formerly called M. frontalis)

A' Correct incision just before ear. Frontal branch of N.VII preserved, Frontal portion of M. epicranius –*m*– not paretic

B Incorrect. Galea and cutis detached from periosteum, periosteum left bone. Thus detachment of periosteum from bone is no longer possible without demage to periosteum. In addition galea has been incorrectly detached from cutis for grafting

B' Correct. Cutis, galea and periosteum detached from skull in one piece. As second step, periosteum loosened from galea –arrow–; thus a thickwalled defect-free periosteum-layer is available. M. epicranius preserved

C Incorrect: Situation **B,** sagittal transection

C' Correct: Situation **B',** sagittal transection

C, C' Broken line: trepanation

Abbreviation:

m M. epicranius, Pars frontalis (formerly: M. frontalis)

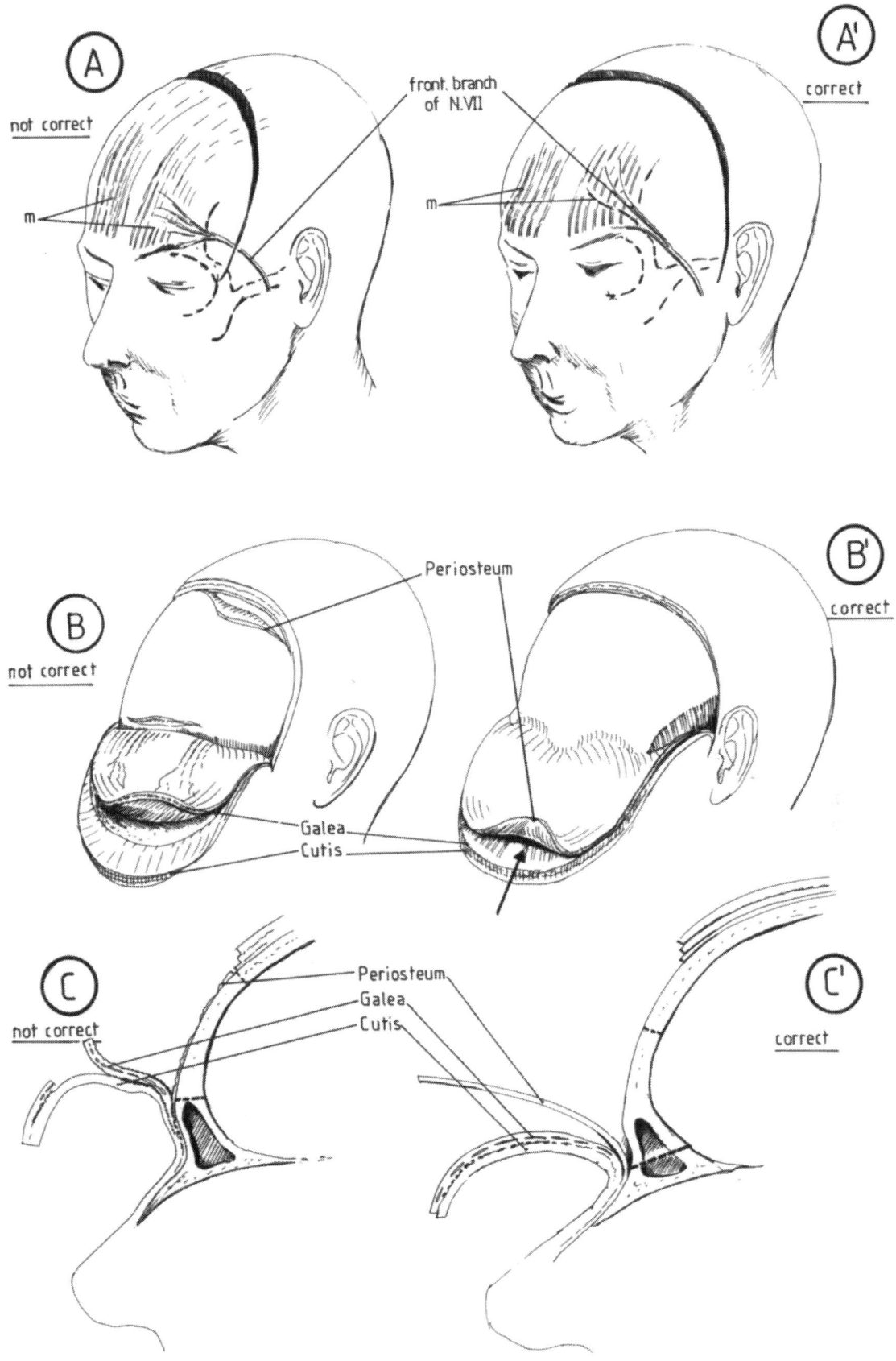
A
not correct
m
front. branch
of N.VII
A'
correct
m
B
not correct
Periosteum
Galea
Cutis
B'
correct
C
not correct
Periosteum
Galea
Cutis
C'
correct

Fig. 120. Frontobasal operations.
Frontobasal fracture with liquor fistula
Preparation of periosteum and fracture zone

A **1a + 1b** Pushing away periosteum together with cutis and galea from bone in a **single** layer
2 Lifting periosteum from galea
3a + 3b Detachment of periosteum from galea using sharp and/or blunt instruments

B Periosteum is pushed away as far as orbita edges. Fracture zones can be recognized between orbitae
1a + 1b Loosening of scar adhesions between fragments and Squama frontalis
Broken line: bone structures (projection)

C Sectional detail from **B,** microsurgical site
1a + 1b Blunt loosening of fragments
2 Sharp separation of adhesions

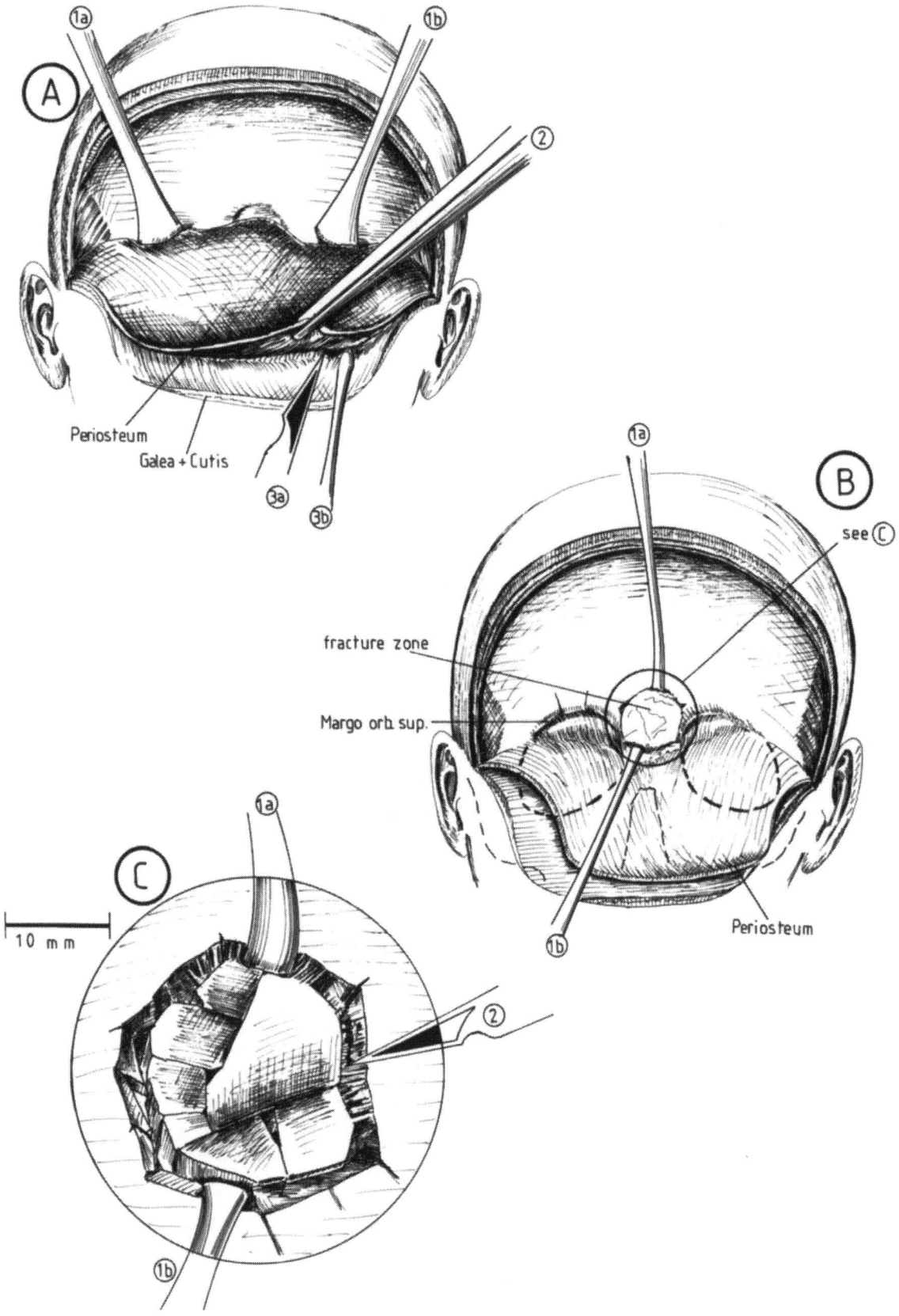
A
1a
1b
2
Periosteum
Galea + Cutis
3a
3b
B
1a
see C
fracture zone
Margo orb. sup.
Periosteum
1b
C
1a
10 mm
2
1b

Fig. 121. Frontobasal operations.
Frontobasal fracture with liquor fistula
Trepanation

A Trepanation as small and as far basally as possible. Cosmetically disfiguring burr holes must be filled with drill shavings at reimplanation

A' **2a – 2d** Sequence of drilling. Midline area is the last to be drilled

B Microsurgical detail from **A**

1a – 1d Loosening and removal of mucosa remnants from right Sinus frontalis

2a As **1a – 1d**

C Enlargement of **B**

1a Loosening of dura from bone spur, which had led to small dura injury *–g–*

1b Detachment of dura from base

2a + 2b Detachment of dura from medial bone fragments

Abbreviation:

g Dura injury

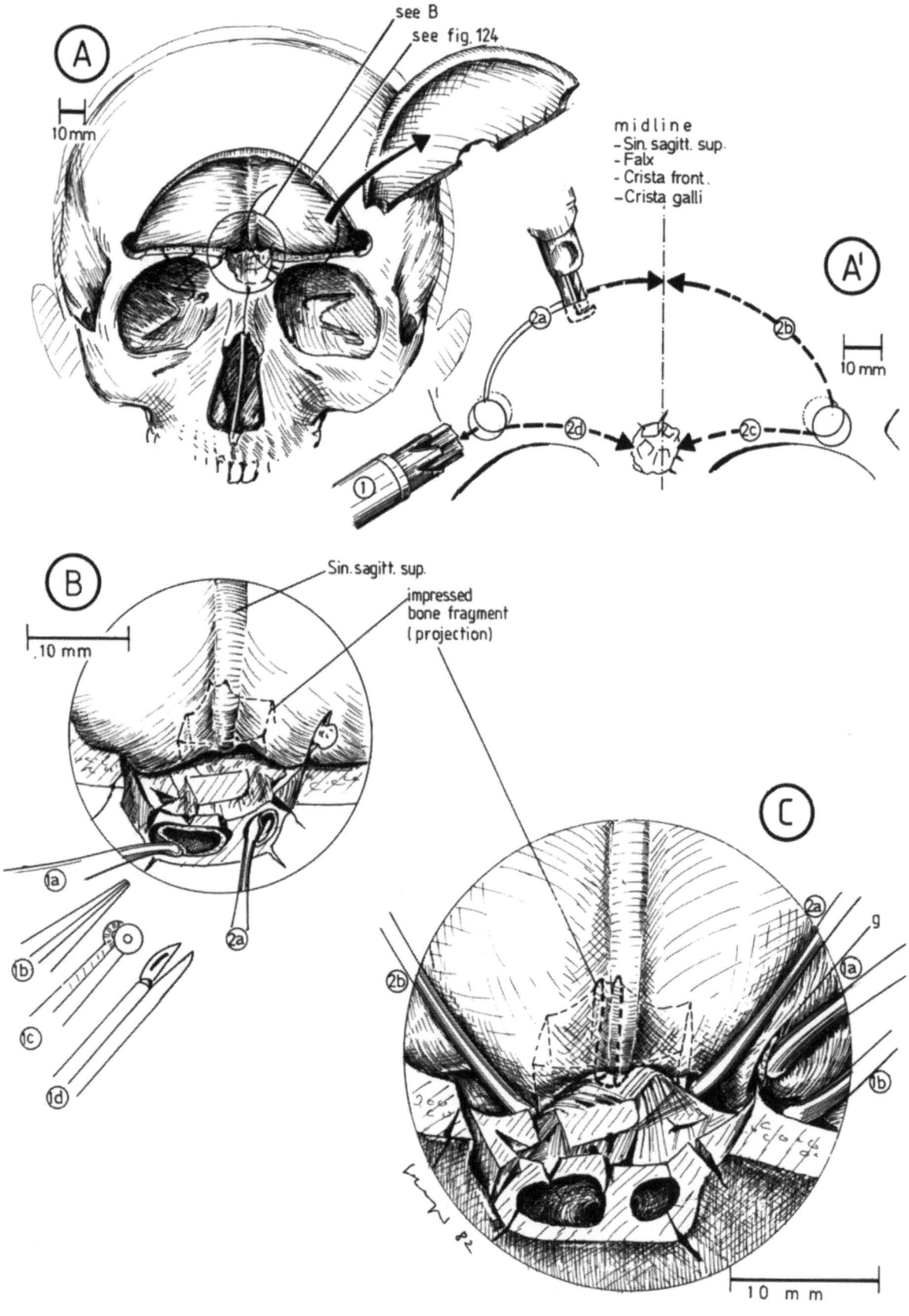
A
10mm
see B
see fig. 124
midline
- Sin. sagitt. sup.
- Falx
- Crista front.
- Crista galli
A'
10 mm
2a
2b
2c
2d
1
B
10 mm
Sin. sagitt. sup.
impressed
bone fragment
(projection)
1a
1b
1c
1d
2a
C
2a
g
1a
2b
1b
10 mm

Fig. 122. Frontobasal operations.
Frontobasal fracture with liquor fistula
Closure of both Sinus frontalis remnants by muscle grafting

A Overview, operation site **B** and **F** drawn in
B Incision of fascia temporalis
C **1** Holding back fascia temporalis
2 Holding incised Aponeurosis temporalis in place
3 Detachment of Aponeurosis temporalis from M. temporalis
D Removal of muscle piece
D' Corresponding to varying sizes of the small Sinus frontalis remnants, muscle piece is divided in two appropriate-sized portions
E Fascia and Aponeurosis temporalis are sutured
F **1** Muscle piece, soaked with thrombin/calcium, is positioned in Sinus frontalis and squirted from below with fibrinogen concentrate *
2 Immediately after squirting, muscle piece is pressed firmly into place
G **1** Principle of dura opening and attaching of resulting dura flaps to periosteum at the root of the nose

* Immuno.

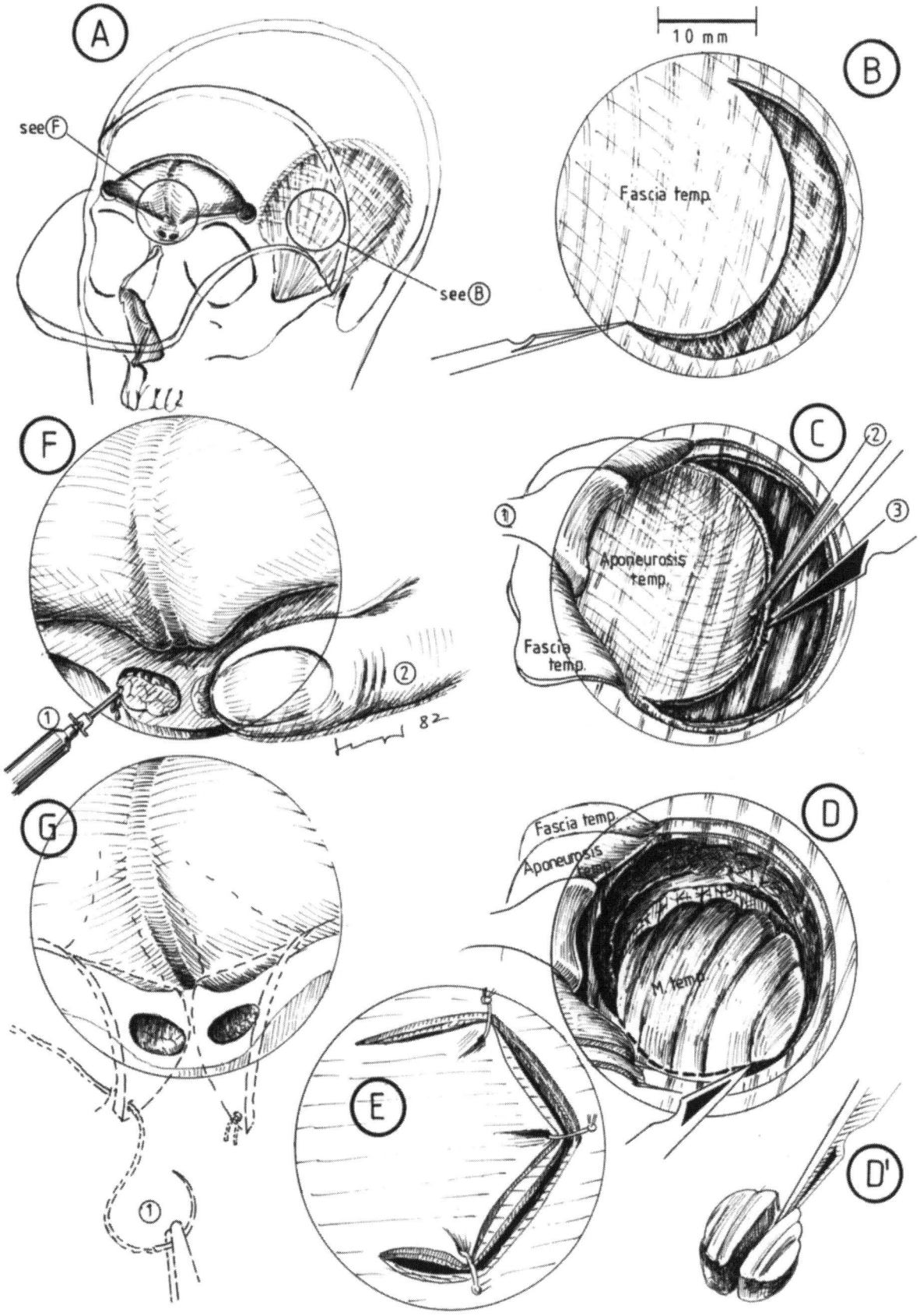
A
see F
see B
10 mm
B
Fascia temp.
F
1
2
82
C
1
2
3
Aponeurosis temp.
Fascia temp.
G
1
D
Fascia temp.
Aponeurosis temp.
M. temp.
E
D'

Fig. 123. Frontobasal operations.
Frontobasal fracture with liquor fistula
Dura opening and brain retraction; possible mistakes

A Incorrect

1 Ligature and separation of Sinus sagittalis sup. and Falx

2a, 2b Too forceful retraction of both Lobi frontales. During reclination Sinus sagittalis sup. and cerebral veins leading thereinto are simultaneously compressed. Danger of brain edema and encephalomalacia

B Correct. Sinus sagittalis sup. preserved. In the presence of major cerebrospinal fluid loss it is possible to eliminate use of spatulas; reclination is carried out solely by use of suction device

A' + A'' Anatomical sketch for **B**

B' + B'' Anatomical sketch for **A**

Arrows: operative approach

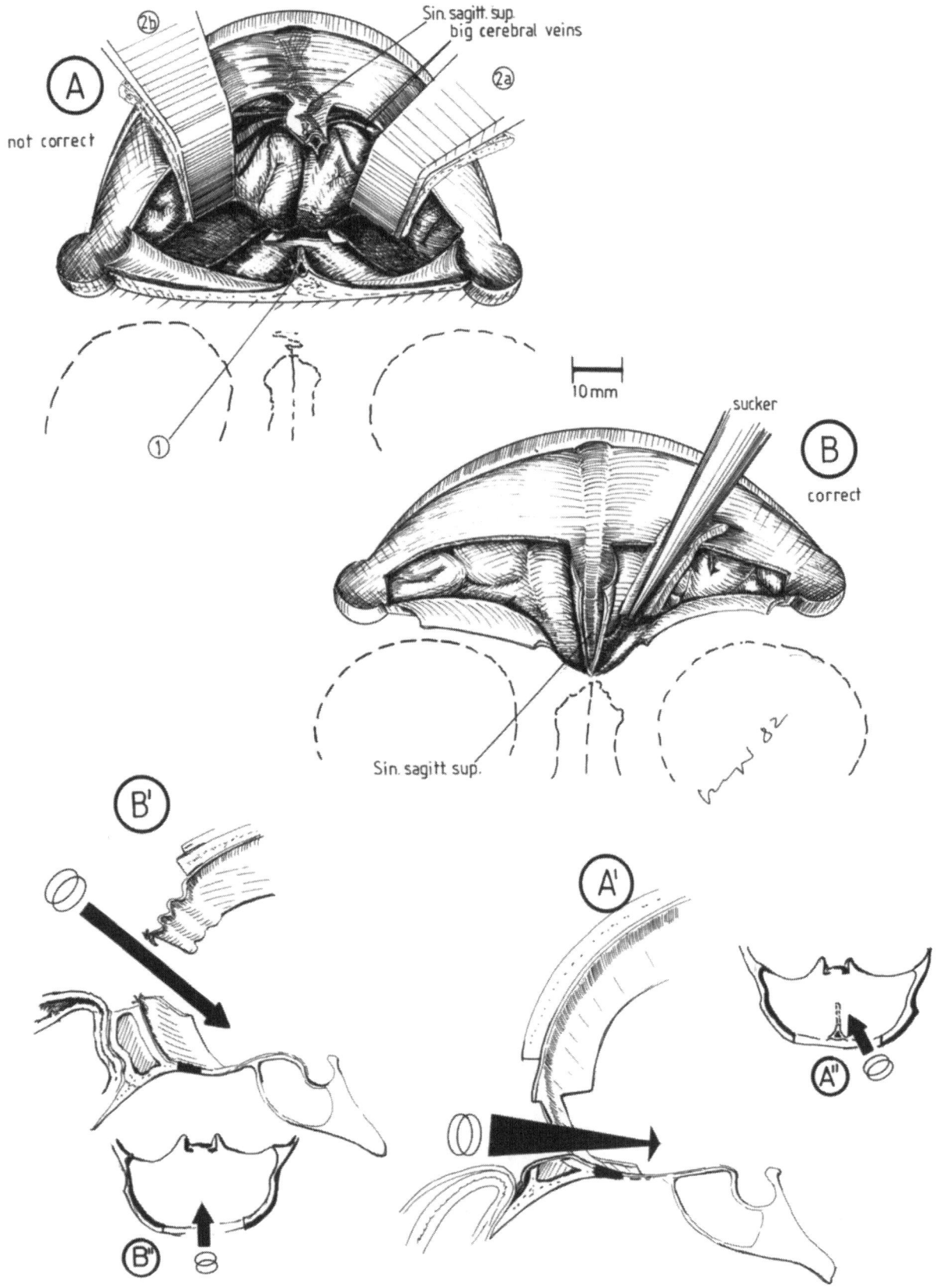
Sin. sagitt. sup.
big cerebral veins
2b
2a
A
not correct
1
10 mm
sucker
B
correct
Sin. sagitt. sup.
B'
B''
A'
A''

Fig. 124. Frontobasal operations.
Frontobasal fracture with liquor fistula
Preparation between dura and cortex

A **1** Dura incision

2a – 2c Light arrows: folding out of dura flaps. Shortly before reaching Sinus a lacuna was opened during dura incision, and closed by suture

A' Closure of incised lacuna at edge of Sinus sagittalis sup.

B **1** Removal of bone splinters which have penetrated dura

2 Blunt detachment of adhesions between dura and brain surface

3 As **2,** with forceps (this instrument preferable to the one shown in **2**)

4 Sharp separation of loosened adhesions

5 Dura incision above and beneath a cerebral vein

B' Enlarged detail from **B.** After dura circumcision, juncture of cerebral vein to Sinus sagittalis sup. remains undisturbed

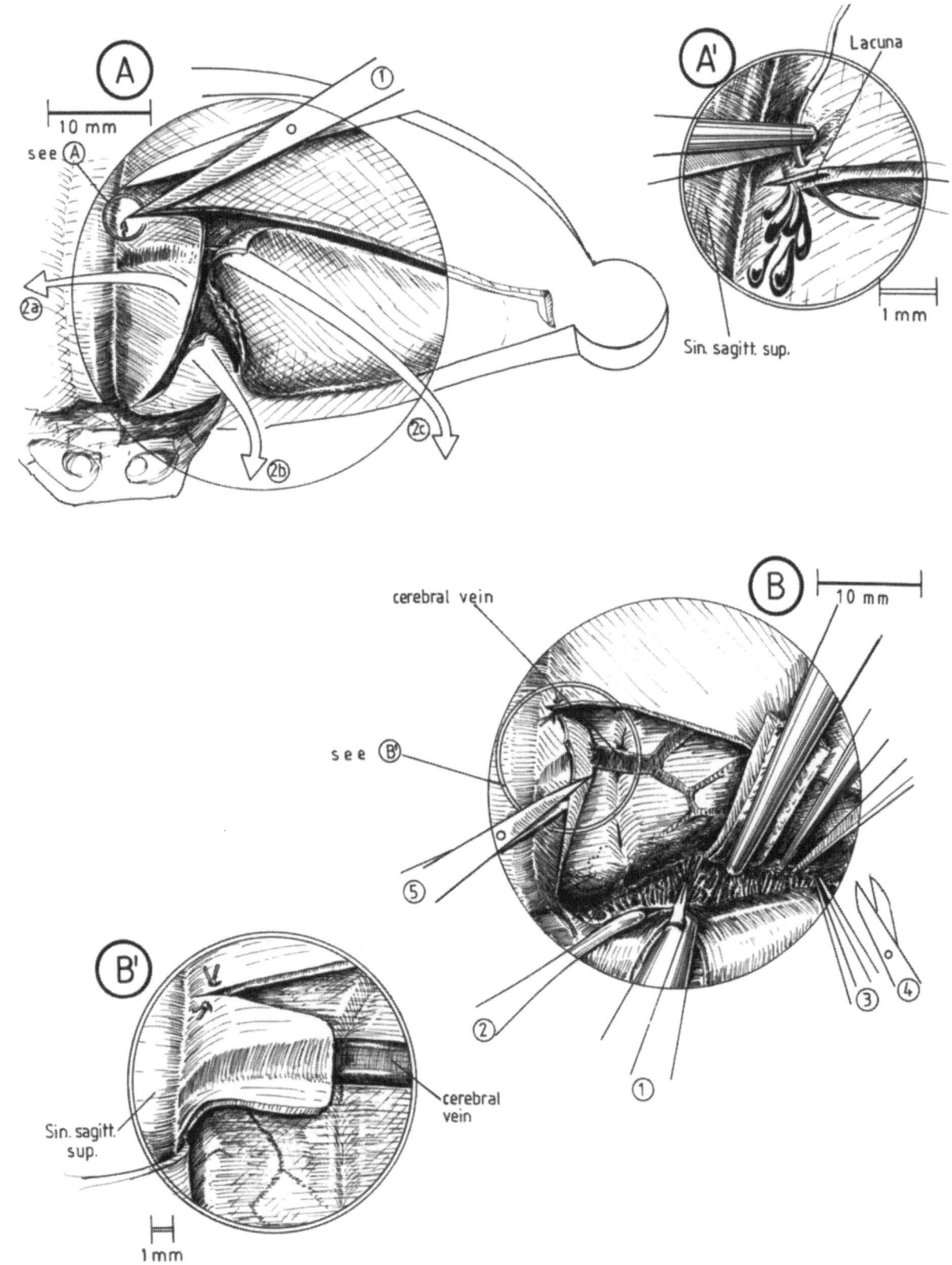
A
10 mm
see A
1
2a
2b
2c
A'
Lacuna
1 mm
Sin. sagitt. sup.
B
10 mm
cerebral vein
see B'
5
2
1
3
4
B'
Sin. sagitt. sup.
cerebral vein
1 mm

Fig. 125. Frontobasal operations.
Frontobasal fracture with liquor fistula
Removal of basal bone fragments in Sinus sphenoidalis area, particularly in the area of Crista galli and Falx

A Microsurgical site after loosening basal leptomeningeal adhesions. Baso-medial brain reclination amounts to approximately 1 cm. Spatula unnecessary after liquor outflow. Holding back of brain with sucker (with cotton wool beneath it). Nn. olfactorii on both sides are no longer identifiable

B Enlarged detail from **A**

- **1** Reclination of medio-basal frontal brain portions
- **2** Reducing impressed bone fragments, after loosening adjoining adhesions
- **3a + 3b** After falx incision with scalpel, falx resection follows; in case of bleeding, suturing (see clinical example of olfactorius meningioma)

C Resection of impressed bone fragments below incised falx through to the other side

C' Anatomical topographical sketch for **C**

Abbreviation:

ss Sinus sagittalis sup.

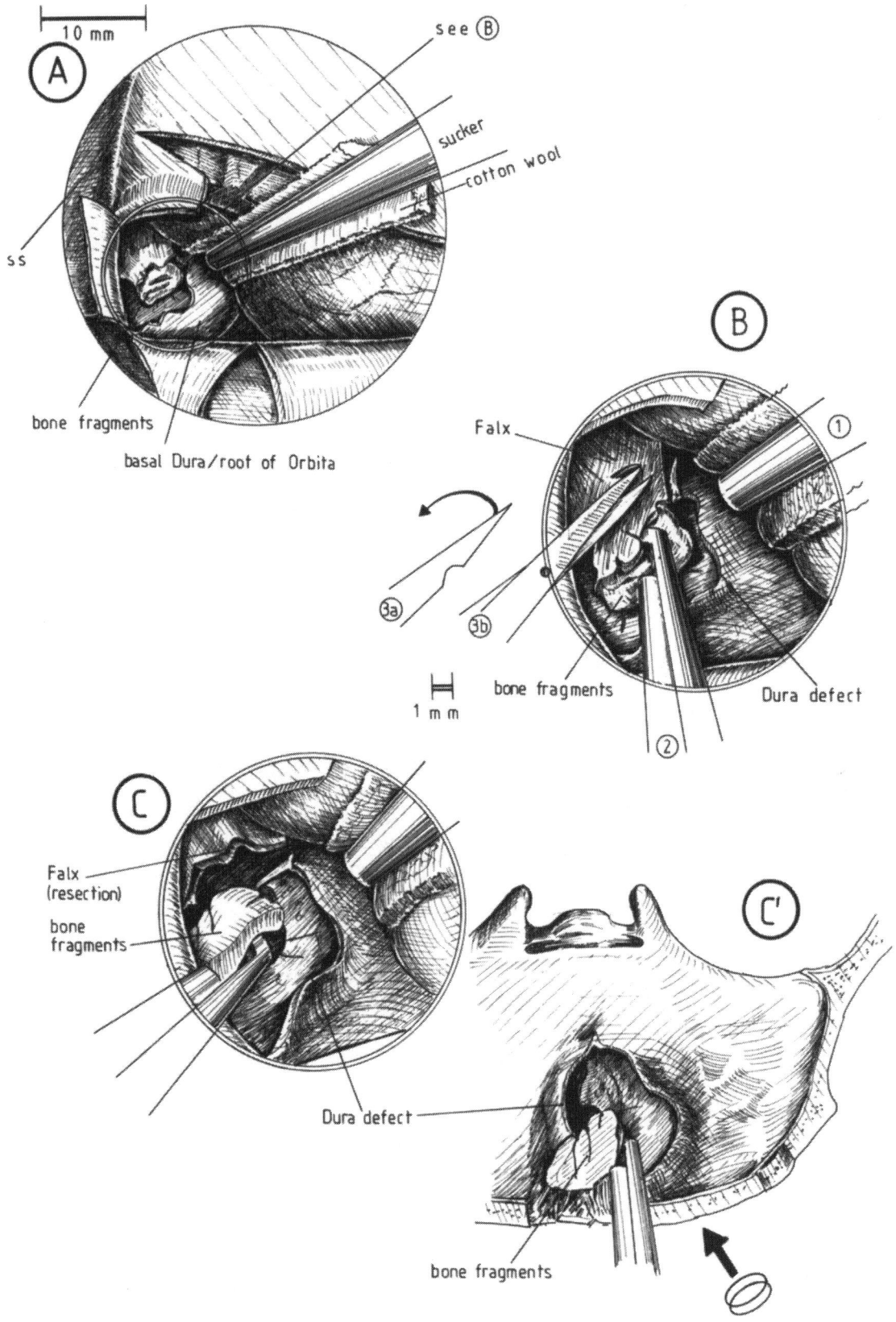
10 mm
A
see B
sucker
cotton wool
ss
bone fragments
basal Dura/root of Orbita
B
Falx
1
3a
3b
1 mm
bone fragments
Dura defect
2
C
Falx
(resection)
bone
fragments
Dura defect
C'
bone fragments

Fig. 126. Frontobasal operations.
Frontobasal fracture with liquor fistula
Removal of basal bone fragments

A Anatomical topographical sketch for **B.** Operative approach on right side. Arrow: microsurgical approach **B**

B Although fractures are more extensive on right side than on left, only a few leptomeningeal adhesions are found on the right

1 Dura opening on right side

2 Pulling back of frontal brain

3a – 3c Loosening of adhesions between Gyrus rectus and Dura of skull base

C Enlarged detail from **B.** After loosening of leptomeningeal adhesions

1a Sucker pushed forward (arrow), and

1b (arrow) farther pulling back of Gyrus rectus from base

2 Removal of bone fragments on right side

Abbreviation:

ss Sin. sagitt. sup.

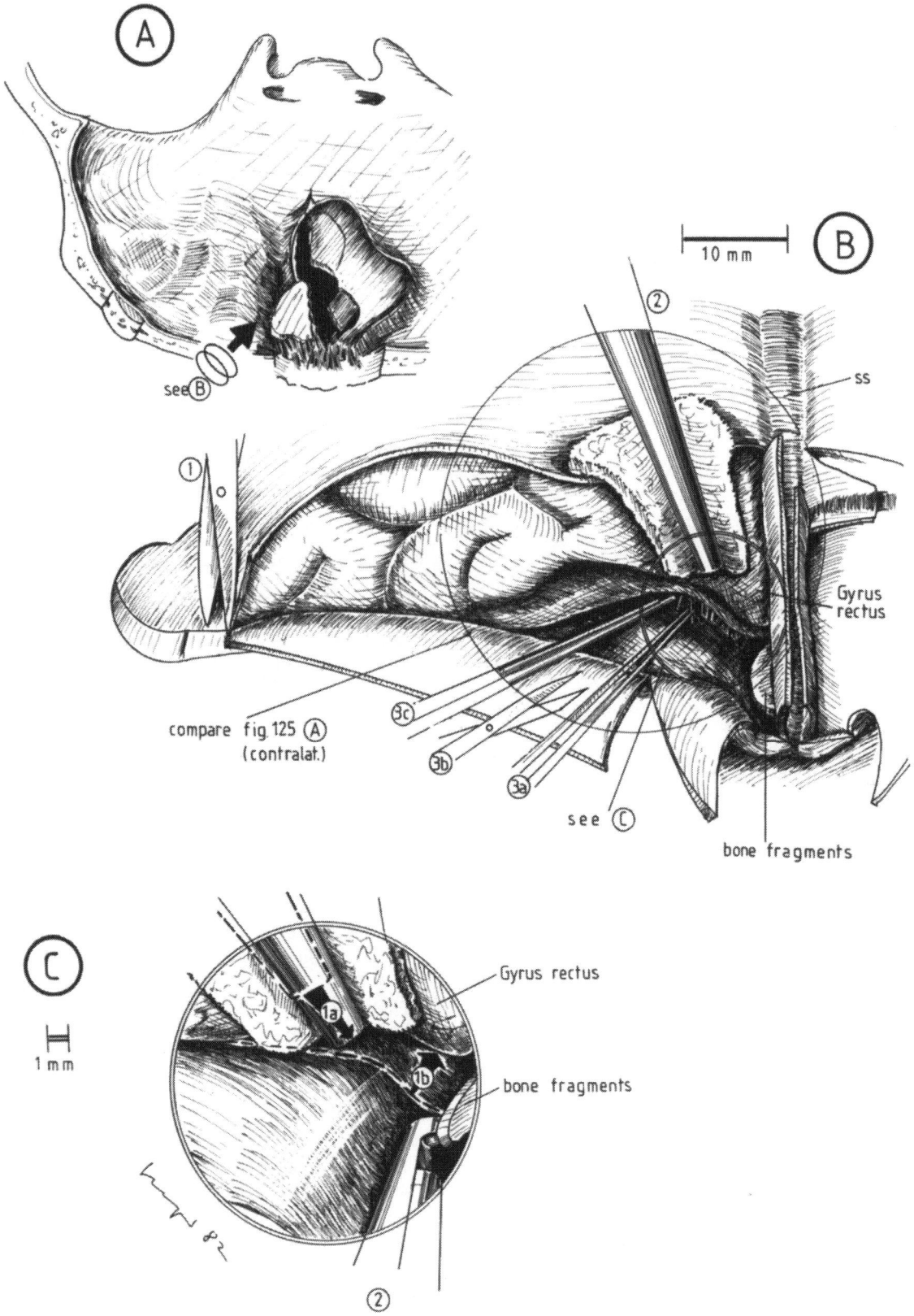
A
see B
B
10 mm
2
ss
1
Gyrus rectus
compare fig. 125 A (contralat.)
3c
3b
3a
see C
bone fragments
C
1 mm
Gyrus rectus
1a
1b
bone fragments
2

Fig. 127. Frontobasal operations.
Frontobasal fracture with liquor fistula
Exposure of liquor fistula and exclusion of additional fistulas

A Localization of microsurgical approach, skull sketch

B Microsurgical site with exposure of right medial liquor fistula

1 Spatula insertion is necessary for frontal base overview

2 Below torn falx, after removal of bone fragments, dura-bone gap becomes visible. Opening communicates with ethmoid cells

3 In the presence of extensive fracturing, area between both Nn. optici is examined by bulb headed probe (or dental mirror) to ascertain whether dura cover of anterior sella wall below Tuberculum sellae is intact. **This area cannot often be directly visualized.** Since posterior wall of Sinus frontalis has been removed as far as base, good bilateral inspection is possible.

B' Exclusion of liquor fistula of anterior sella wall, corresponding to **B 3,** shown in anatomical sagittal section sketch. Site of ethmoidal liquor fistula also drawn in

B'' Enlarged detail from **B'.** Because instruments lie so close to Infundibulum, there is risk of Diabetes insipidus. Arachnoid layer was preserved* served*

---

* In one case author observed the complication of Diabetes insipidus of long duration, without additional findings. Liquor fistula was diagnosed by the above method and was closed by grafting.

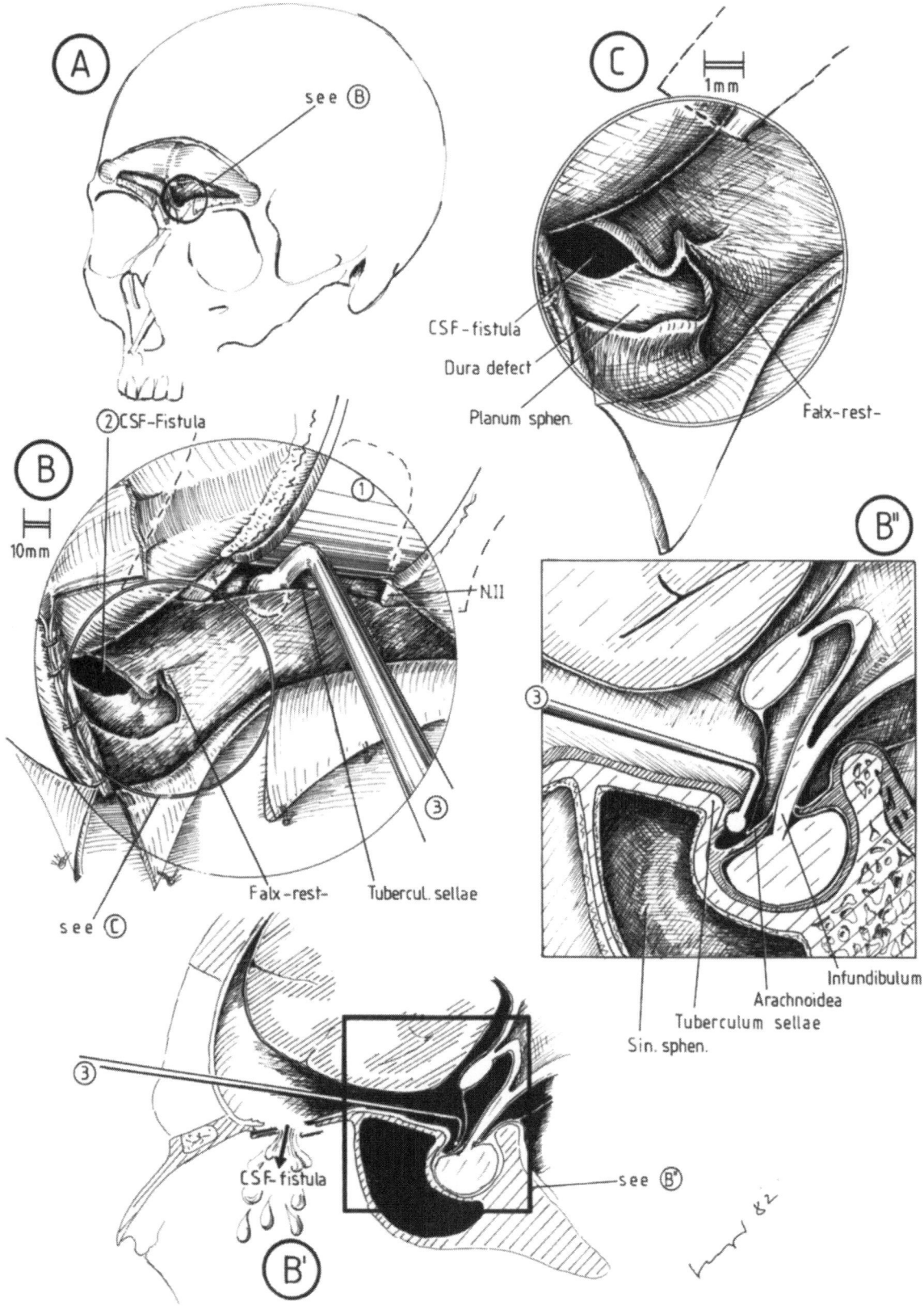
A
see B
C
1mm
CSF-fistula
Dura defect
Planum sphen.
Falx-rest-
B
10mm
2 CSF-Fistula
1
N.II
3
Falx-rest-
Tubercul. sellae
see C
B''
3
Infundibulum
Arachnoidea
Tuberculum sellae
Sin. sphen.
3
CSF-fistula
see B''
B'

Fig. 128. Frontobasal operations.
Frontobasal fracture with liquor fistula
Closure of liquor fistula

A Dura is loose after extensive bone fracturing. Therefore, dura gap can be made smaller by suture

B Situation after dura suture. Small falx remnant included in suture

C Anatomical sketch for **B.** Light arrow: principle of additional covering of incompletely closed dura, using periosteum

D Anatomical model of periosteum graft. Light arrows: direction in which sutures are pulled

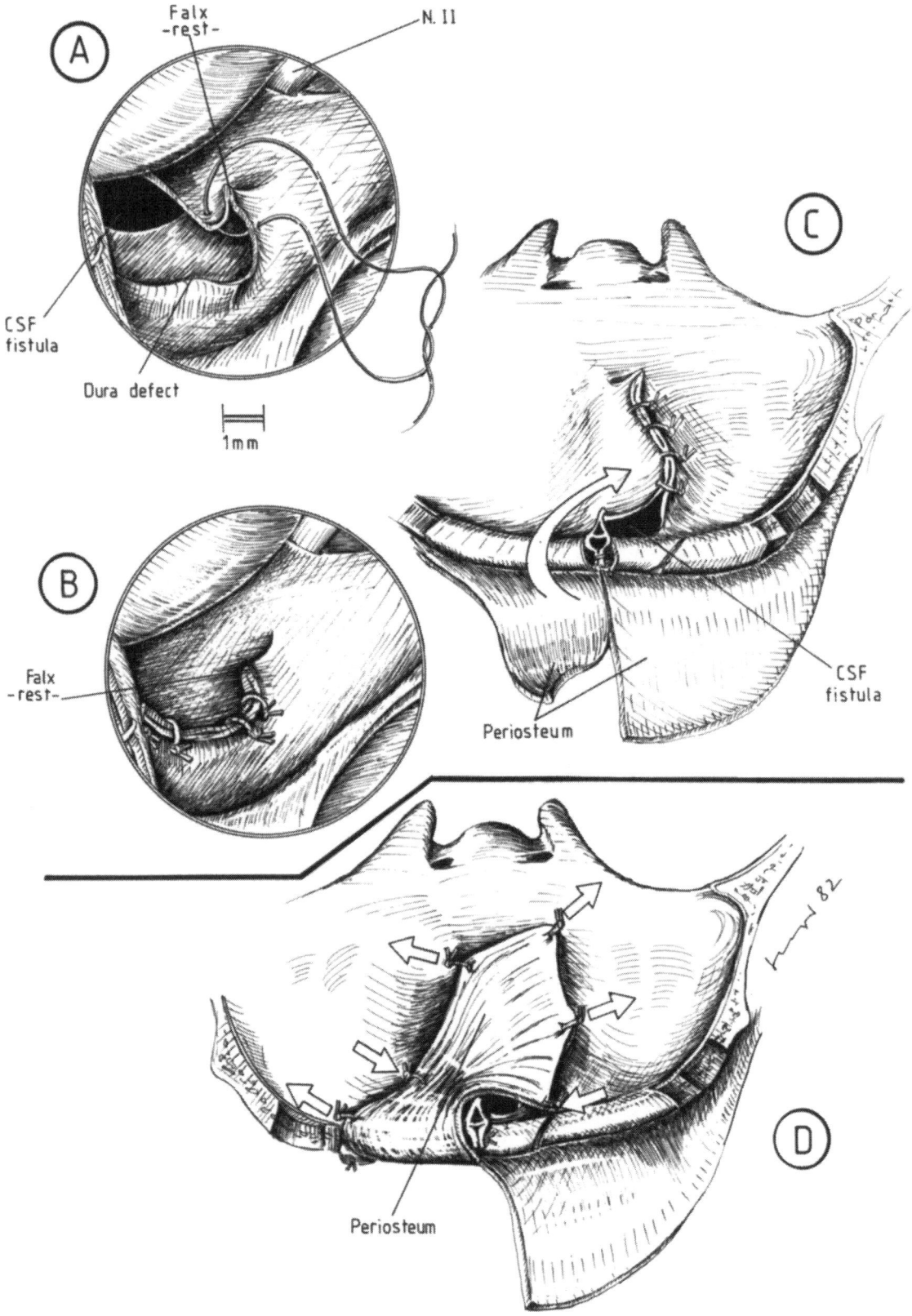
A
Falx
-rest-
N. II
CSF
fistula
Dura defect
1mm
B
Falx
-rest-
C
CSF
fistula
Periosteum
D
Periosteum

Fig. 129. Frontobasal operations.
Frontobasal fracture with liquor fistula
Anatomical model of liquor fistula closure by grafting

A Light arrow: positioning of left periosteum flap onto base

B Situation after fixation of both periosteum flaps. Liquor fistula is covered from both sides, Sinus sagittalis sup. not compressed

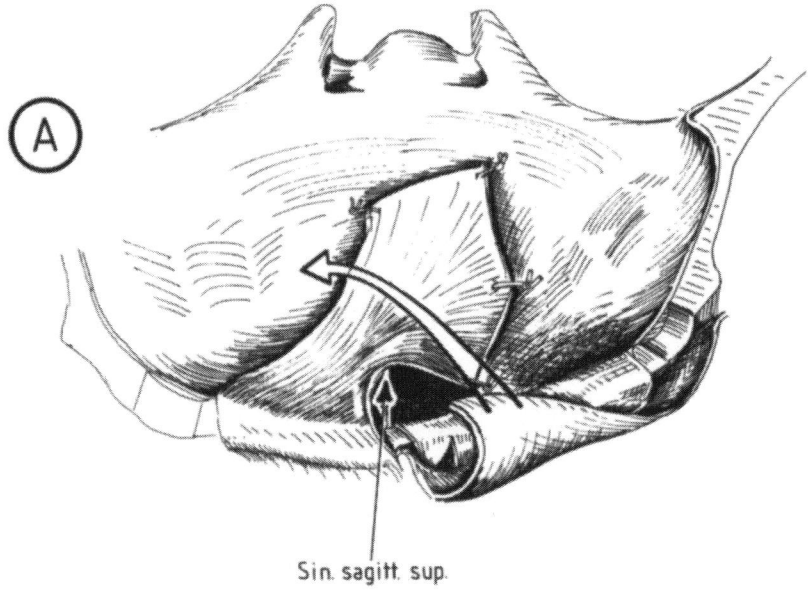
A
Sin. sagitt. sup.

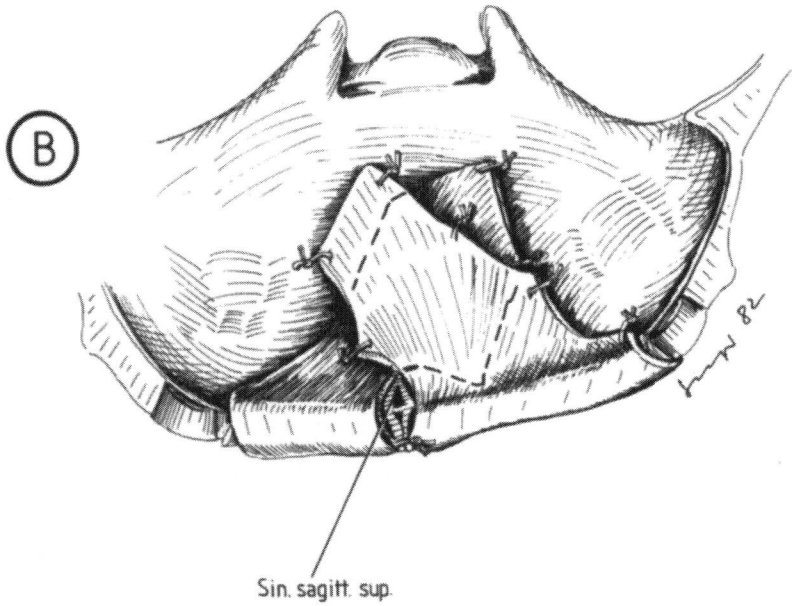
B
Sin. sagitt. sup.

Fig. 130. Frontobasal operations.
Frontobasal fracture with liquor fistula
Closure of liquor fistula

A Median splitting of periosteum flap

B **1** Basal dura portions are fastened by suture to periosteum

2 Medial dura portions from both sides are joined together over Sinus sagittalis sup.

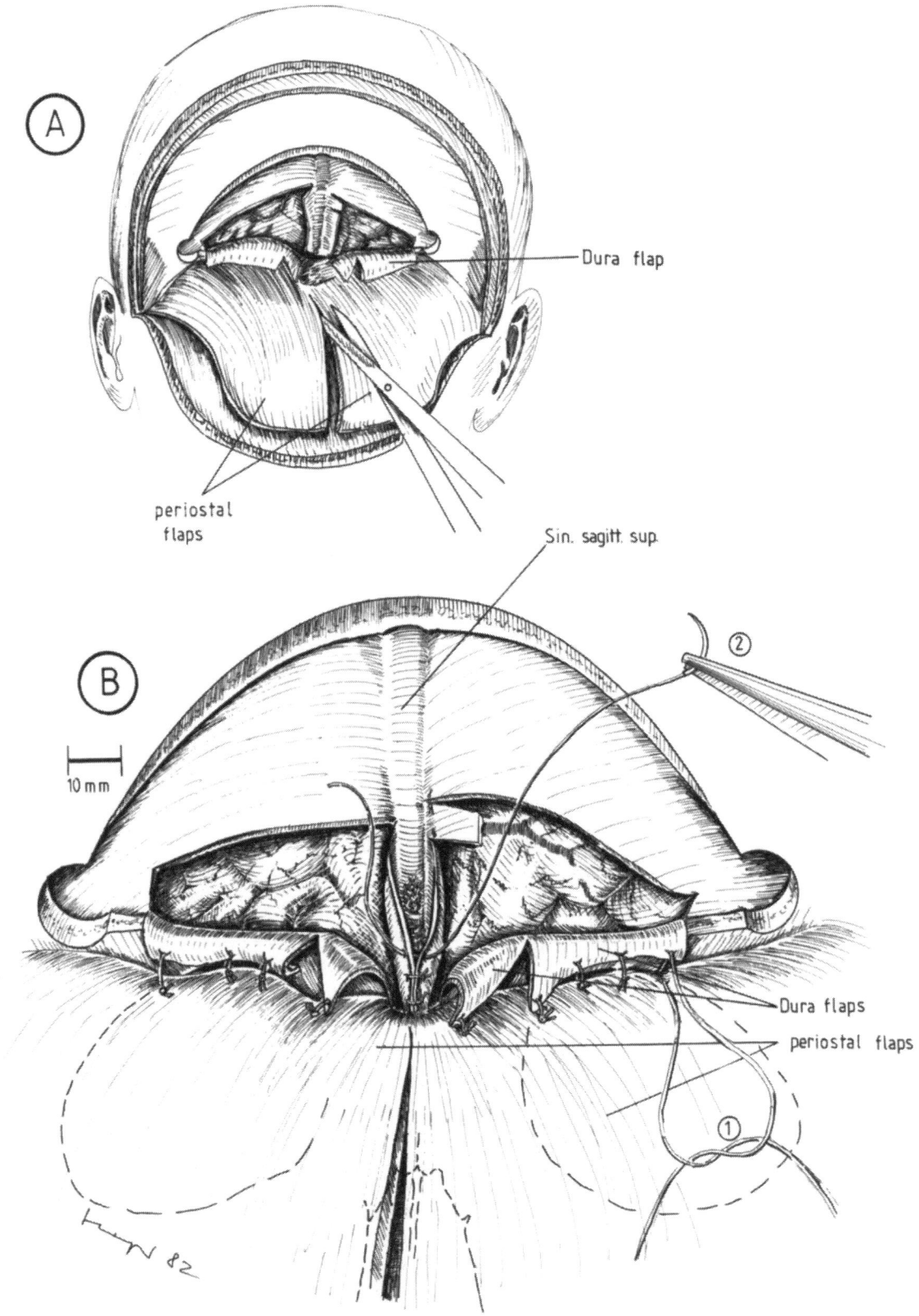
A
Dura flap
periostal
flaps
Sin. sagitt. sup.
B
10 mm
②
Dura flaps
periostal flaps
①
82

Fig. 131. Frontobasal operations.
Frontobasal fracture with liquor fistula
Closure of liquor fistula

A Position sketch of microsurgical operation site **A'** – left side –

A' Periosteum graft is pushed in from the right, then from left microsurgical site it is fastened to base by suture

B As **A,** contralateral – right side – approach

B' Microsurgical site, right side. Right periosteum graft, already fastened contralaterally (see **A'**), now is fastened to the base on the right by suture, using moderate tension

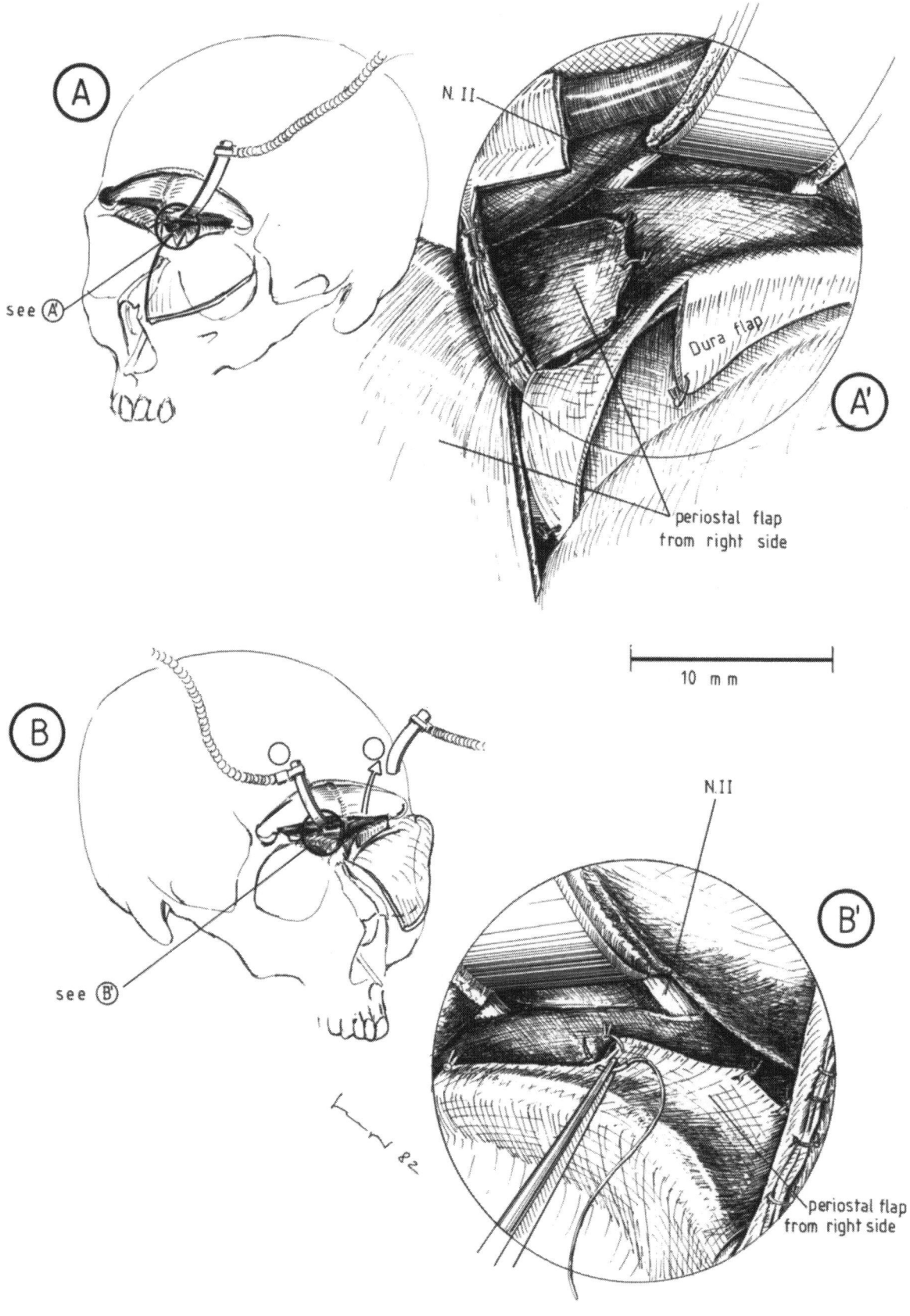
A
see A'
N. II
Dura flap
A'
periostal flap
from right side
10 mm
B
see B'
N.II
B'
periostal flap
from right side

Fig. 132. Frontobasal operations.
Frontobasal fracture with liquor fistula
Closure of liquor fistula

A Microsurgical site, overview sketch. Operative approach is changed once again to left side (see **A'**)

B As **A,** again changing side of operative approach – to right –

B' Left sided periosteum graft is now fastened contralaterally – right – by suture, using slight tension

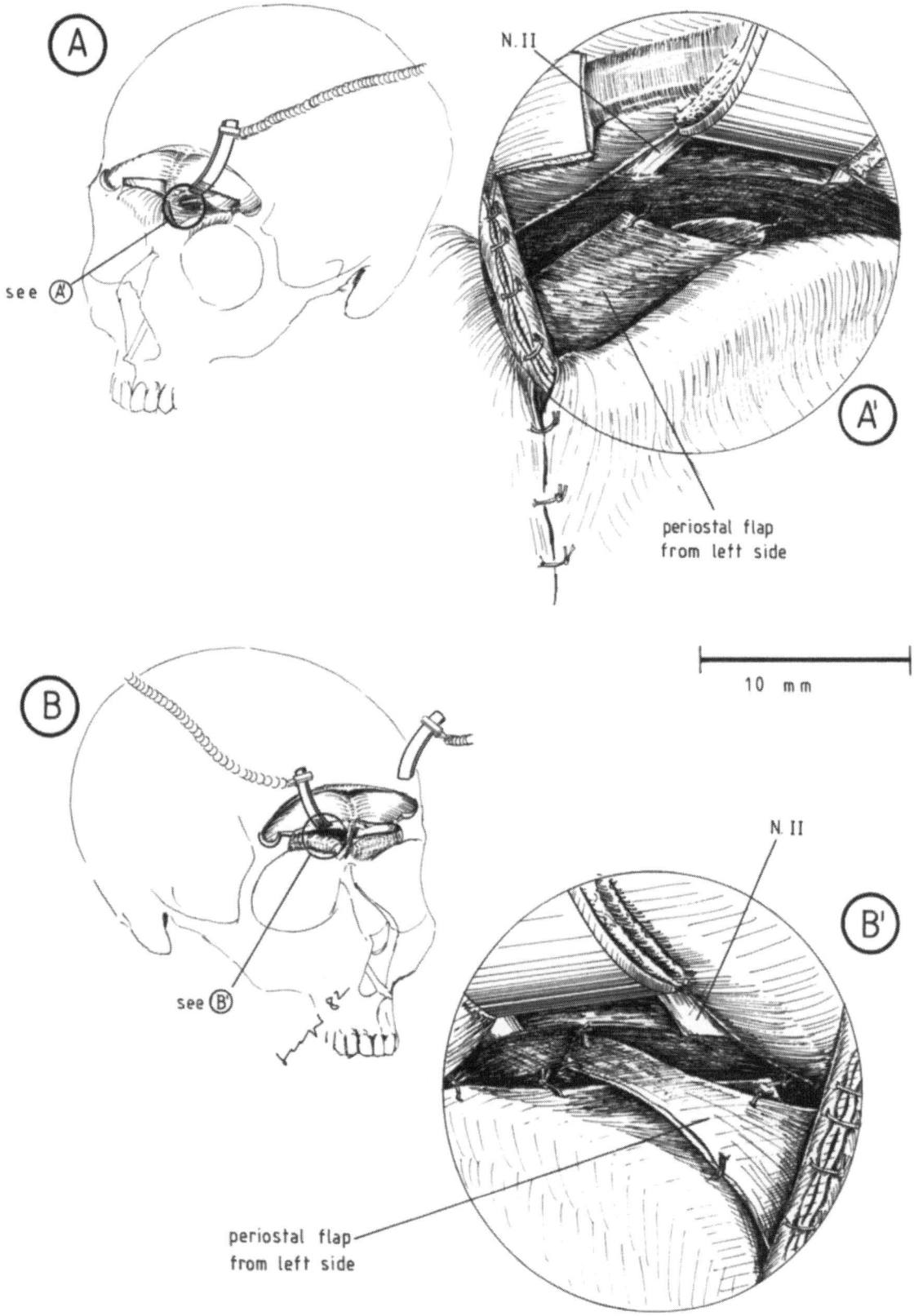
A
see A'
N. II
A'
periostal flap
from left side
10 mm
B
see B'
N. II
B'
periostal flap
from left side

Fig. 133. Frontobasal operations.
Frontobasal fracture with liquor fistula
Closure of liquor fistula

A Anatomical topographical sketch, after fastening of both periosteal grafts by suture. Sinus sagittalis sup. preserved. Additional securing by tissue glue*

1a + 1b The grafts are squirted from beneath on both sides with thrombin/calcium solution and then with fibrinogen concentrate

2 Immediately after injection of fibrin glue, grafts are pressed against skull base using sponge (in case of ample space and good overview, use of finger also possible).

The closer the contact surfaces lie to one another and the thinner the glue film is, the more reliable is the result because a thin fibrin layer is more quickly grown through by connective tissue than a thick fibrin layer

A' + A'' Sketch of anatomical longitudinal section for **A**

B Dura suture

---

* Fibrinogen concentrate Immuno.

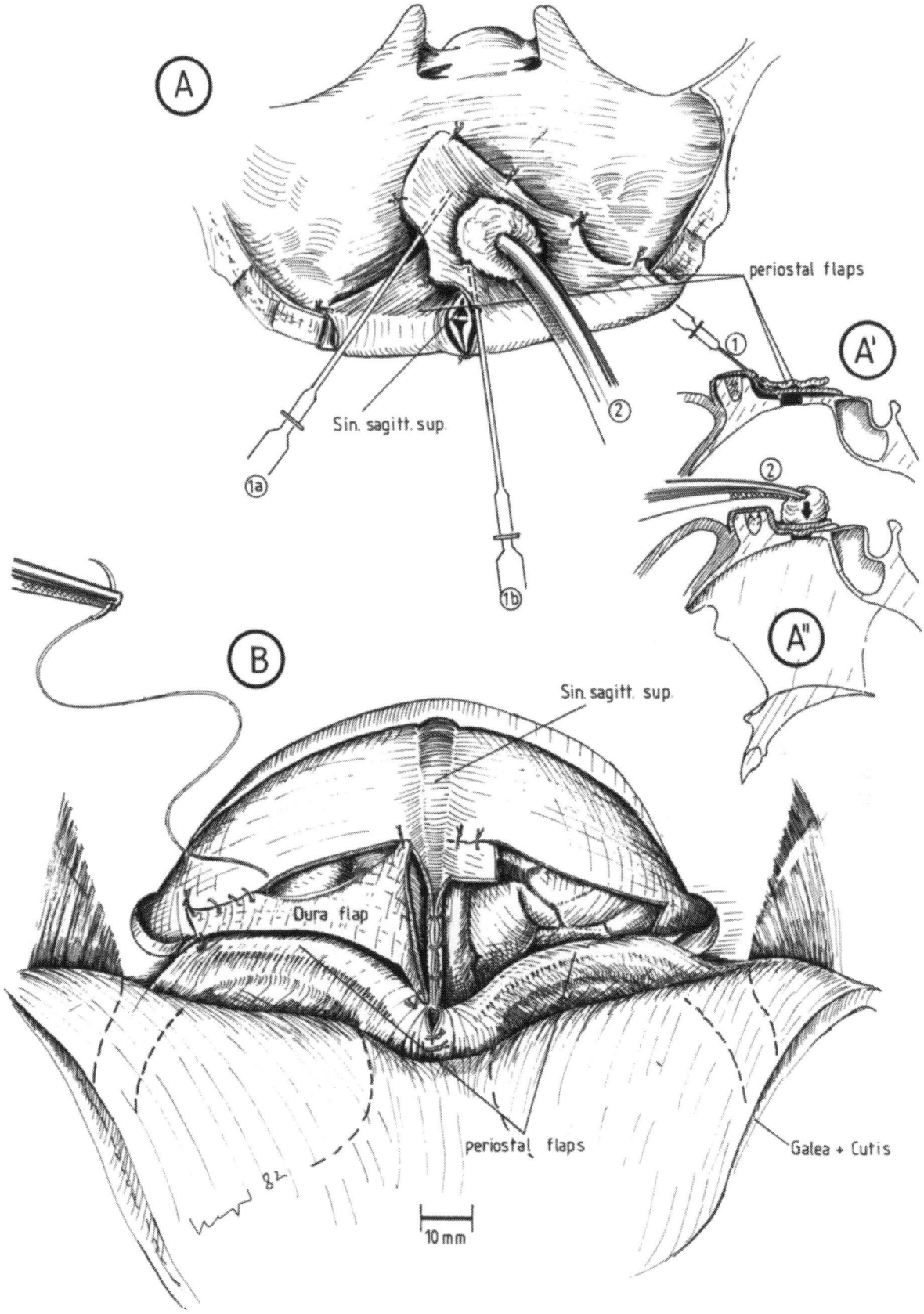
A
periostal flaps
A'
1
2
Sin. sagitt. sup.
1a
1b
A''
B
Sin. sagitt. sup.
Dura flap
periostal flaps
Galea + Cutis
10 mm

Fig. 134. Frontobasal operations.
Frontobasal fracture with liquor fistula
Wound closure

A **1a** Making burr holes at bone edge
1b Protection of dura and brain from drill
2 Insertion of bone flap

A' After creating small burr holes along edge of bone flap, follows:
3 Fastening of bone flap by sutura

A'' **4** For cosmetic reason bone shavings, preserved from operation's beginning, are put in bone gaps (and soaked with fibrinogen concentrate)*
5 Insertion of drain
6 Galea- and skin suture

---

* Immuno.

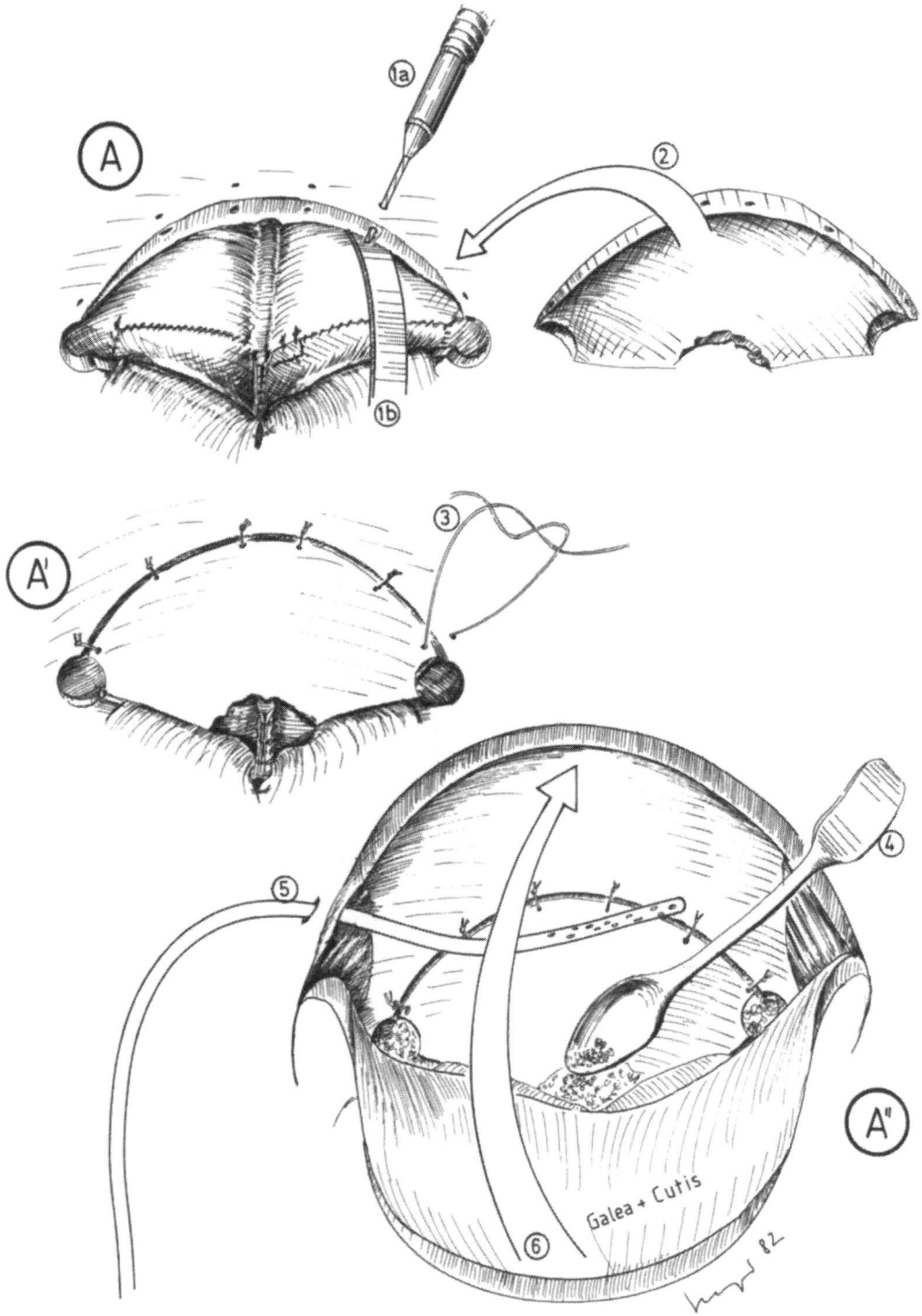
A
1a
2
1b
A'
3
4
5
A''
Galea + Cutis
6

Chapter 4
Extra-intracranial Bypass
(Figs. 135 to 167)

"STAMCA" (Figs. 135 to 156)

Figs. 135–156. Extra-intracranial bypass supratentorial: bypass between Ramus parietalis of A. temporalis superficialis and branch of A. cerebri media (**s**uperficial **t**emporal **a**rtery – **m**iddle **c**erebral **a**rtery – "STAMCA")

Fig. 135. Extra-intracranial bypass "STAMCA"
Clinical example of total occlusion of left A. carotis int. with TIA's. Additionally, stenosis of Truncus brachiocephalicus with vertebral steal syndrome. For months, progressive stenosis of right A. carotis int. also, without clinical findings*.
Postoperatively, no neurological deficits.
Diagnostic procedures

A Arrow: left sided angiogram shows occlusion of A. carotis int. at its origin

B Right A. carotis int. supplies Aa. carot. intt. areas on both sides

C X-ray confirms trepanation site. Because the Doppler sonogram** showed clearly patency of anastomosis, angiography was superfluous

---

* Operation performed by Dr. W. Hassler, author's coworker.
** Microvascular Doppler MF 20, Fa. EME medical electronic, D-7770-Überlingen, Christophstrasse 36, Federal Republic of Germany. The clinical application was developed by Dr. J. Gilsbach, author's coworker. See Fig. 113–154.

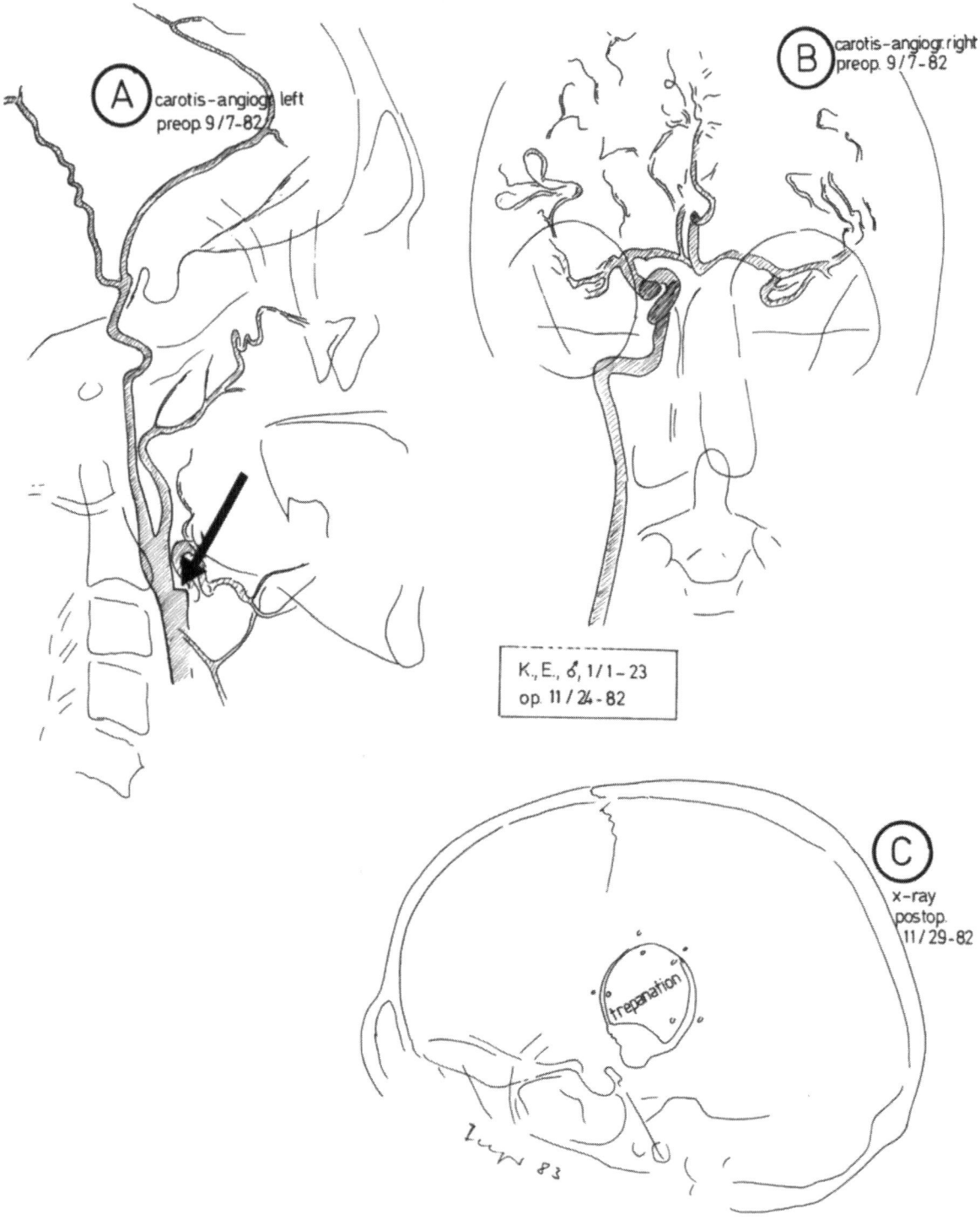
A
carotis-angiogr. left
preop. 9/7-82
B
carotis-angiogr. right
preop. 9/7-82
K., E., ♂, 1/1-23
op. 11/24-82
C
x-ray
postop.
11/29-82
trepanation

Fig. 136. Extra-intracranial bypass "STAMCA"
Mapping of A. temp. superfic. and Fissura lat. Sylvii

A Projection upon external skull surface of Fiss. lat. Sylvii and its anatomical topographical relation to A. temp. superfic. and its branches

B Sketch of Doppler ultrasonographic localization of A. temp. superfic. and of its branches upon external skull surface

- **1a** Localization of Ramus front. of A. temp. superfic.
- **1b** Doppler sonographic localization of Ramus pariet. of A. temp. superfic.
- **1c, 1d** Further localization points of Ramus pariet. using Doppler sonograph

Abbreviations:

(fl) Fissura lat. Sylvii (projection)
rf Ramus front. of A. temp. superfic.
rp Ramus pariet. of A. temp. superfic.
US Ultrasonograph
(US) Ultrasonograph (projection)
zo Ramus zygomaticus of A. temp. superfic.

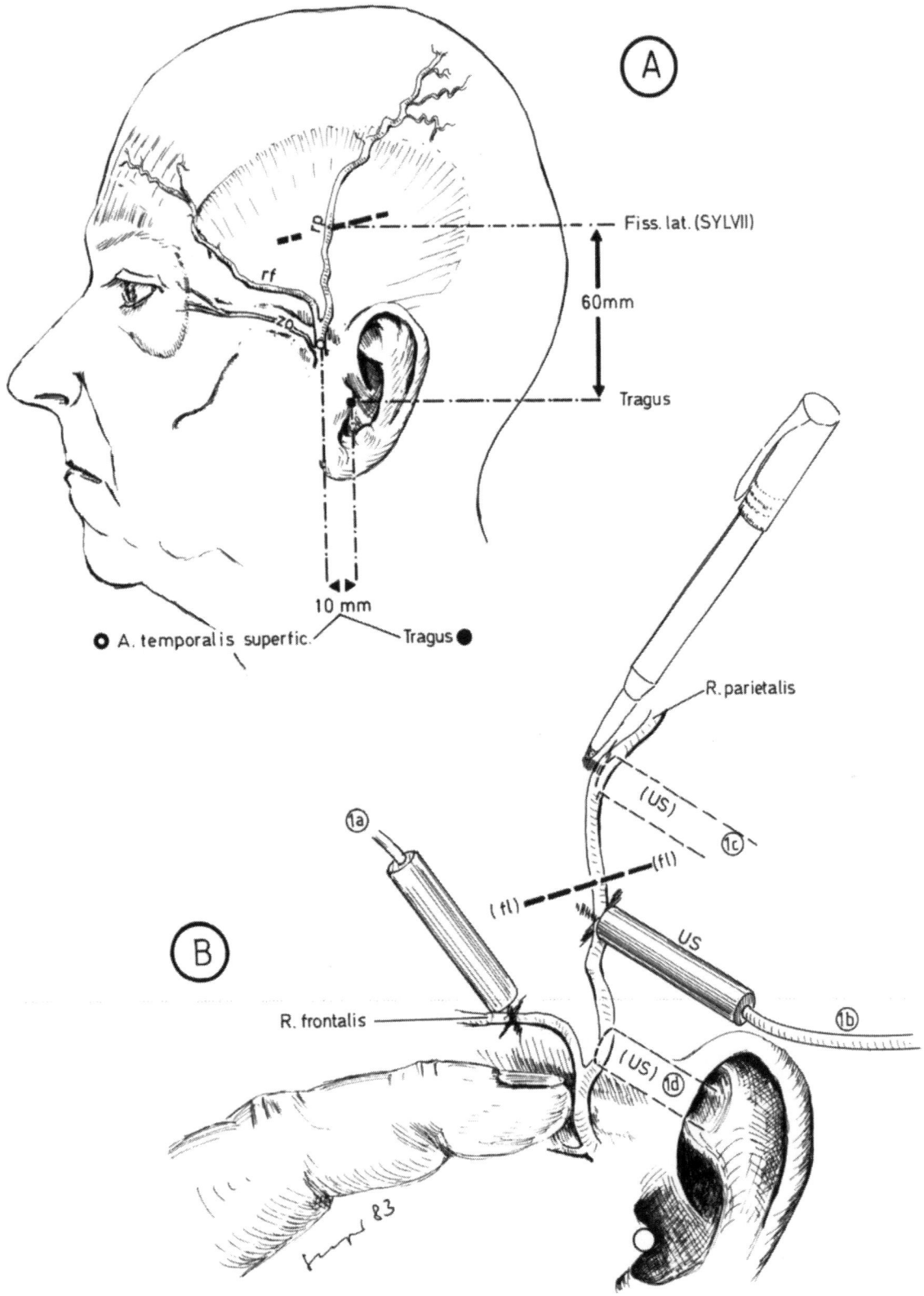
A
Fiss. lat. (SYLVII)
60mm
Tragus
rf
za
10 mm
A. temporalis superfic.
Tragus
B
R. parietalis
(US)
1c
1a
(fl)
(fl)
US
1b
R. frontalis
(US)
1d

Fig. 137. Extra-intracranial bypass "STAMCA"

A **1** Localization of main trunk of A. temp. superfic. by Doppler sonograph

2 Path of arteries drawn upon external skull surface by felt tip pen, corresponding to Doppler sonographic markings

B Examination of Ramus front. and Ramus angularis using Doppler sonograph. Result: normal blood flow in Ramus front. and Ramus angularis-"external type"

1 + 2 Normal direction of blood flow in Ramus front.

B' Reversed in the direction of carotis siphon, so-called "internal type"; indications of cerebro-vascular insufficiency with blood flow reversal in A. ophthalmica. Examination of Ramus front. and Ramus angularis using Doppler sonograph.

Open arrows: blood flow direction. Black graphs: ultrasonograms

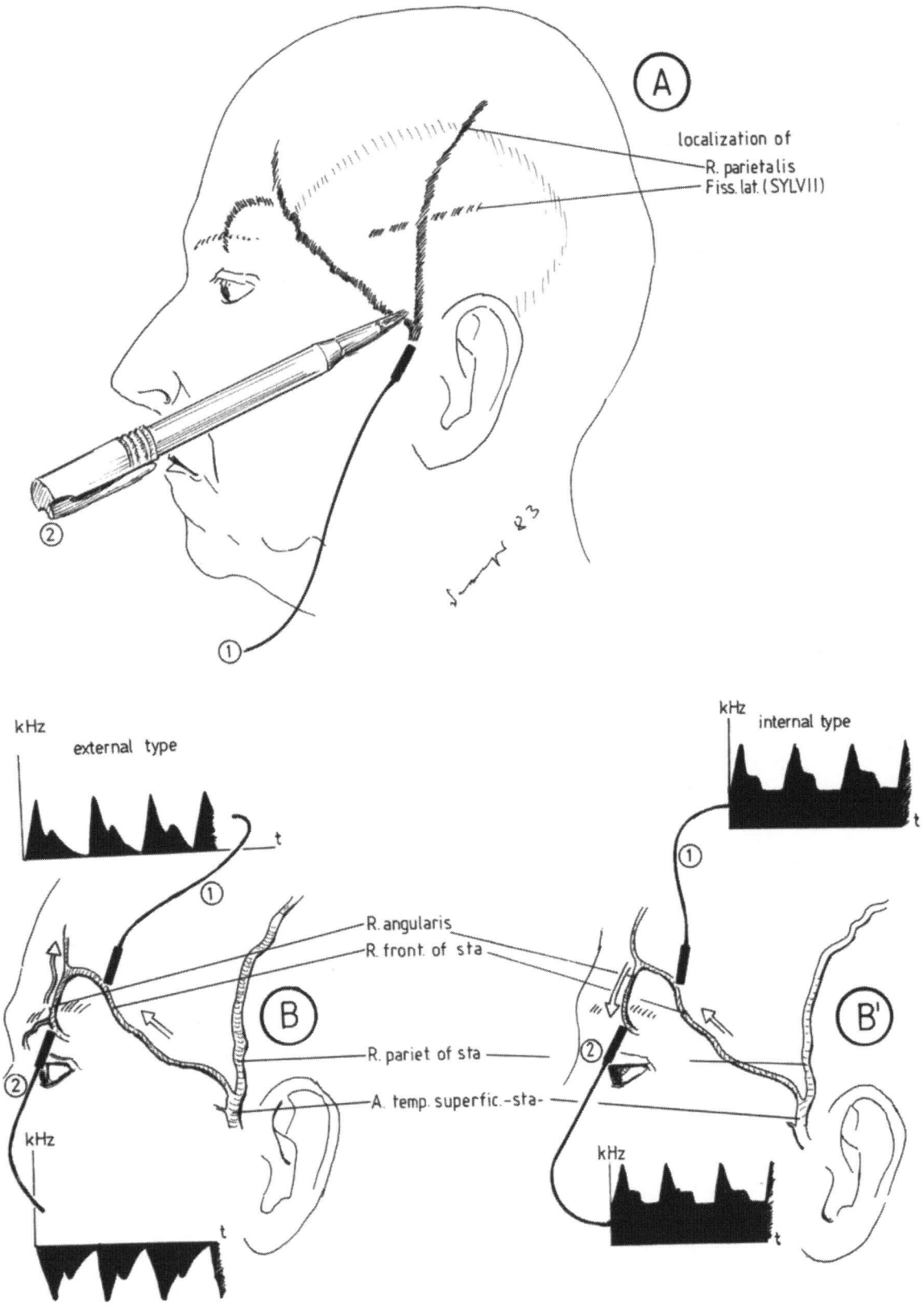
A
localization of
R. parietalis
Fiss. lat. (SYLVII)
kHz
external type
t
kHz
internal type
t
R. angularis
R. front. of sta
B
B'
R. pariet of sta
A. temp. superfic.-sta-
kHz
t
kHz
t

Fig. 138. Extra-intracranial bypass "STAMCA"
Skin incision

A Position of skin incision – approx. 100 mm long – corresponding to Doppler ultrasonic localization of artery

B **1a – 1d** Incision of skin and subcutaneous fatty tissue is carried out in several consecutive steps, whereby only skin and subcutaneous fatty tissue, but not Galea, is incised

C **1** Detachment of subcutis from galea. One sees that Ramus pariet. and Ramus front. of A. temp. superfic. run partly above and partly beneath galea, thereby contacting subcutis

2 Insertion of wound spreader

C' Anatomical section sketch for **C**

1 As in **C**

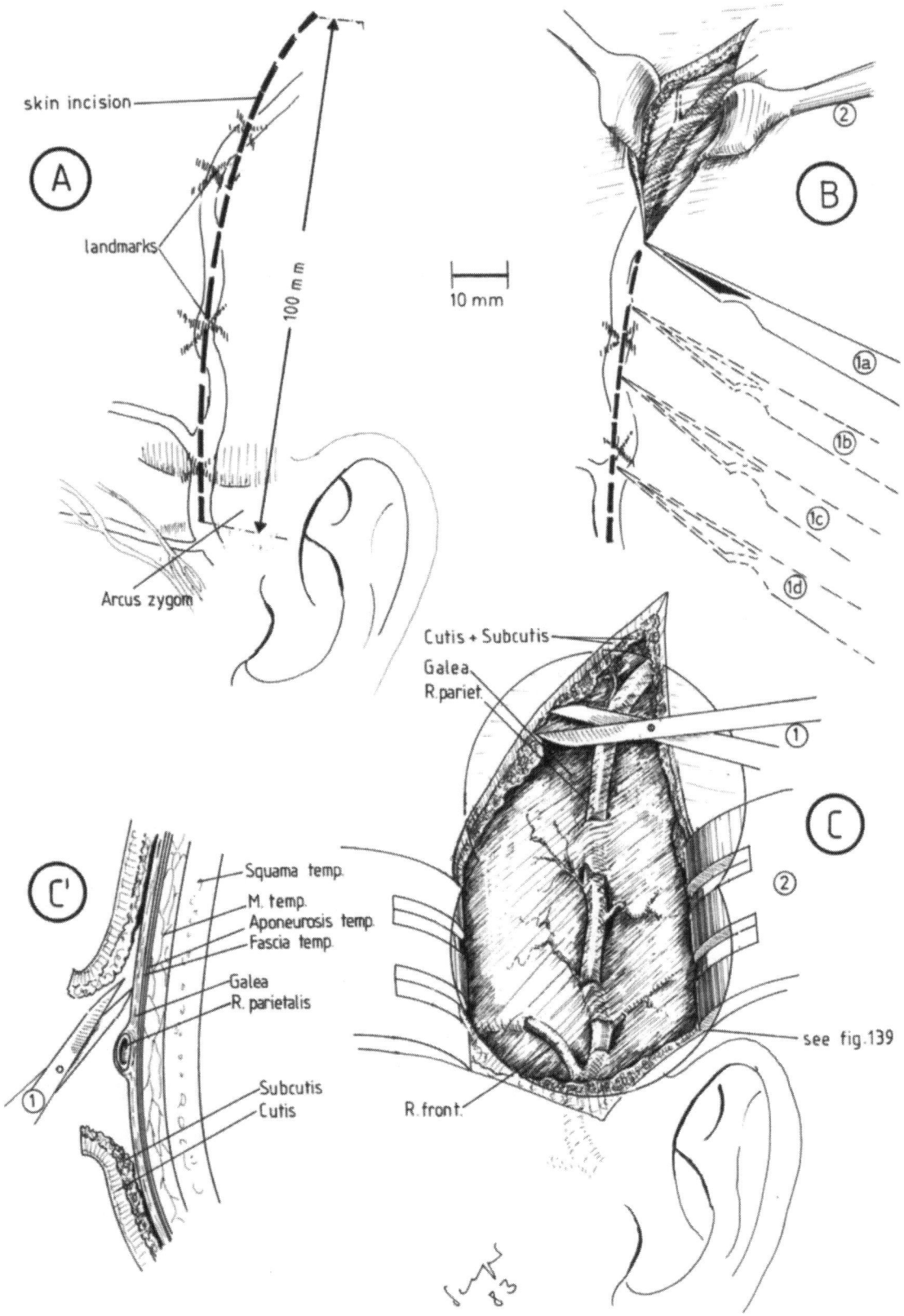
skin incision
A
landmarks
100 mm
Arcus zygom
10 mm
B
2
1a
1b
1c
1d
Cutis + Subcutis
Galea
R.pariet.
1
C
2
see fig.139
R.front.
C'
Squama temp.
M. temp.
Aponeurosis temp.
Fascia temp.
Galea
R. parietalis
Subcutis
Cutis
1

Fig. 139. Extra-intracranial bypass "STAMCA"
Preparation of Ramus par. of A. temp. superf.

A **1** Coagulation of small branches of the artery, but not too close to arterial trunk
2 Cutting of coagulated small branches
3 Incision of galea parallel to arterial path

A' Anatomical section sketch, corresponding to **A**, indications as in **A**

B **1** Lengthening of incision started in **A 3**, after interruption of small side branches
2 + 3 Coagulation and interruption of small arteries alternating with further galea incision
–1–
4a + 4b Further insertion of wound spreader

B' Anatomical section sketch, corresponding to **B**, indications as in **B**

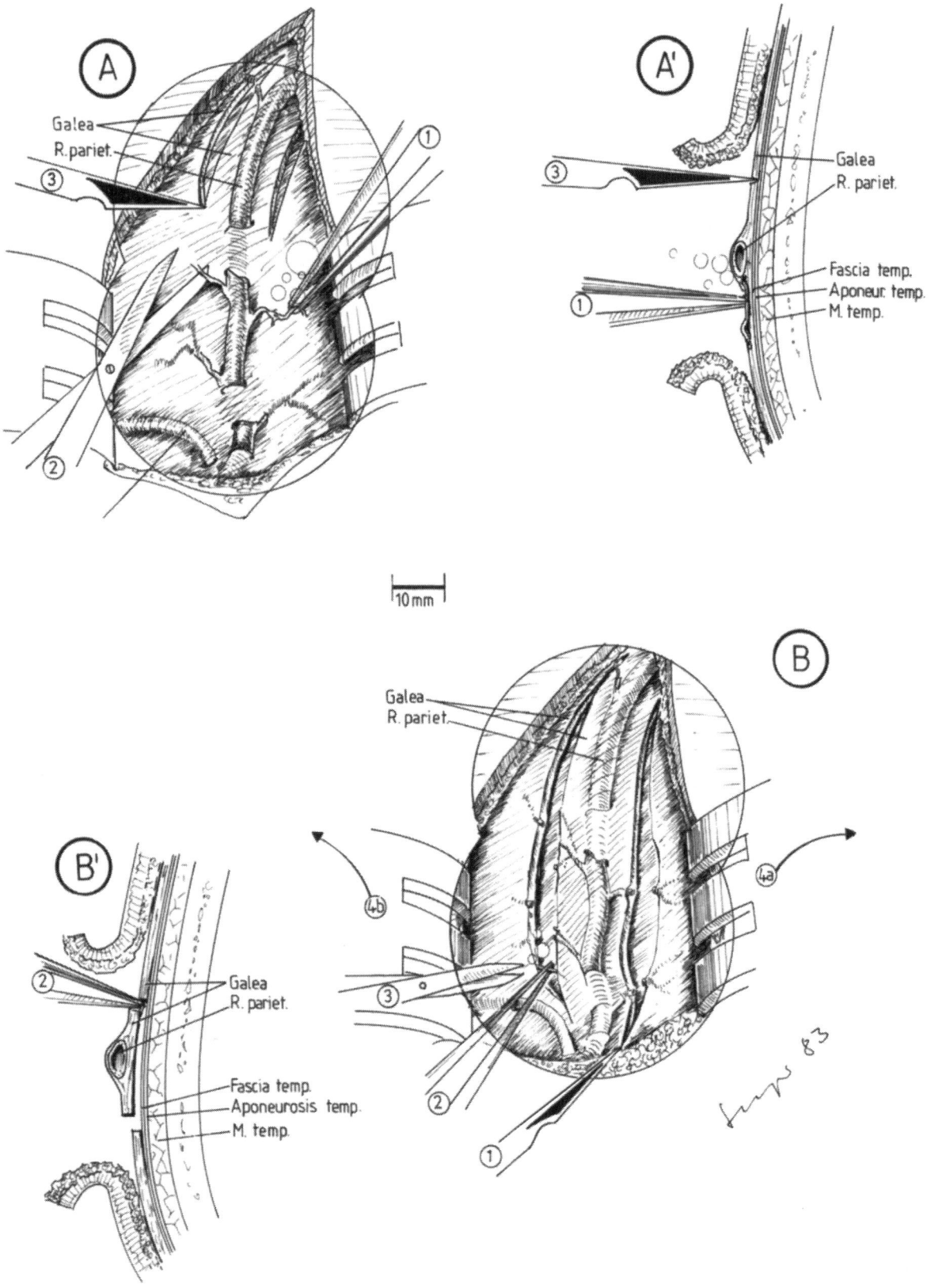
A
Galea
R. pariet.
3
1
2
A'
3
Galea
R. pariet.
Fascia temp.
Aponeur. temp.
M. temp.
1
10 mm
B
Galea
R. pariet.
4b
4a
3
2
1
B'
2
Galea
R. pariet.
Fascia temp.
Aponeurosis temp.
M. temp.

Fig. 140. Extra-intracranial bypass "STAMCA"

A Incision of M. temporalis

A' Preparation of M. temporalis, anatomical model. Anterior muscle portion *–x–*, together with Ramus parietalis is folded forward, the muscle thus covering this artery

B Detachment of muscle

B' Spreader holds back portions of M. temporalis. Anterior muscle portions cover Ramus parietalis of A. temporalis superficialis. Broken line: Fissura lateralis *–(fl)–* (projection)

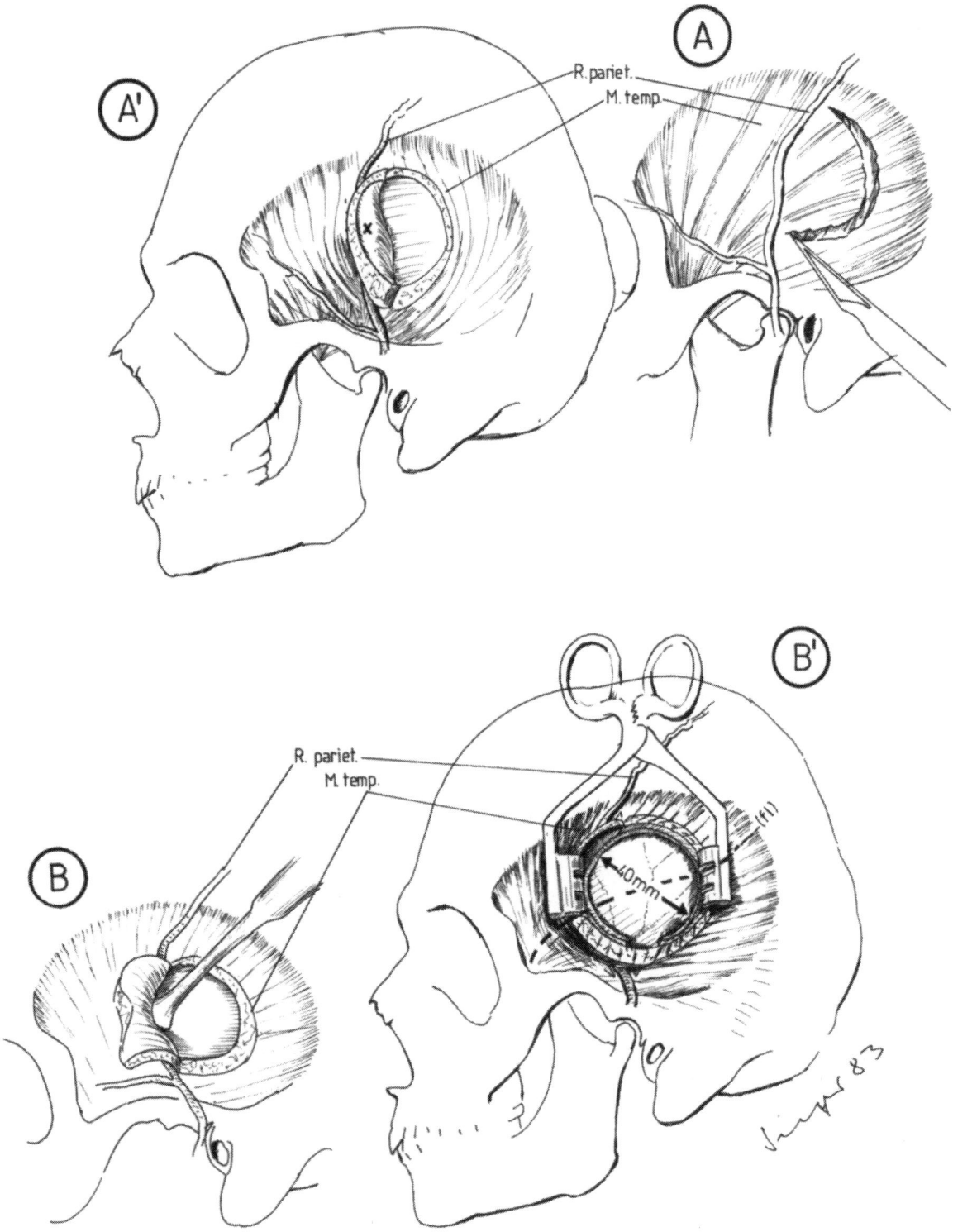
A'
A
R. pariet.
M. temp.
x
B'
B
R. pariet.
M. temp.
40mm
(f1)

Fig. 141. Extra-intracranial bypass "STAMCA"
Preparation of M. temporalis, microsurgical preparation

A **1a** Holding back posterior M. temporalis portion with spatula
1b + 1c Holding back Ramus parietalis and the Galea strip containing artery
2 Curved incision of M. temporalis
3 Detachment of muscle and periosteum from Squama temporalis

A' Anatomical section sketch, corresponding to **A**

B **1a – 1c** Removal of spatula
2a, 2b Insertion of spreader. Ramus parietalis of A. temporalis superficialis is protected from spreader by M. temporalis

B' Anatomical section sketch, corresponding **B**

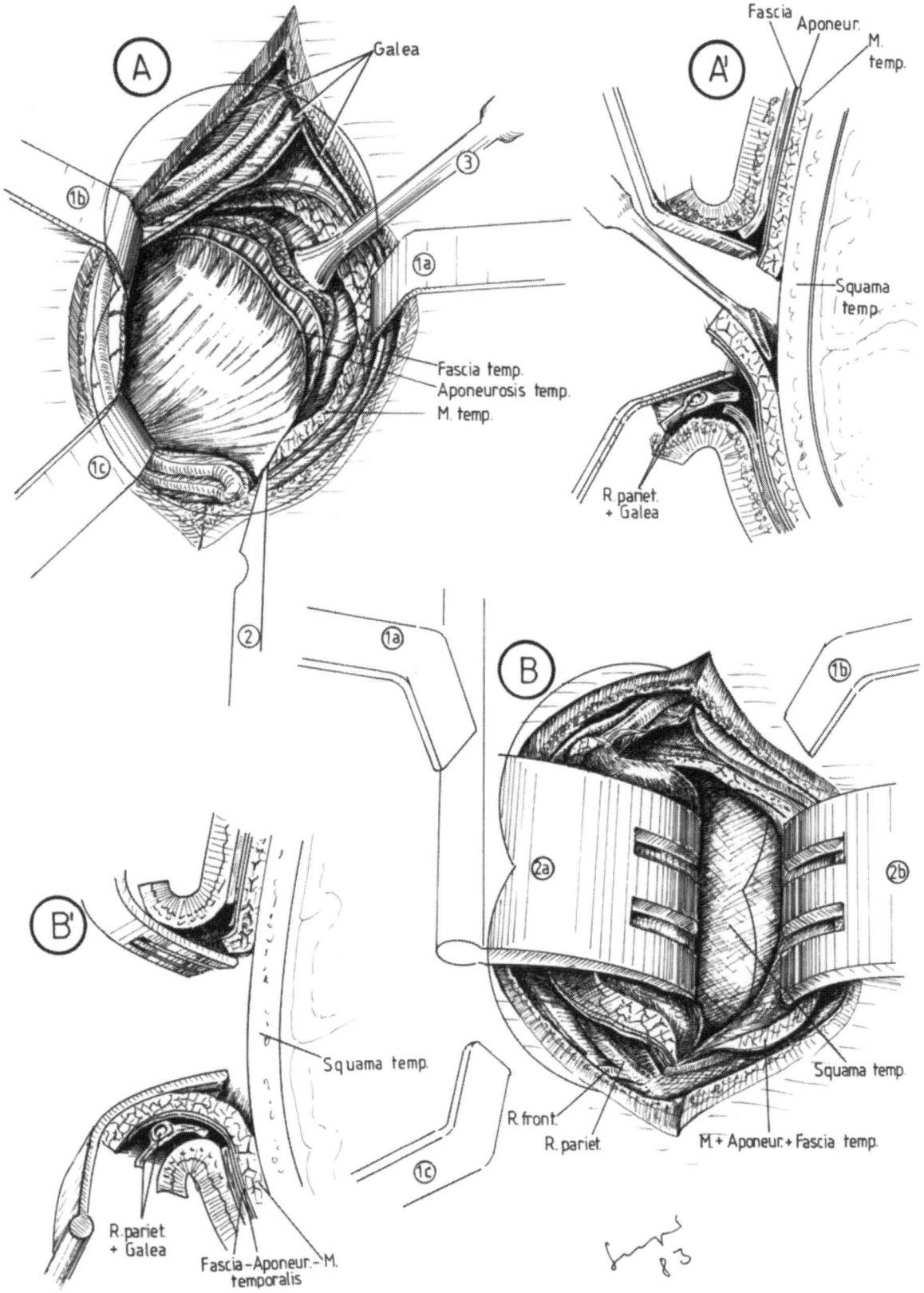
A
Galea
1b
3
1a
Fascia temp.
Aponeurosis temp.
M. temp.
1c
2
A'
Fascia
Aponeur.
M. temp.
Squama temp.
R. pariet. + Galea
1a
B
1b
2a
2b
Squama temp.
R. front.
R. pariet.
M. + Aponeur. + Fascia temp.
1c
B'
Squama temp.
R. pariet. + Galea
Fascia - Aponeur. - M. temporalis

Fig. 142. Extra-intracranial bypass "STAMCA"
A Trepanation
A' Anatomical transection sketch for **A**
B Bone flap removed. Dura incision (broken line)
B' Anatomical transection sketch for **B**

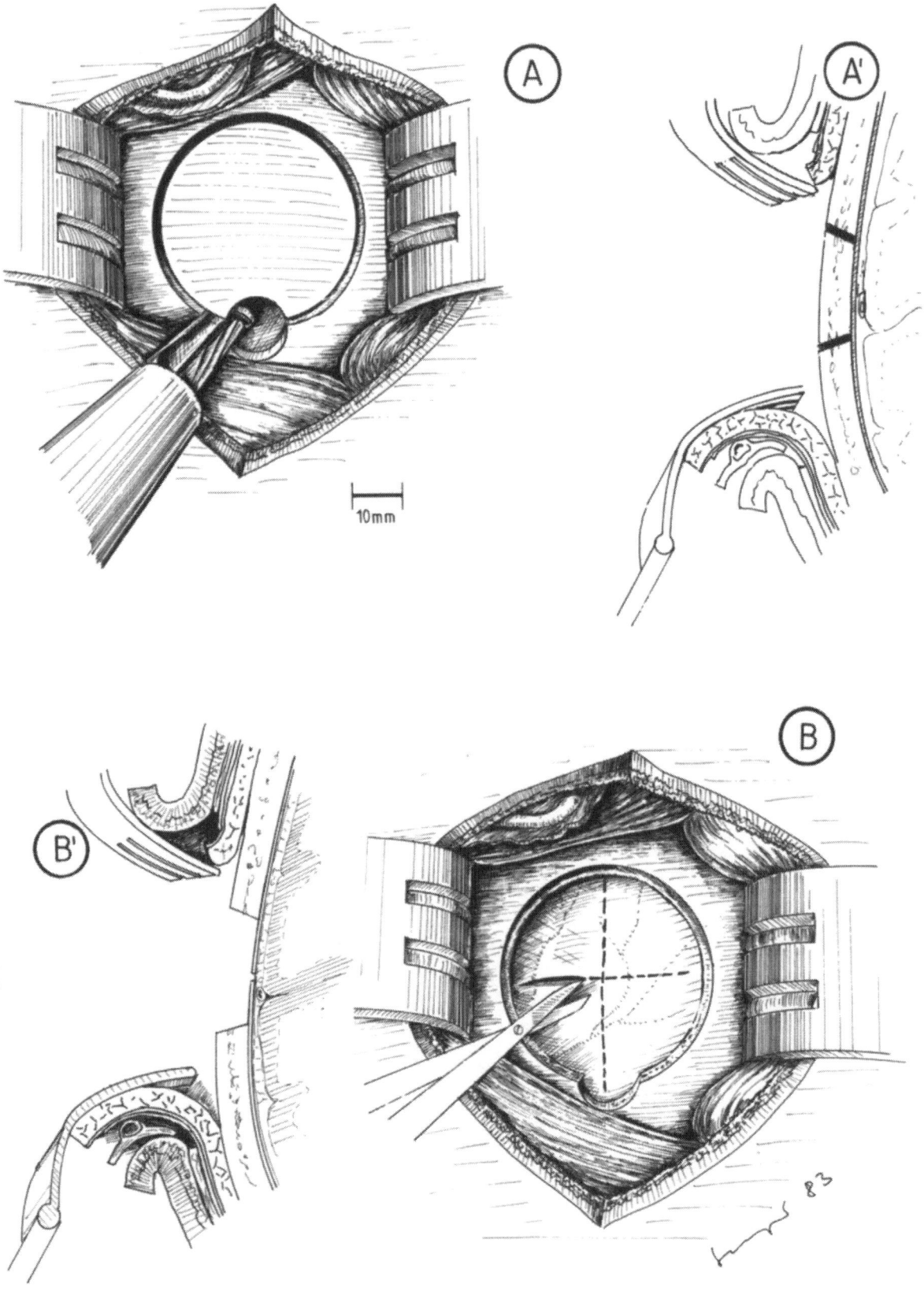
A
A'
10mm
B
B'

Fig. 143. Extra-intracranial bypass "STAMCA"
Site after dura opening

A Fissura lateralis Sylvii with temporal branch of A. cerebri media is exposed

A' Anatomical transection sketch for **A**

B Enlarged detail from **A**

1 Doppler ultrasonographic check* of various exposed arteries, in this case, a parietal branch of A. cerebri media

2 The same check of A. cerebri media branch shown in **A** and **A'**

3 Having verified that temporal branch of artery has the best blood flow (which is usually the case), arachnoidea is opened over this vessel. Light arrow: flow direction verified by Doppler sonograph

* Method of Dr. J. Gilsbach, author's coworker.

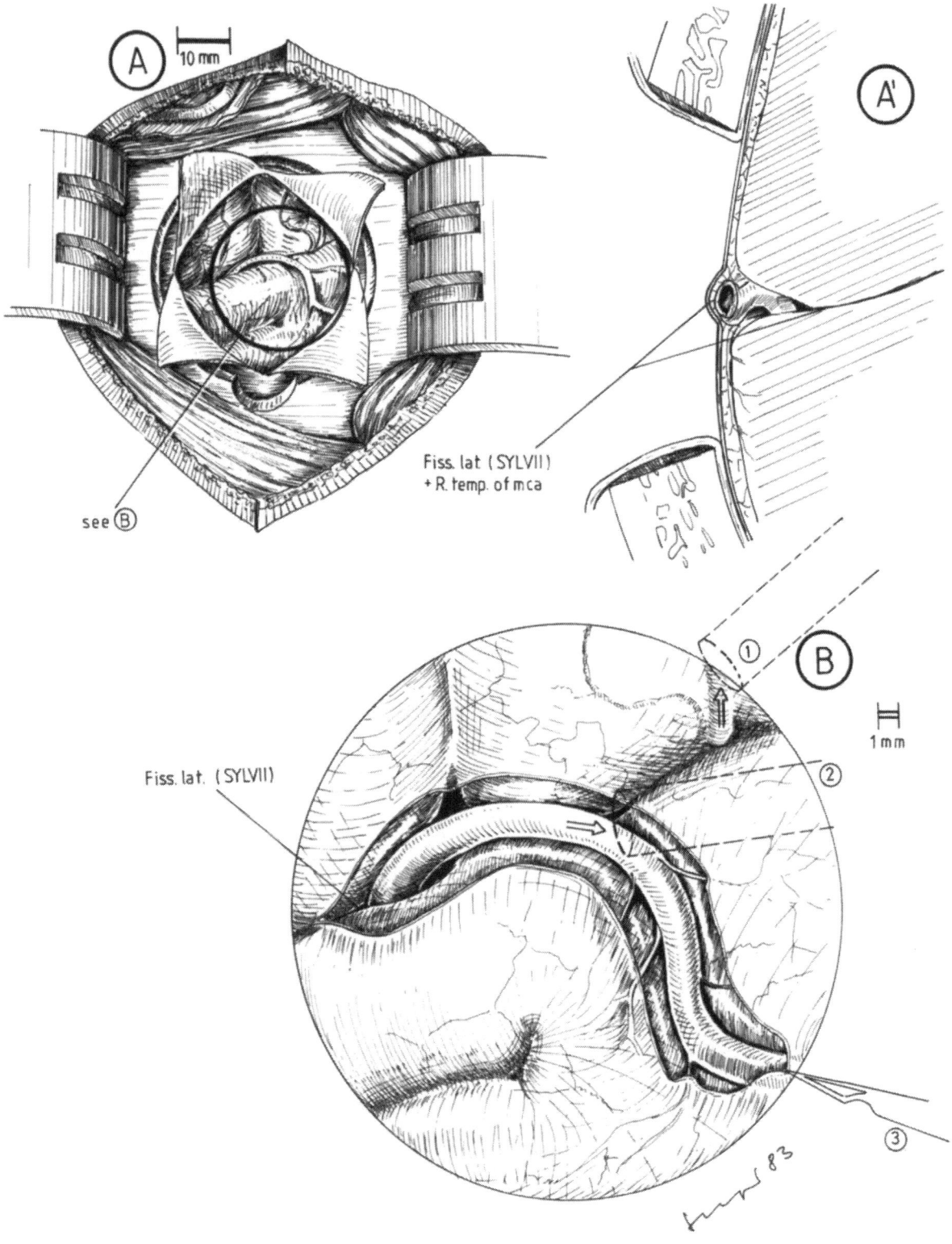
A
10 mm
see B
A'
Fiss. lat (SYLVII)
+ R. temp. of m.ca
B
1 mm
Fiss. lat. (SYLVII)
1
2
3

Fig. 144. Extra-intracranial bypass "STAMCA"
Preparation of Ramus temporalis of A. cerebri media

1 Detachment of arachnoidea

2a Coagulation of smallest cerebral arterial branches

2b Cutting of these branches

3 Check by Doppler sonograph, to see whether manipulation caused spasms

A' Anatomical transection sketch for **A,** Indications as in **A**

B **1a + 1b** Introduction of small piece of rubber foil between Ramus temporalis of A. cerebri media and cortex

2 Check of blood flow by Doppler sonograph
Light arrow: flow direction, verified by Doppler sonograph.
Light arrow: flow direction, verified by Doppler sonograph

B' Anatomical transection sketch, corresponding to **B**

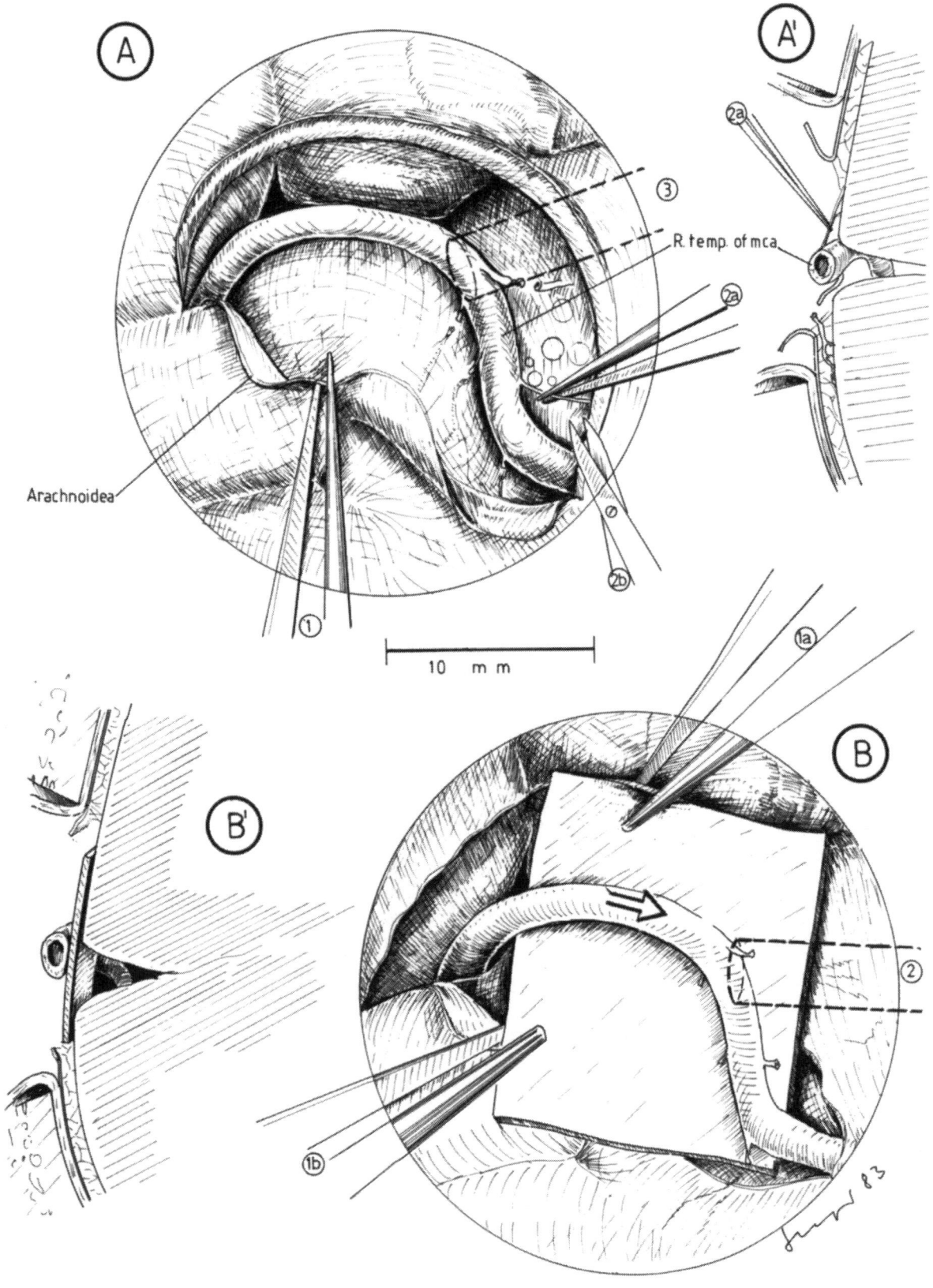
A
A'
B
B'
3
R. temp. of mca
2a
2a
Arachnoidea
2b
1
10 mm
1a
2
1b

Fig. 145. Extra-intracranial bypass "STAMCA"
Preparation of Ramus parietalis of A. temporalis superficialis

A **1a + 1b** After removal and reinsertion of spreader, freed Ramus parietalis of A. temporalis superficialis slides over and beyond M. temporalis and now lies over trepanation area

A' As **A.** Arrow shows dislocation of Ramus parietalis corresponding to **A**

B Galea resection along distal path of Ramus parietalis

B' **1** Distal ligation of Ramus parietalis of A. temporalis superficialis

2 Proximal temporary clipping of Ramus parietalis

3 Distal cutting of Ramus parietalis

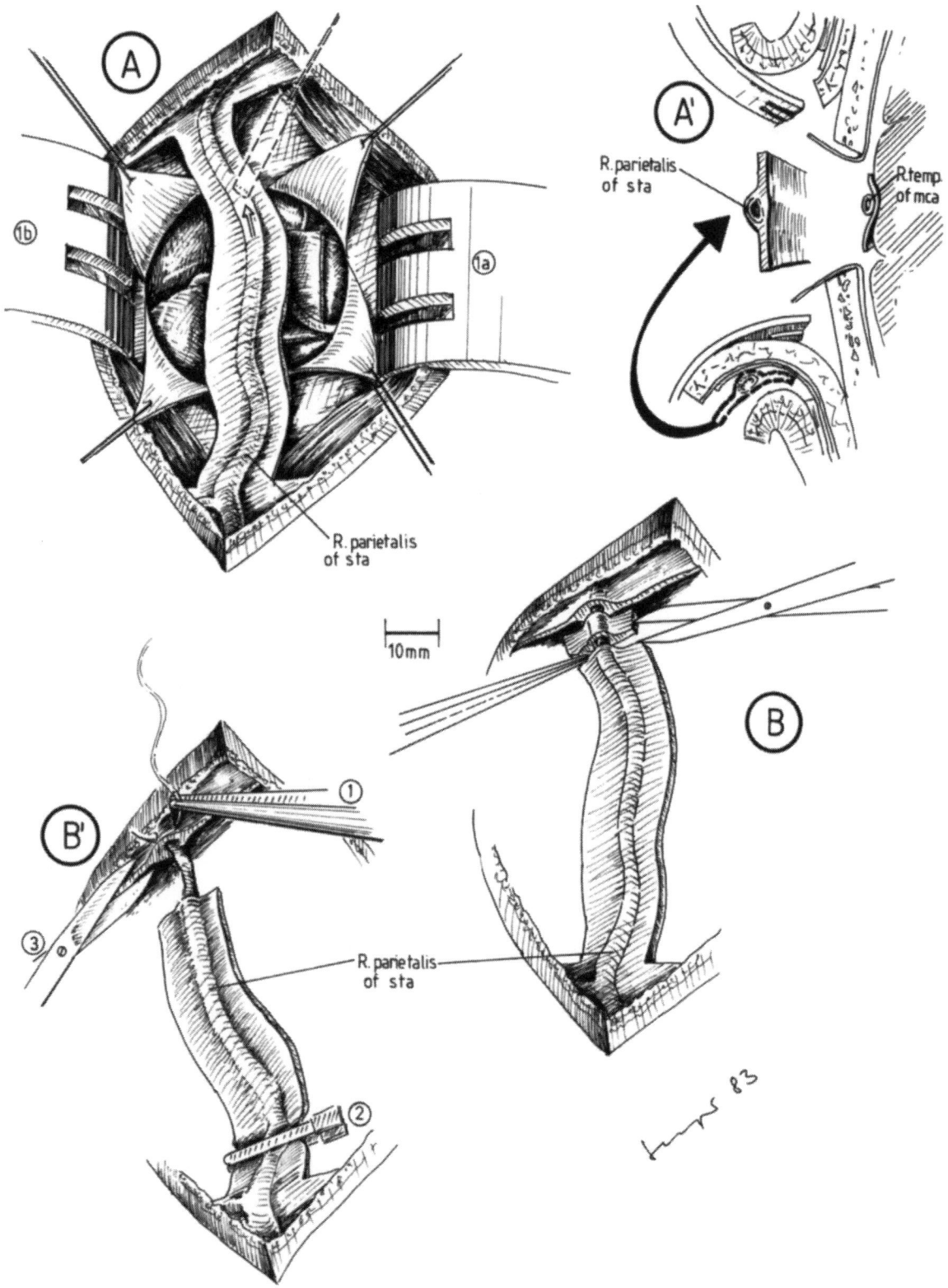
A
1b
1a
R. parietalis
of sta
A'
R. parietalis
of sta
R. temp.
of mca
10mm
B
B'
1
2
3
R. parietalis
of sta

Fig. 146. Extra-intracranial bypass "STAMCA"
Preparation of Ramus parietalis of A. temporalis superficialis

A **1** Removal of temporay clip
2 Measurement of blood flow per/min.

B **1** Proximal temporary clipping of Ramus parietalis again
2 Remaining blood is washed out of artery with saline solution. Abocat plastic cannula is used

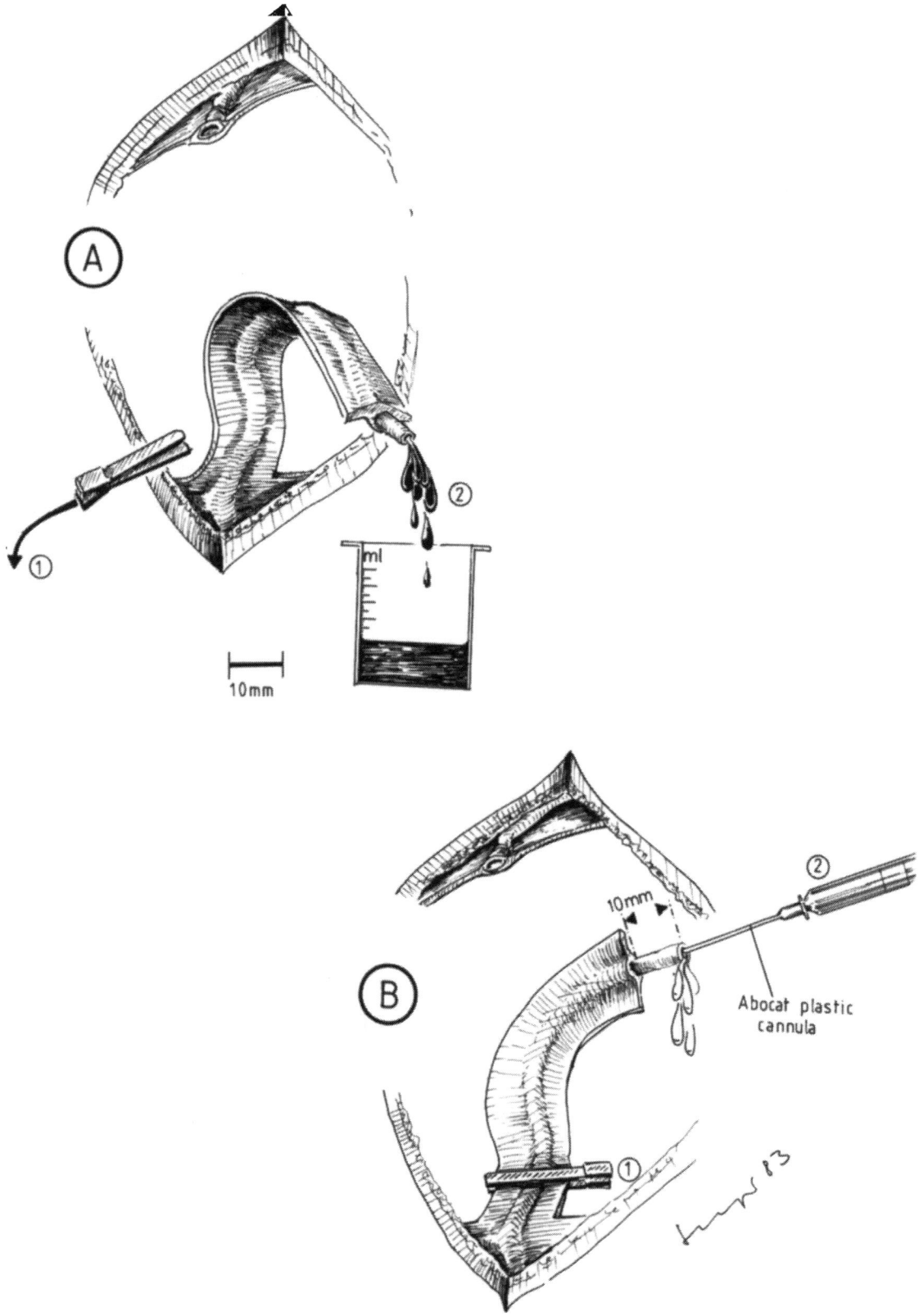
A
1
2
ml
10mm
B
1
2
10mm
Abocat plastic cannula

Fig. 147. Extra-intracranial bypass "STAMCA"
Vascular anastomosis

A Ramus parietalis is positioned on cortical surface

B Enlarged detail from **A.** Doppler ultrasonographic check of blood flow direction in cerebral vessels (arrows). Blood is flowing from Fissura Sylvii in a distal direction. Normally, Doppler ultrasonographic check is done against blood flow direction (see curve at **1b**). The reverse procedure **1a** (check in the direction of blood flow) may be appropriate, given limited space

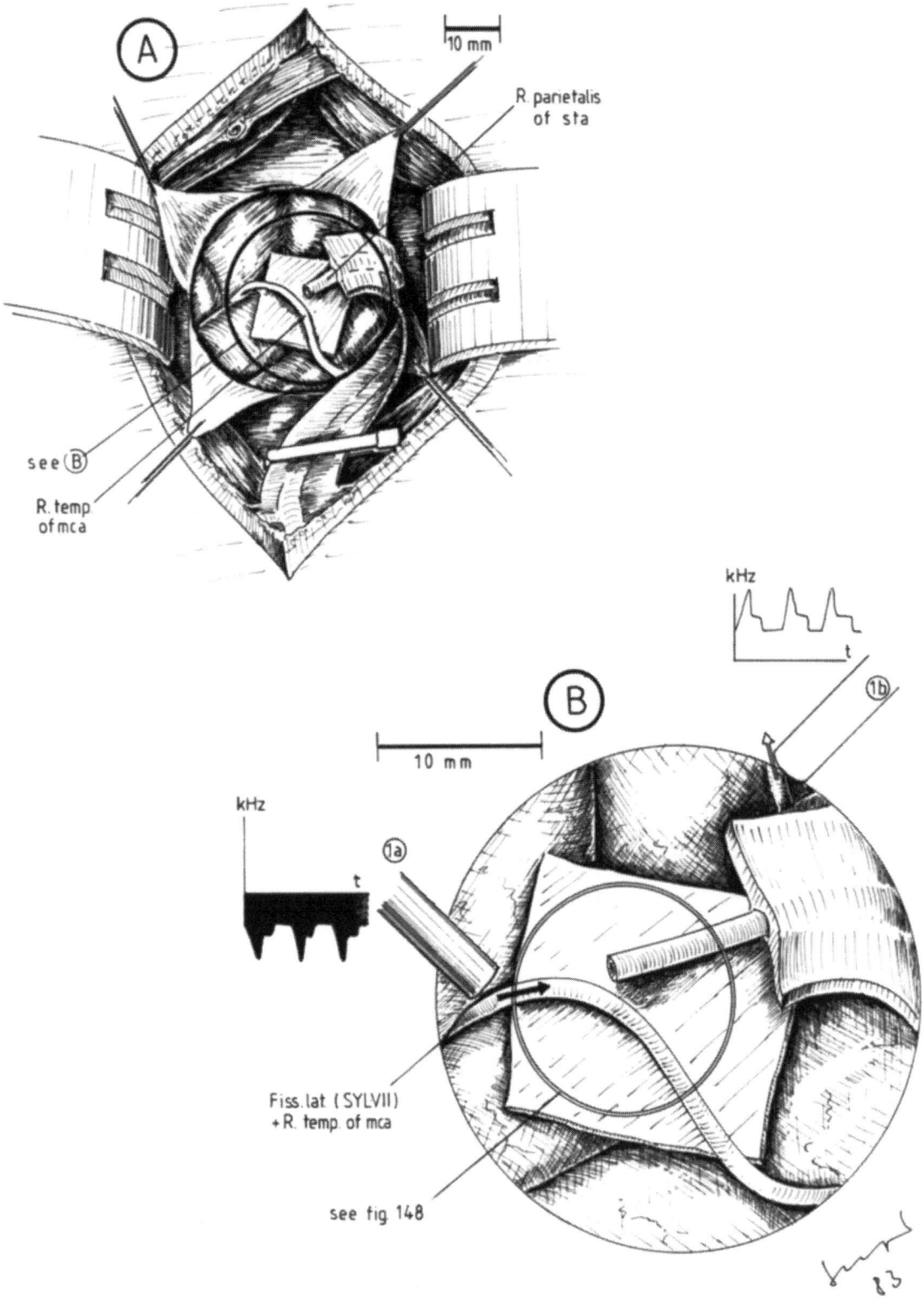
A
10 mm
R. parietalis
of sta
see B
R. temp.
of mca
kHz
t
B
1b
10 mm
kHz
t
1a
Fiss. lat. (SYLVII)
+ R. temp. of mca
see fig. 148
83

Fig. 148. Extra-intracranial bypass "STAMCA"
Vascular anastomosis

A Enlarged detail from Fig. 147 **B.** End of donor vessel (Ramus parietalis) is cut obliquely

B Additionally, this vessel is incised lengthwise **–1–**

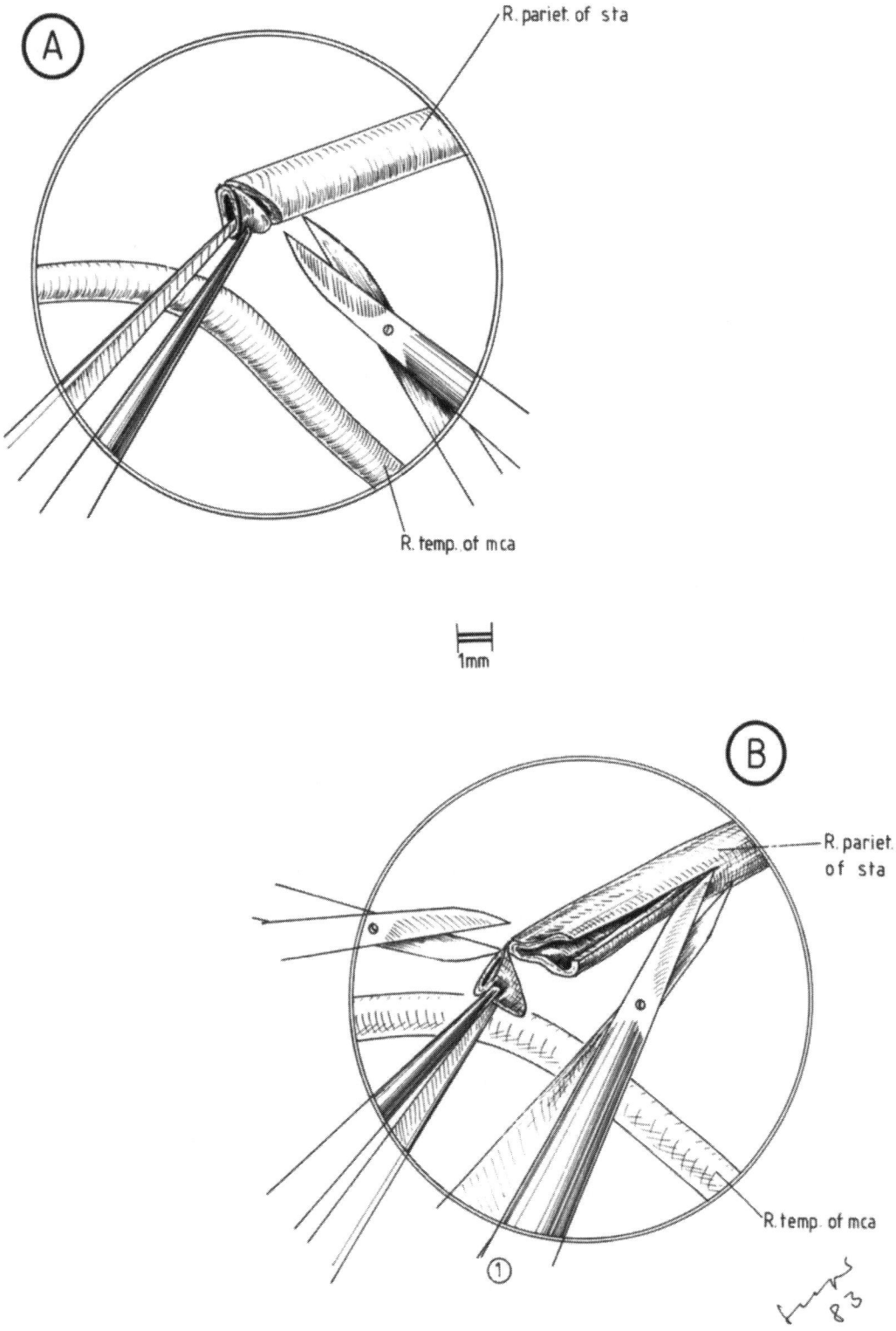
A
R. pariet. of sta
R. temp. of mca
1mm
B
R. pariet.
of sta
R. temp. of mca
1

Fig. 149. Extra-intracranial bypass "STAMCA"
Continuation from Fig. 148. Vascular anastomosis

A **1a + 1b** Temporary clipping of Ramus temporalis of A. cerebri media

2 Incision of Ramus temporalis of A. cerebri media. Incisions –*a*– of Ramus parietalis and –*a'*– of Ramus temporalis of A. cerebri media are of equal length

B Donor vessel – Ramus parietalis – is positioned along the receiver vessel – light arrow – against receiver's blood flow direction. First suture is applied

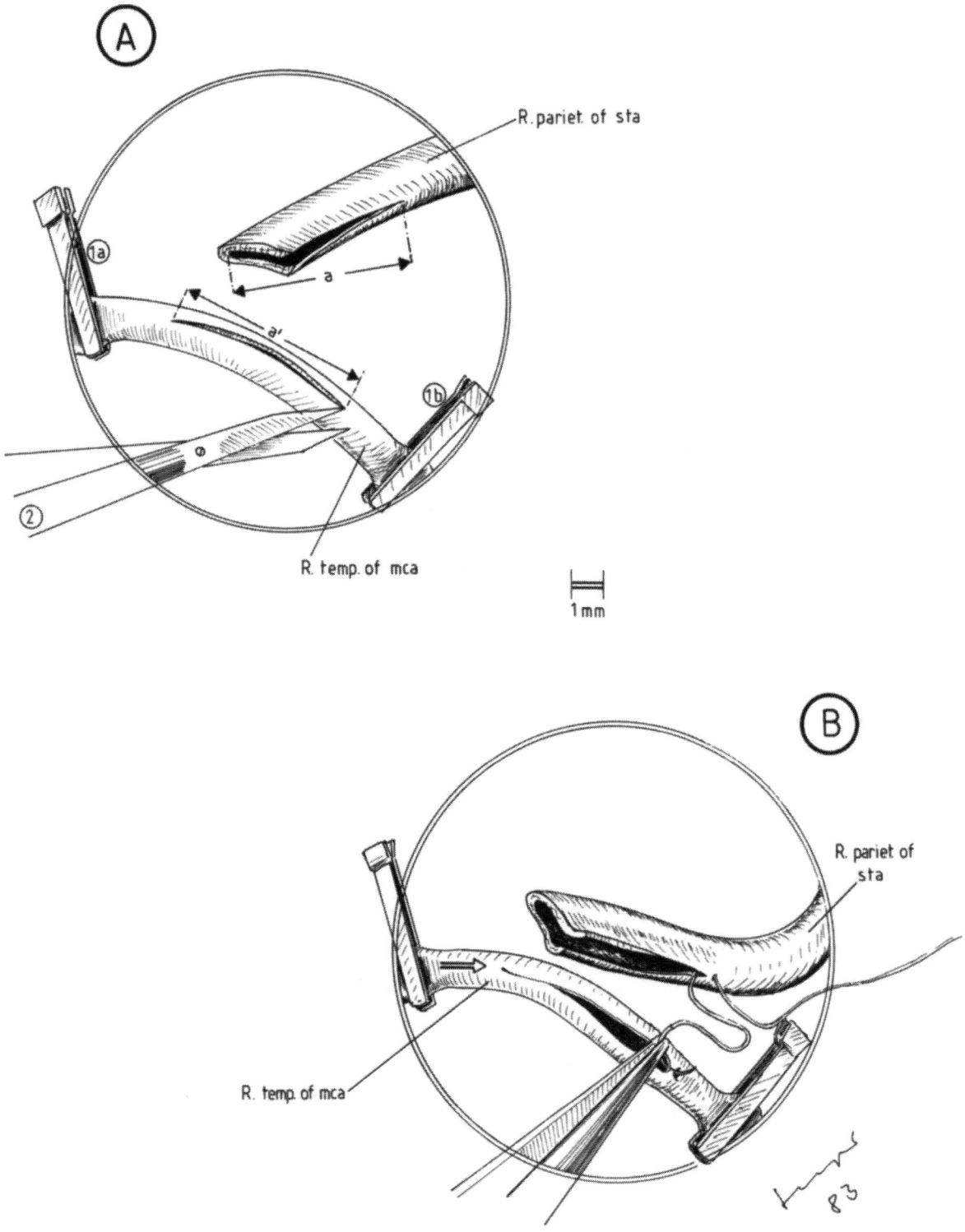
A
R. pariet. of sta
1a
a
a'
1b
2
R. temp. of mca
1 mm
B
R. pariet of sta
R. temp. of mca

Fig. 150. Extra-intracranial bypass "STAMCA"

A Application of second suture

B **1** Donor vessel – Ramus parietalis – is folded downwards (light arrow)

2 First row of stitches is applied at back side of vessels

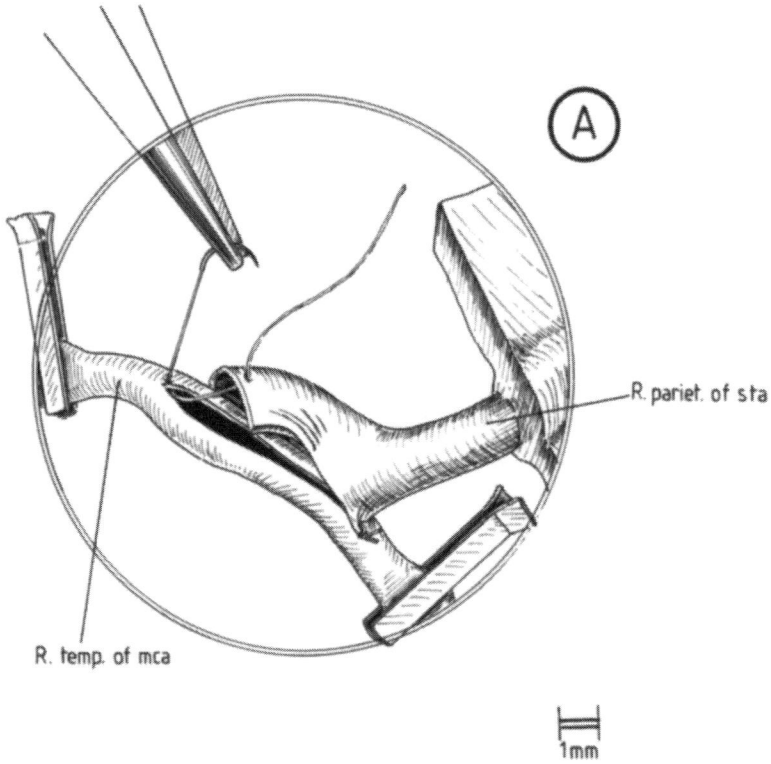
A
R. pariet. of sta
R. temp. of mca
1mm

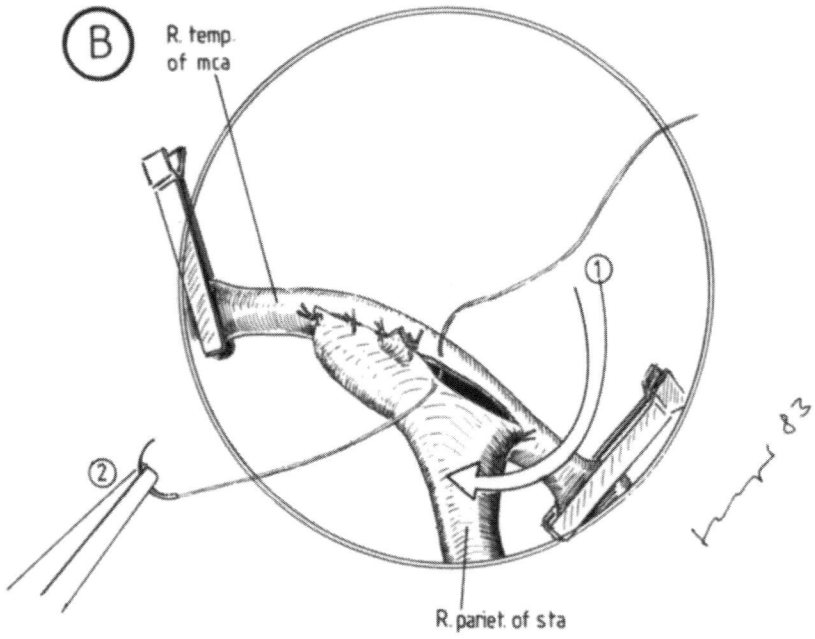
B
R. temp.
of mca
1
2
R. pariet. of sta

Fig. 151. Extra-intracranial bypass "STAMCA"

A **1** Folding of donor vessel (Ramus parietalis) back to original position (light arrow)

2 First row of stitches is applied at vessel's front side. A total of approximately 15 sutures 0-00- is applied

B **1a** Removal of temporary clip from donor artery – Ramus parietalis – (light arrow)

1b + 1c Removal of temporary clip from receiver artery – Ramus temporalis – (light arrows)

2a – 2c Doppler ultrasonographic check of anastomosis. Even if visually inspected suture appears to be correct, stenosis should be assumed, if blood flow is shown to have speeded up. Greatest stenosis risk occurs at the distal anastomosis portion – sonography **2d** –. Black arrows: correct flow direction; blood flow divides in the area of donor vessel – Ramus parietalis – anastomosis; the receiving vessels – Ramus temporalis – shows reversed flow at measurement point **2c**

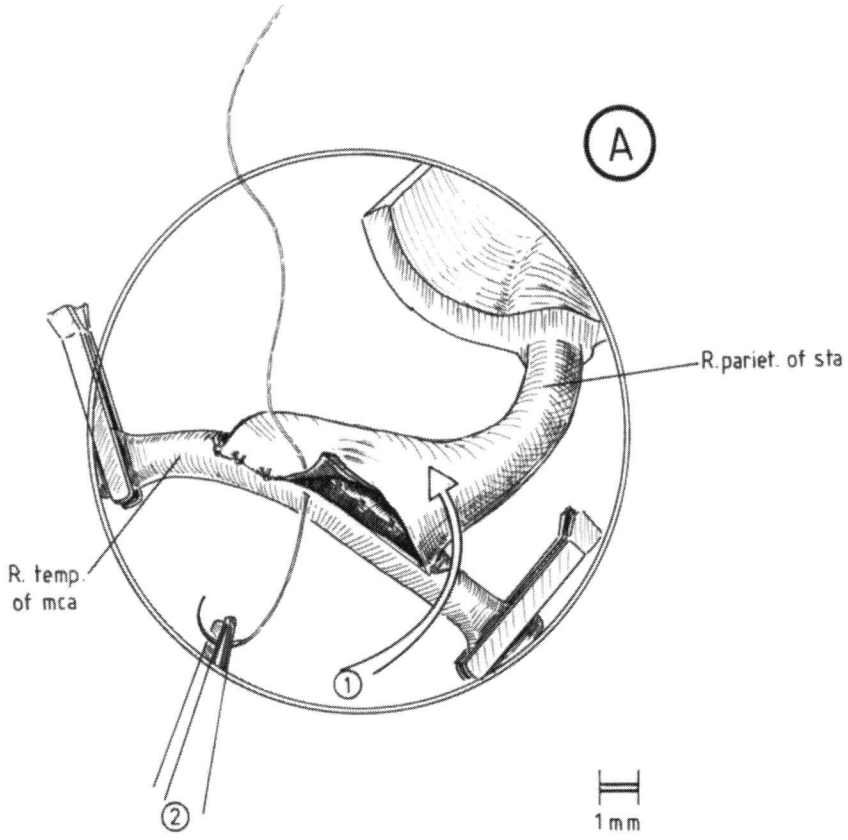
A
R. pariet. of sta
R. temp.
of mca
1
2
1 mm

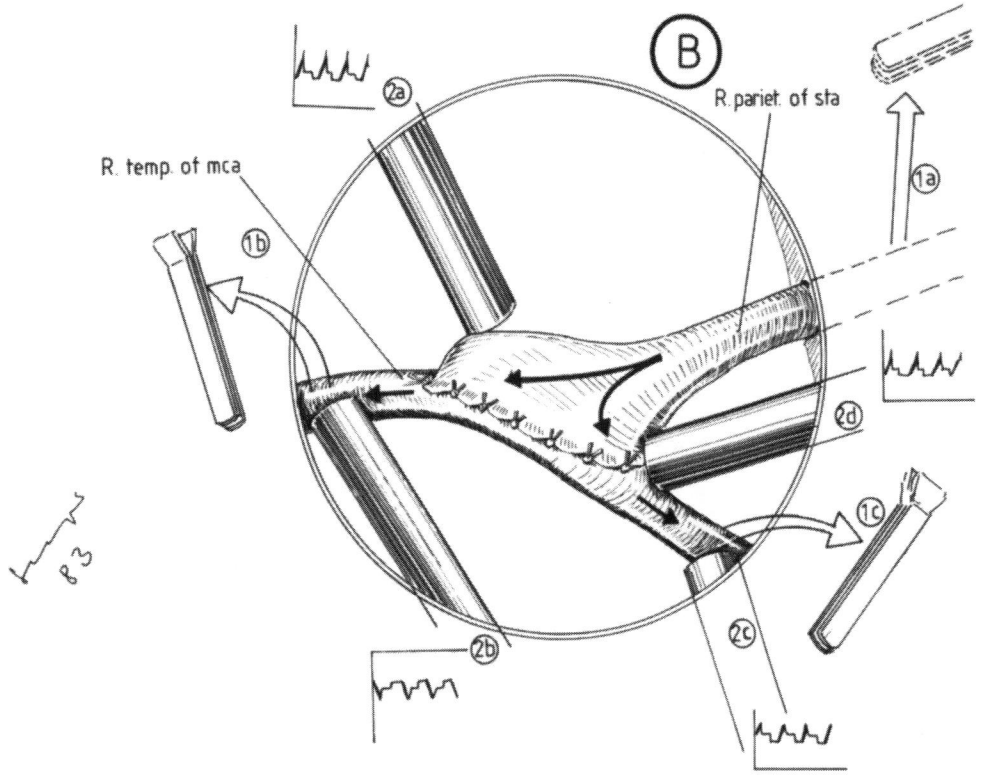
B
R. pariet. of sta
R. temp. of mca
2a
1a
1b
2d
1c
2c
2b
83

Fig. 152. Extra-intracranial bypass "STAMCA"
Wound closure

A Removal of rubber foil (light arrow)

B Operation site, overview

1 Doppler ultrasonographic check of donor vessel – Ramus parietalis – especially at point of previous clipping, to verify that clip caused no flow disturbance

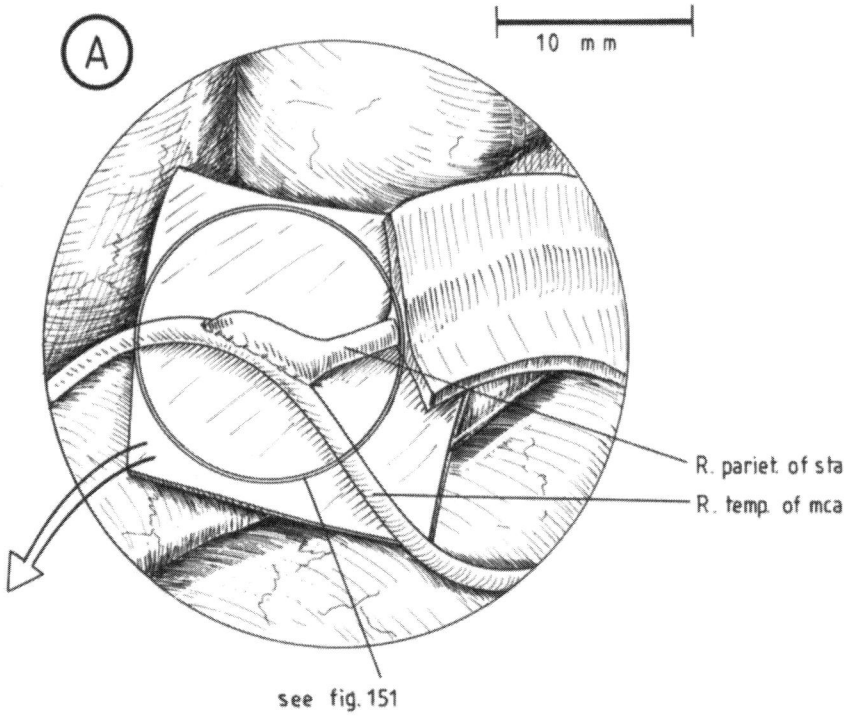
A
10 mm
R. pariet. of sta
R. temp. of mca
see fig. 151

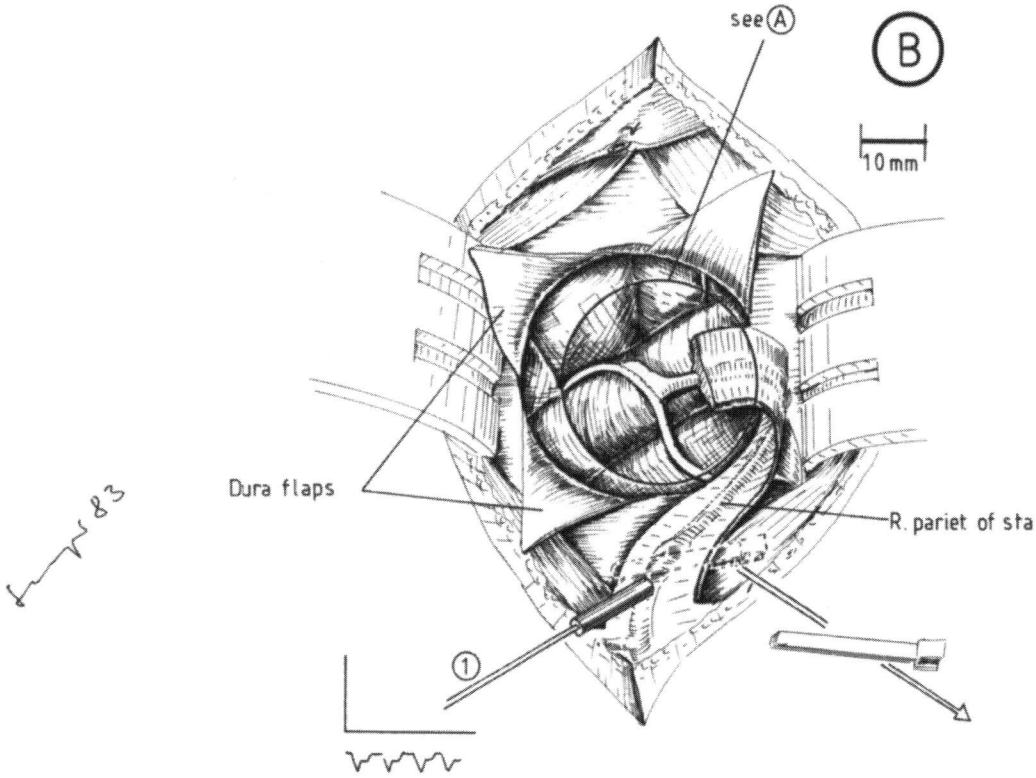
see A
B
10 mm
Dura flaps
R. pariet. of sta
1

Fig. 153. Extra-intracranial bypass "STAMCA"
Wound closure

A Dura suture

B **1** Widening of trepanation at penetration point of Ramus parietalis of A. temporalis superficialis, in order to avoid pinching of vessel

2 Doppler ultrasonographic check of vessel for free passage after dura closure and bone resection

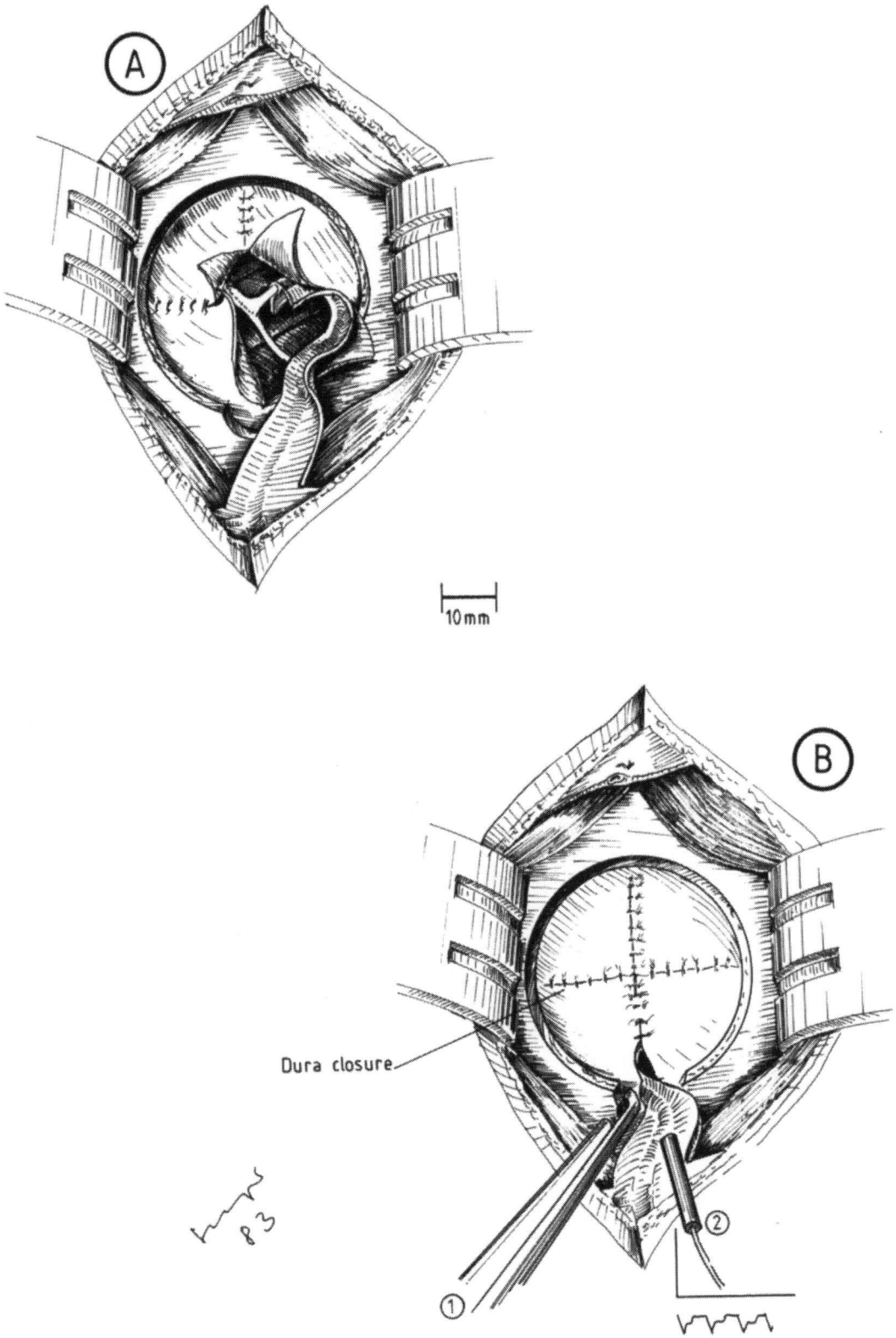
A
10mm
B
Dura closure
1
2

Fig. 154. Extra-intracranial bypass "STAMCA"
Wound closure

A **1** Reinsertion of bone flap
2 Ultrasonographic check of Ramus parietalis for free flow

B **1** After suturing muscle, fascia, gaela and skin, Ramus parietalis is checked again by ultrasonograph, this time through closed skin

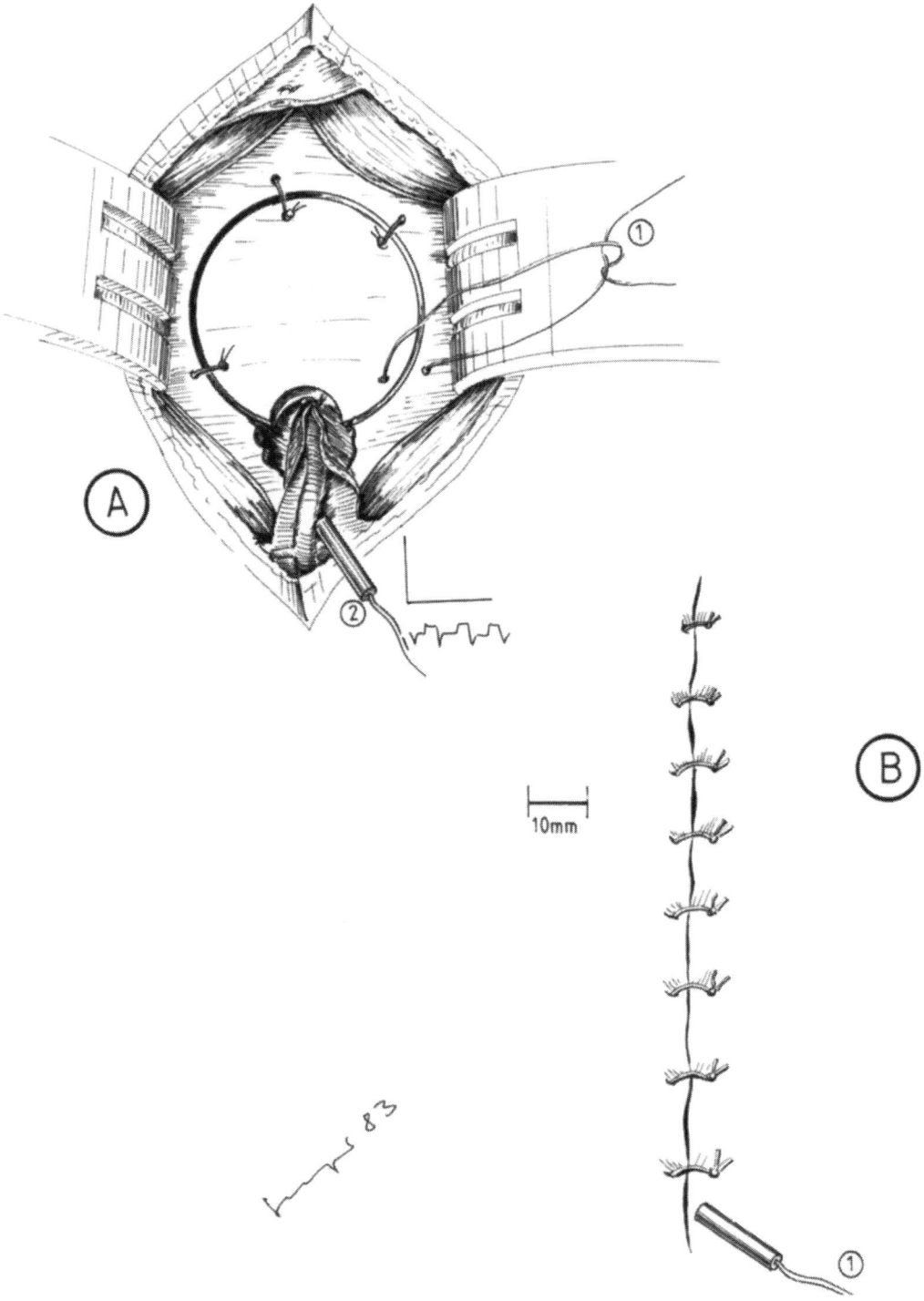
A
1
2
B
10mm
1

Fig. 155. Extra-intracranial bypass "STAMCA"
Appendix. Comparison of various anastomosis techniques

A + B Anastomosis technique according to Yaşargil, Spetzler and others. Classic, most commonly applied method, which, however, as proven in animal experiments, is not ideal*

B' Using this classic technique, stenoses are possible at two points

* J. Gilsbach, Thesis, Freiburg 1983.

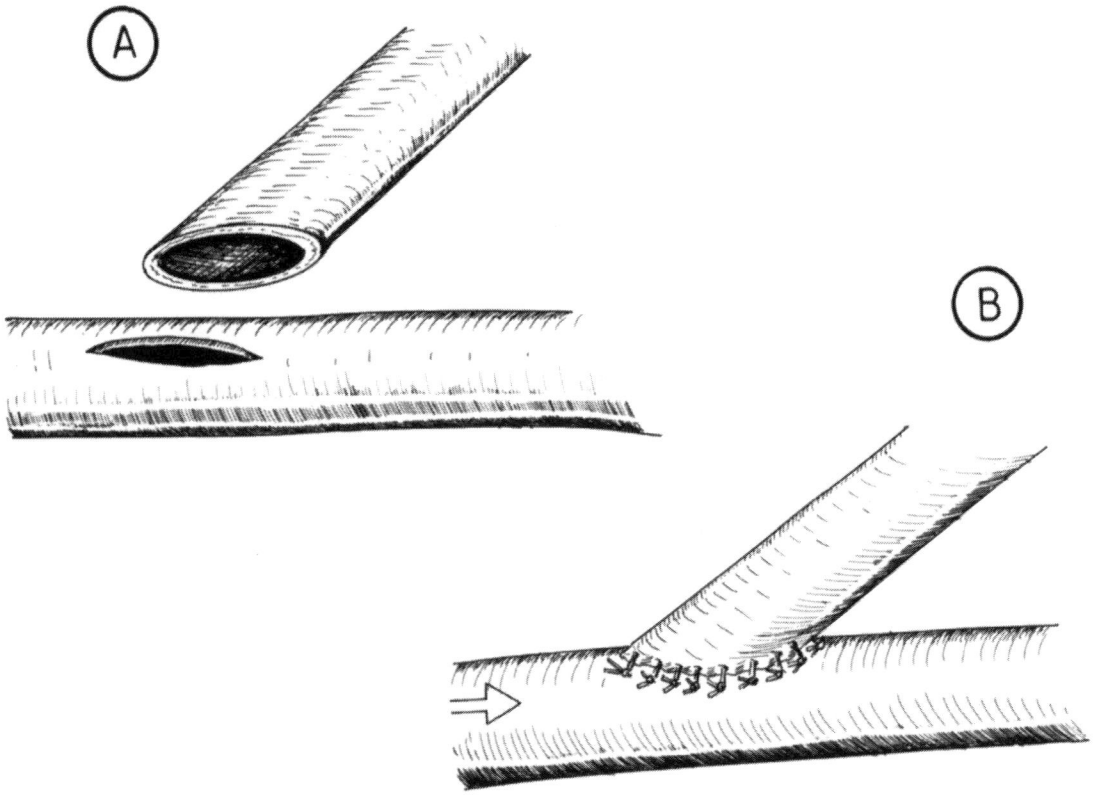

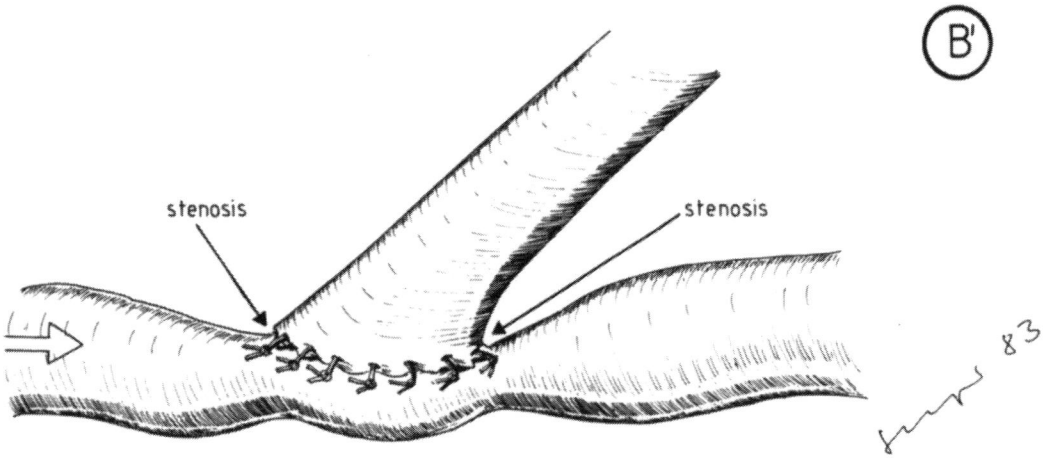

83

Fig. 156. Extra-intracranial bypass "STAMCA"
A + B Patch technique *
B' Stenosis is possible at only **one** point

* Robertson, J. H., Robertson, J. T., 1978, Animal experiments by Rosenbaum and Sundt, 1977.

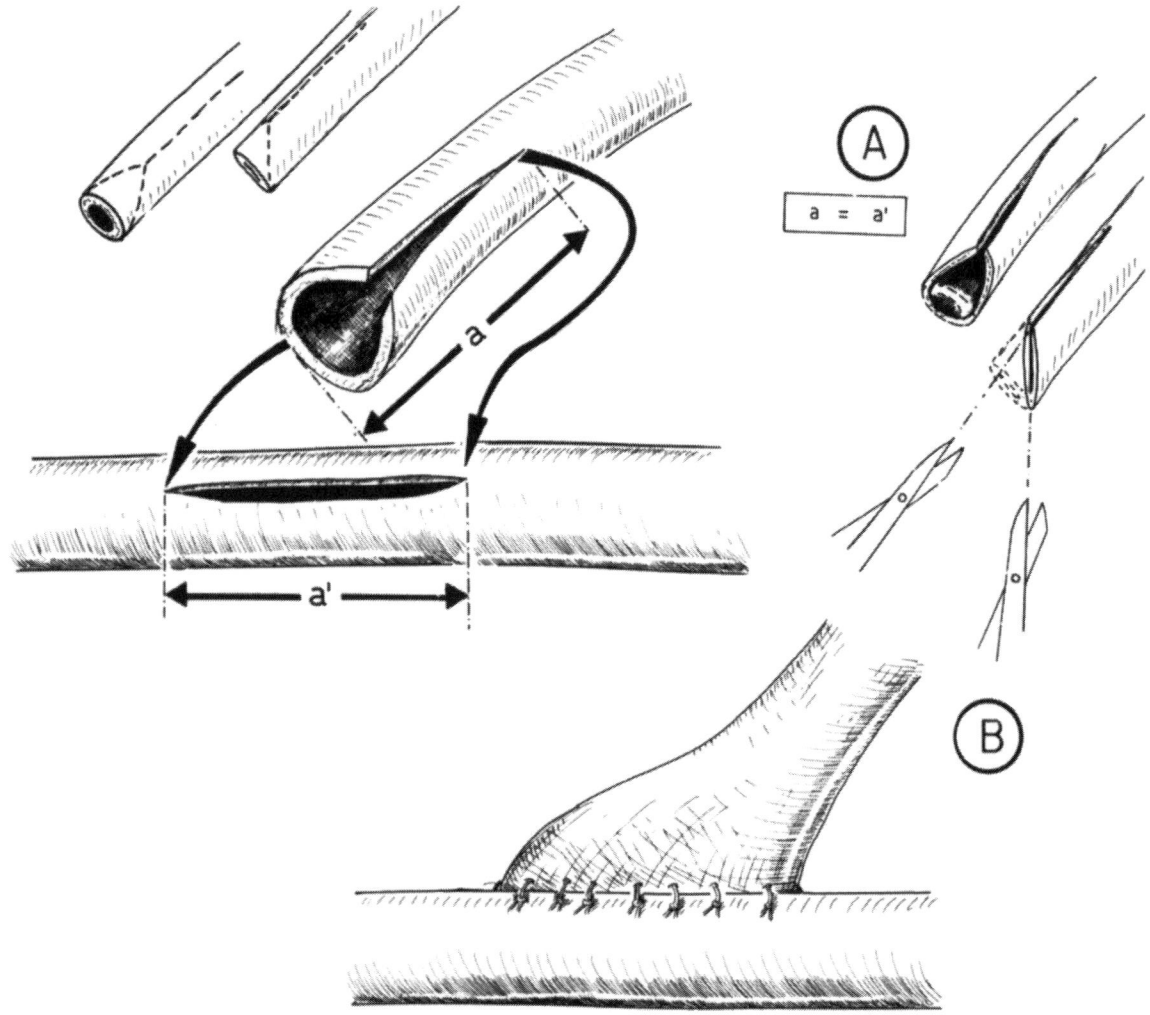
A
a = a'
a
a'
B

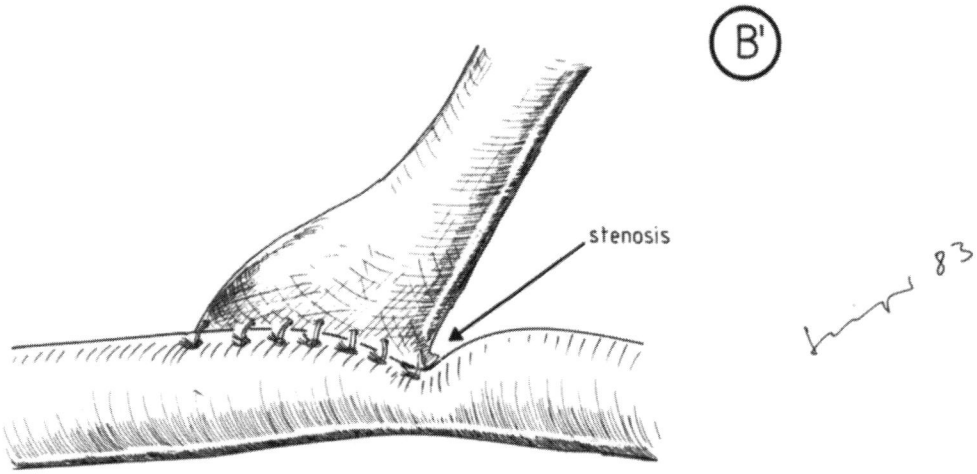
B'
stenosis

Bypass between A. occipitalis and A. cerebelli inf. post. (Figs. 157 to 167)

Fig. 157. Extra-intracranial bypass
Infratentorial: bypass from A. occipitalis and A. cerebelli inf. post.
Clinical example of left sided A. vertebralis occlusion in congenital hypoplasia of right A. vertebralis, which supplies only the right A. cerebelli inf. post. –"PICA"–. Increasing daily attacks of dizziness for 3 months. No pre- and postoperative * neurological deficits **.
Diagnostic procedures

A A. cubitalis angiography, left side: black arrow indicates A. vertebralis occlusion in upper cervical area.
Light arrow: faint contrast appearance of left A. vertebralis above occlusion point.
X: contrast-medium-uptake into A. vertebralis in the nape muscles

B Aortography shows hypoplastic right A. vertebralis continuing directly as A. cerebralis inf. post.-"PICA", without showing intracranial A. vertebralis-basilaris circulation

C Black arrow: operative anastomosis from A. occipitalis to A. cerebelli inf. post. –"PICA"–

D X-ray shows trepanation

---

* Since anastomosis cannot be ascertained through thick nape muscles by Doppler sonograph – in contrast to "STAMCA" – postoperative angiography must be carried out.
** Operation performed by Dr. W. Hassler, author's coworker.

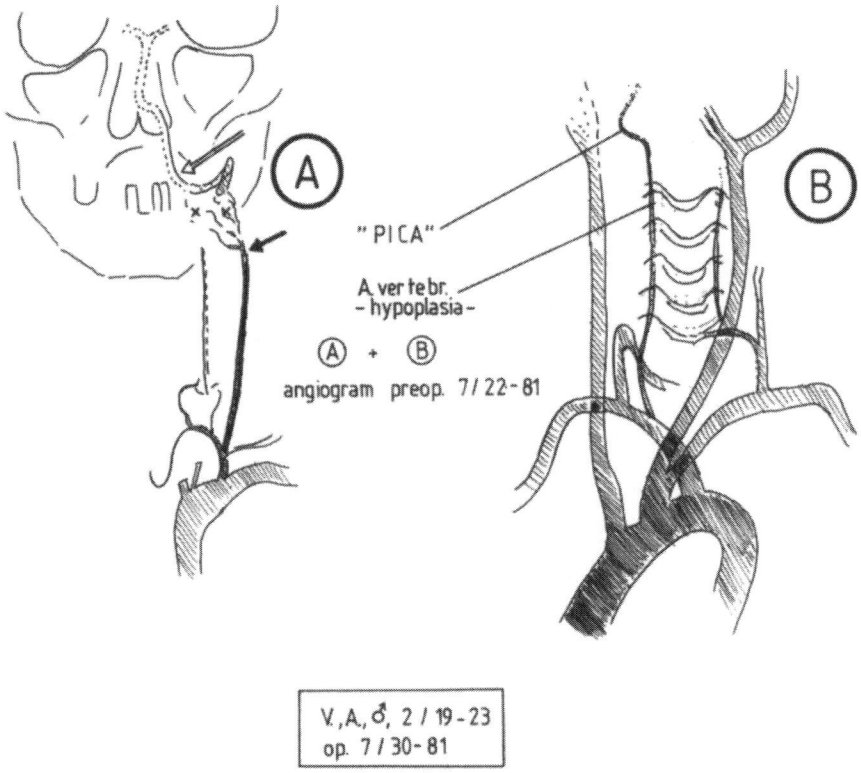
A
B
"PICA"
A. vertebr.
- hypoplasia -
A + B
angiogram preop. 7/22-81
V., A., ♂, 2/19-23
op. 7/30-81

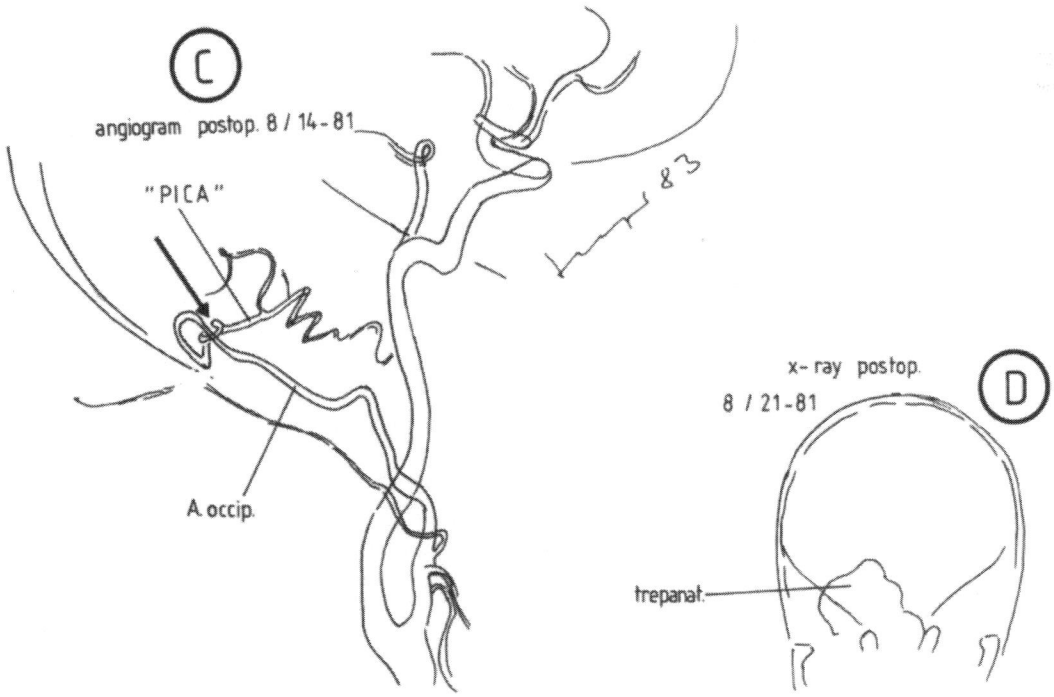
C
angiogram postop. 8/14-81
"PICA"
A. occip.
x-ray postop.
8/21-81
D
trepanat.

Fig. 158. Extra-intracranial bypass
Infratentorial: bypass from A. occipitalis and A. cerebelli inf. post.
Anatomy

A Anatomical topographical relation between N. occipitalis major and A. occipitalis, overview

A' Enlarged detail from **A.** A. occipitalis penetrates Fascia nuchalis approximately 40 mm lateral from midline and there N. occipitalis major crosses over it. Nerve must be saved during artery preparation because of danger of neuralgia

B Anatomical topographical relation of A. occipitalis, Processus mastoideus and middle muscle layer

B' Enlarged detail from **B**

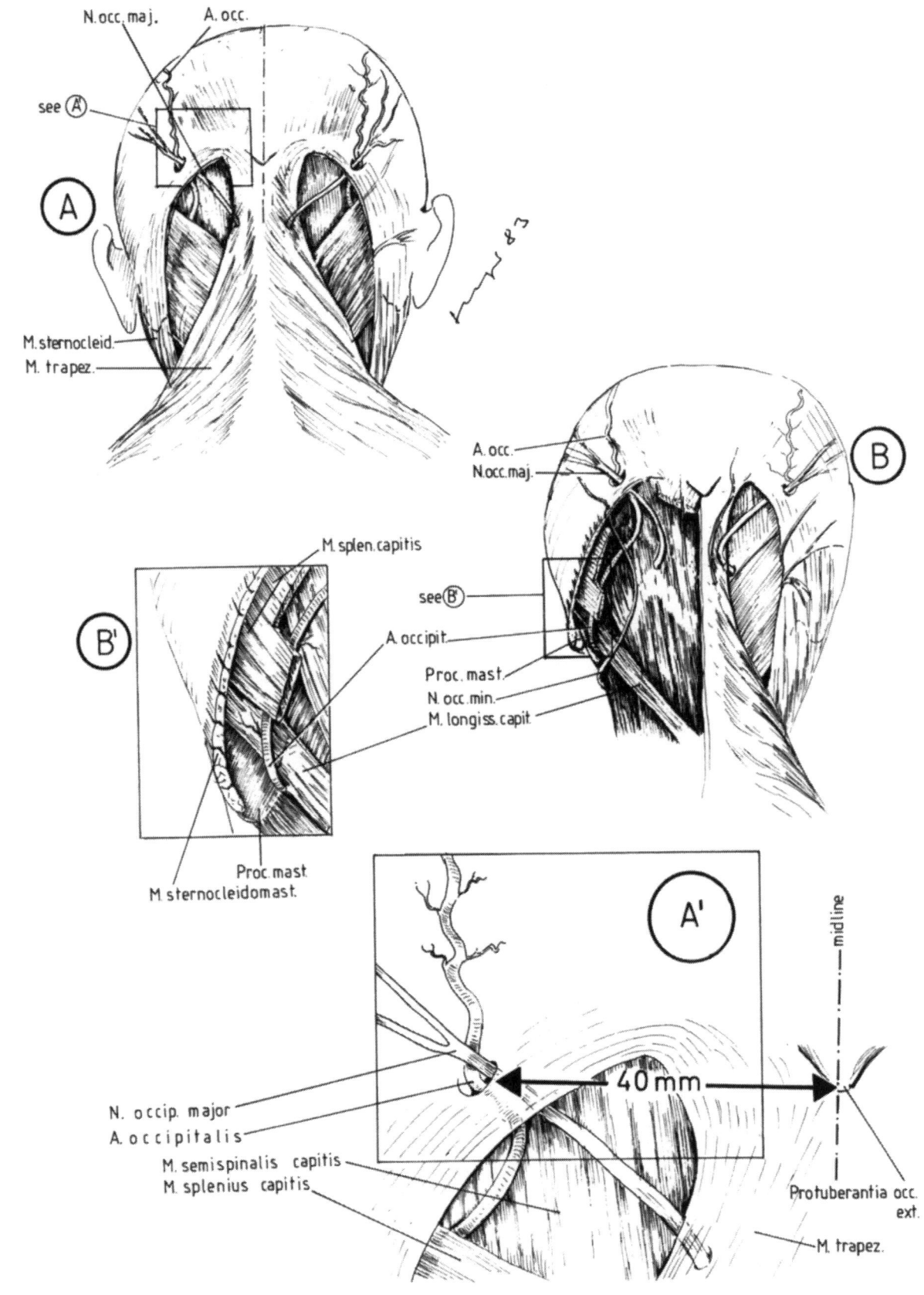
N. occ. maj.
A. occ.
see A'
A
M. sternocleid.
M. trapez.
A. occ.
N. occ. maj.
B
M. splen. capitis
see B'
B'
A. occipit.
Proc. mast.
N. occ. min.
M. longiss. capit.
Proc. mast.
M. sternocleidomast.
A'
midline
40 mm
N. occip. major
A. occipitalis
M. semispinalis capitis
M. splenius capitis
Protuberantia occ. ext.
M. trapez.

Fig. 159. Extra-intracranial bypass
Infratentorial: bypass from A. occipitalis and A. cerebelli inf. post.
Anatomy

A Processus mastoideus, overview

A' Enlarged detail from **A.** Incisura mastoidea: origin of M. digastricus.
Sulcus a. occip.: bony groove for A. occipitalis

A'' As **A'**, deep muscle layer and A. occipitalis drawn in

B Anatomical overview sketch, with position of both Aa. occipitales drawn in, between deep nape muscles

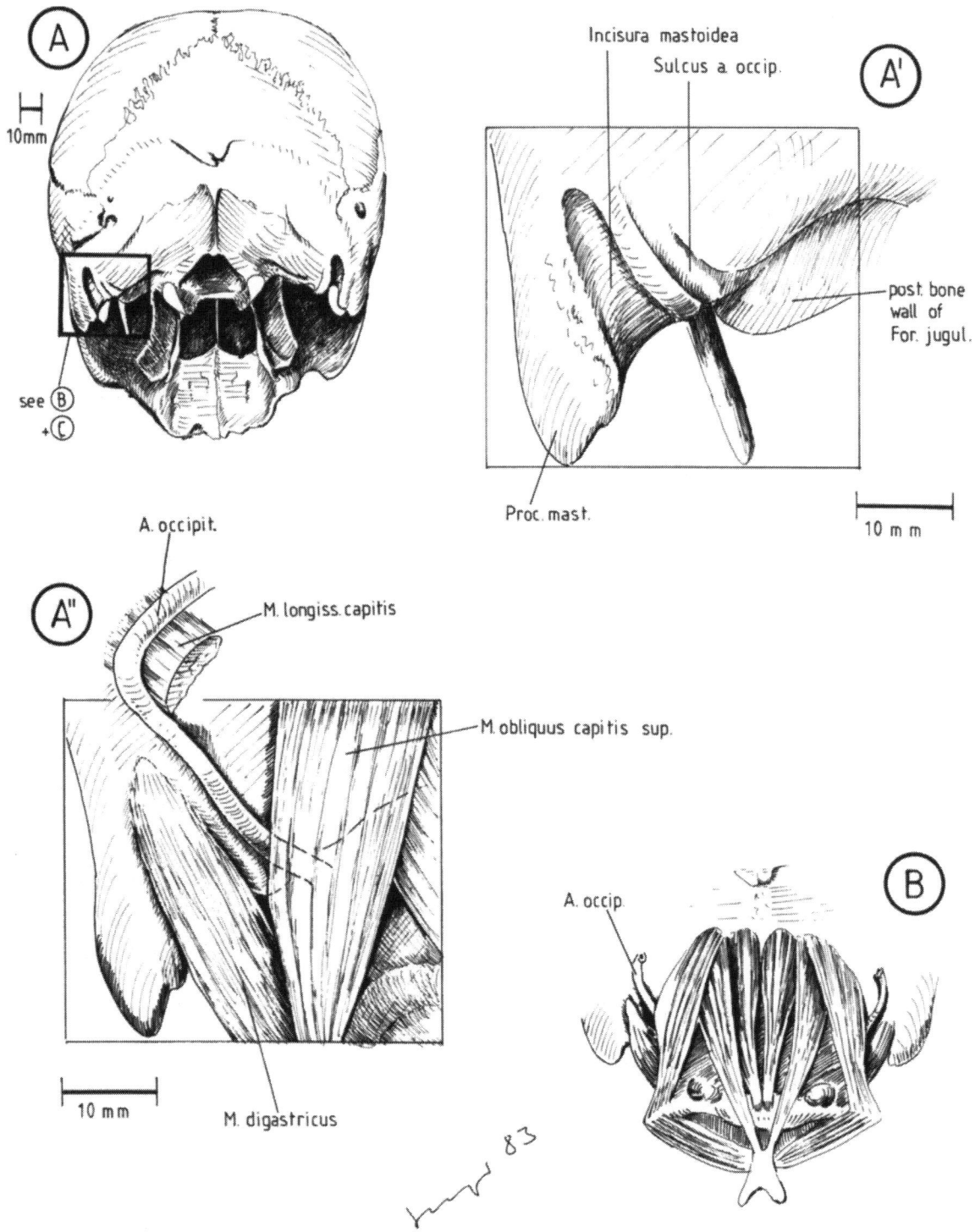
A
10mm
see B
+C
Incisura mastoidea
Sulcus a. occip.
A'
post. bone
wall of
For. jugul.
Proc. mast.
10 mm
A. occipit.
A''
M. longiss. capitis
M. obliquus capitis sup.
10 mm
M. digastricus
B
A. occip.

Fig. 160. Extra-intracranial bypass
Infratentorial: bypass from A. occipitalis and A. cerebelli inf. post.
Operation

A **1** + **2** Localization of midline on the sitting patient
- **1** Palpation of Processus spinosus axis
- **2** Palpation of Protub. occipitalis ext.
- **3** Palpation of Processus mastoideus on both sides
- **4a – 4c** Defining of A. occipitalis path by Doppler sonography
- **5a** + **5b** Skin incision drawn in
- **5a** Portion of skin incision in the midline between Protuberantia occip. ext. and Processus spinosus axis
- **5b** Lateral portion of skin incision nearly parallel to and above path of A. occipitalis (broken lines), defined by Doppler ultrasonogram

B At first, median skin incision only, splitting of Lig. nuchae, exposure of Arcus atlantis post. *–aa–* and exposure of Planum nuchae *–pn–*

C Enlarged detail from **B,** microsurgical site

Abbreviations:

aa Arcus atlantis post.
fo Foramen occipitale (edge)
map Membrana atlanto-occipitalis post.
nm Neck musculature
pn Planum nuchae
vl A. vertebralis over Sulcus a. vertebralis of Arcus atlantis post. (palpable; pulsations visible)

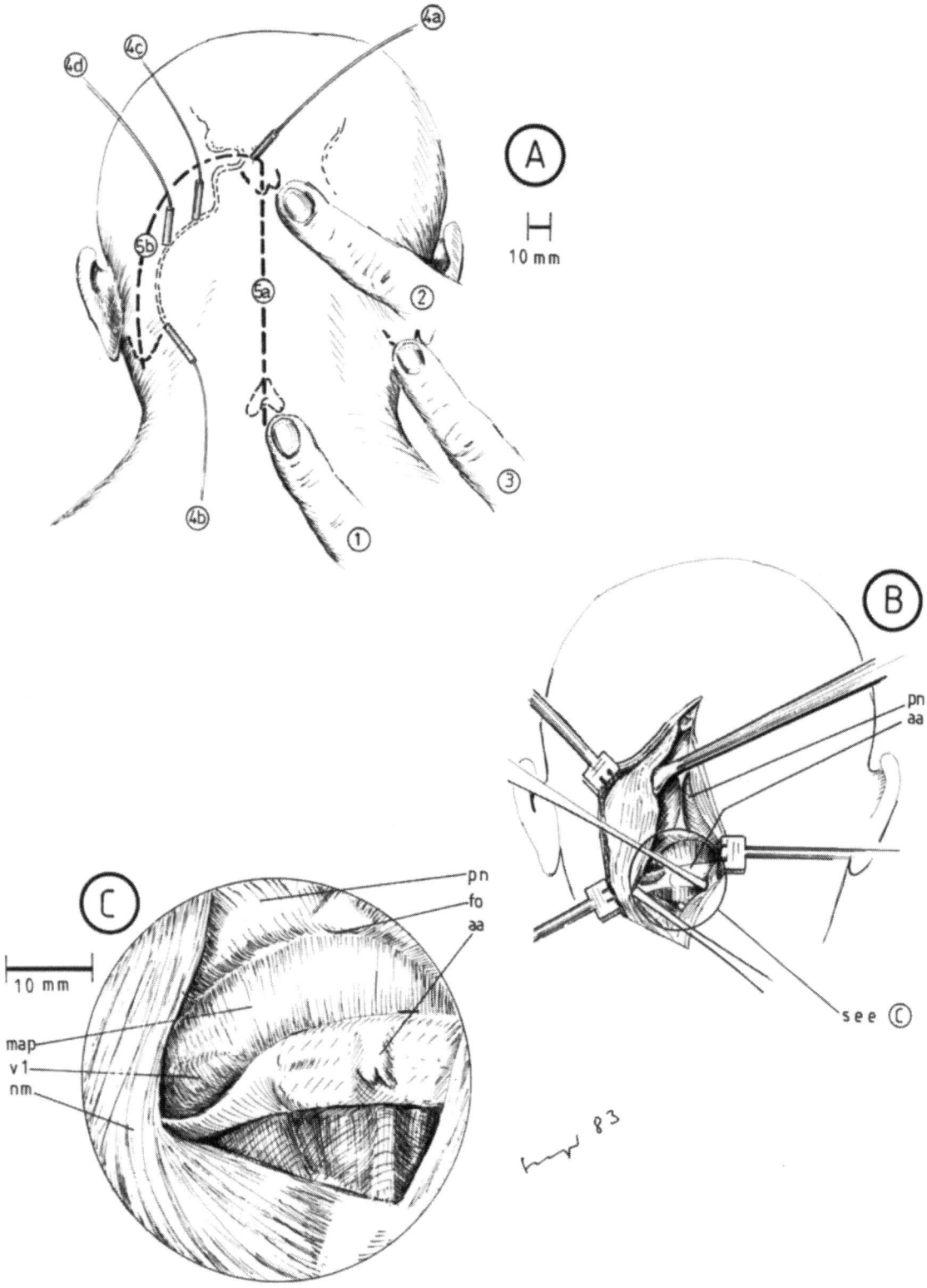
A
10 mm
4a
4c
4d
5b
5a
4b
1
2
3
B
pn
aa
see C
C
10 mm
pn
fo
aa
map
v1
nm
83

Fig. 161. Extra-intracranial bypass
Infratentorial: bypass from A. occipitalis and A. cerebelli inf. post.
Operation

A **1** Skin incision is extended laterally. Skin and muscle flap are folded outwards. Ligation and cutting of A. occipitalis, see **A'**

A' **2a** A. occipitalis ligated distally
2b A. occipitalis temporarily clipped proximal to penetration point
3 After ligation and clipping of A. occipitalis, it is cut
4 (arrow) clipped stump of A. occipitalis is pulled downwards under N. occipitalis major; then, preserving N. occipitalis major, musculature is sectioned to the bone (see **A**)

B + C Composite microsurgical site presentation
1 Incision of periosteum and deep muscle layer almost to A. occipitalis.
Arrow: direction of artery preparation.
Broken lines: projection of artery upon exposed periosteum

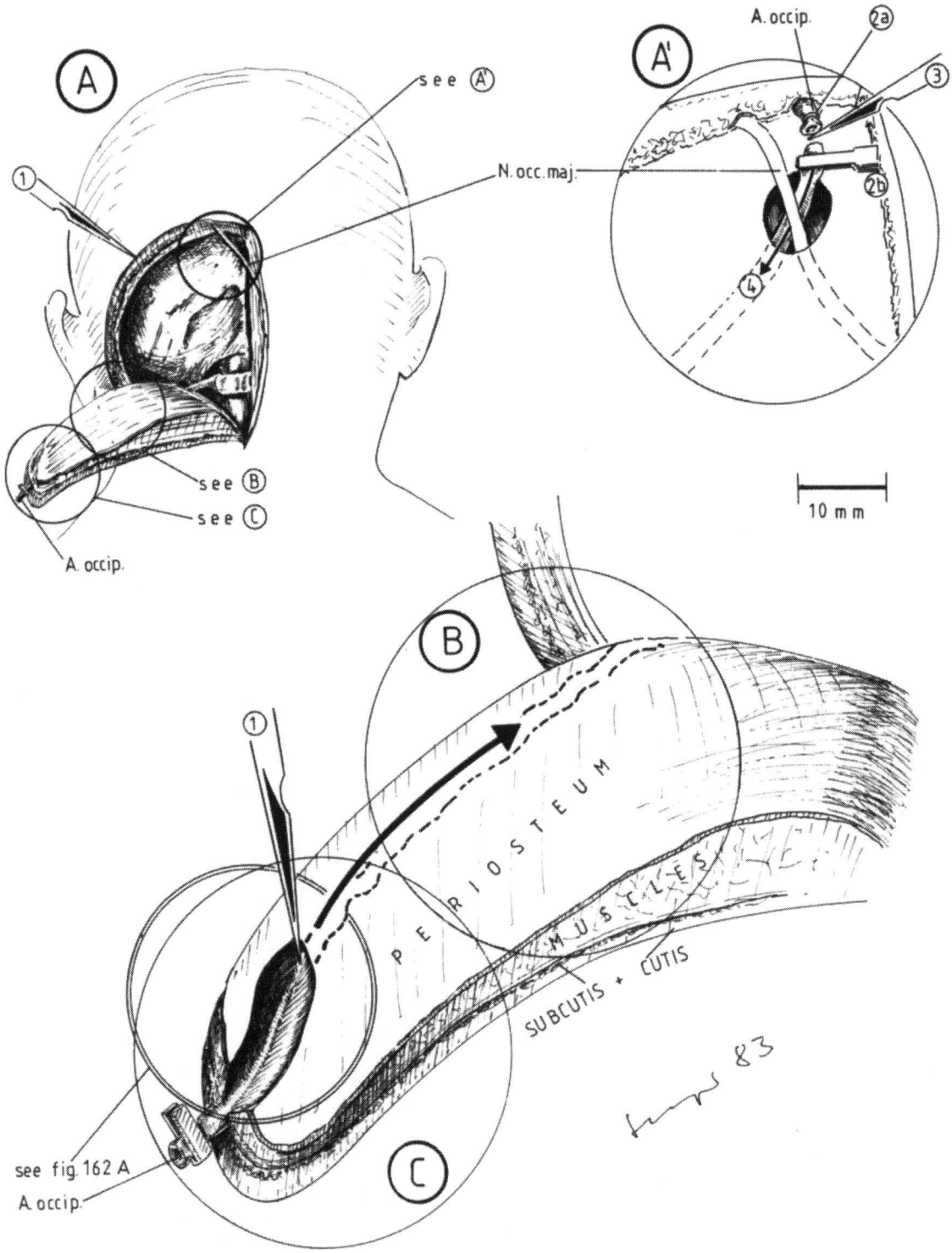
A
A'
see A'
N. occ. maj.
A. occip.
2a
3
2b
4
1
see B
see C
A. occip.
10 mm
B
C
1
PERIOSTEUM
MUSCLES
SUBCUTIS + CUTIS
see fig. 162 A
A. occip.
83

Fig. 162. Extra-intracranial bypass
Infratentorial: bypass from A. occipitalis and A. cerebelli inf. post.
Operation

A Microsurgical site. Enlarged detail from Fig. 161 **C**
- **1** Extension of incision of periosteum and musculature over artery path (arrow)
- **2a + 2b** Incisions of periosteum and musculature parallel to path of artery, and deeper
- **3** Artery, with surrounding musculature and periosteum, is detached from periosteum and nape muscles. Cutis and subcutis are preserved
- **4a + 4b** Interruption of smaller vessels in nape musculature

B
- **1** Removal of temporary clip
- **2** Measurement of blood flow/min.

C Sketch
- **1** Application of temporary clip to A. occipitalis, very proximal and close to skull base
- **2** Irrigation of A. occipitalis with isotonic saline solution.

Starting at the cut end of A. occipitalis for a length of approx. 20 mm the periosteum muscle envelope must be detached from vessel

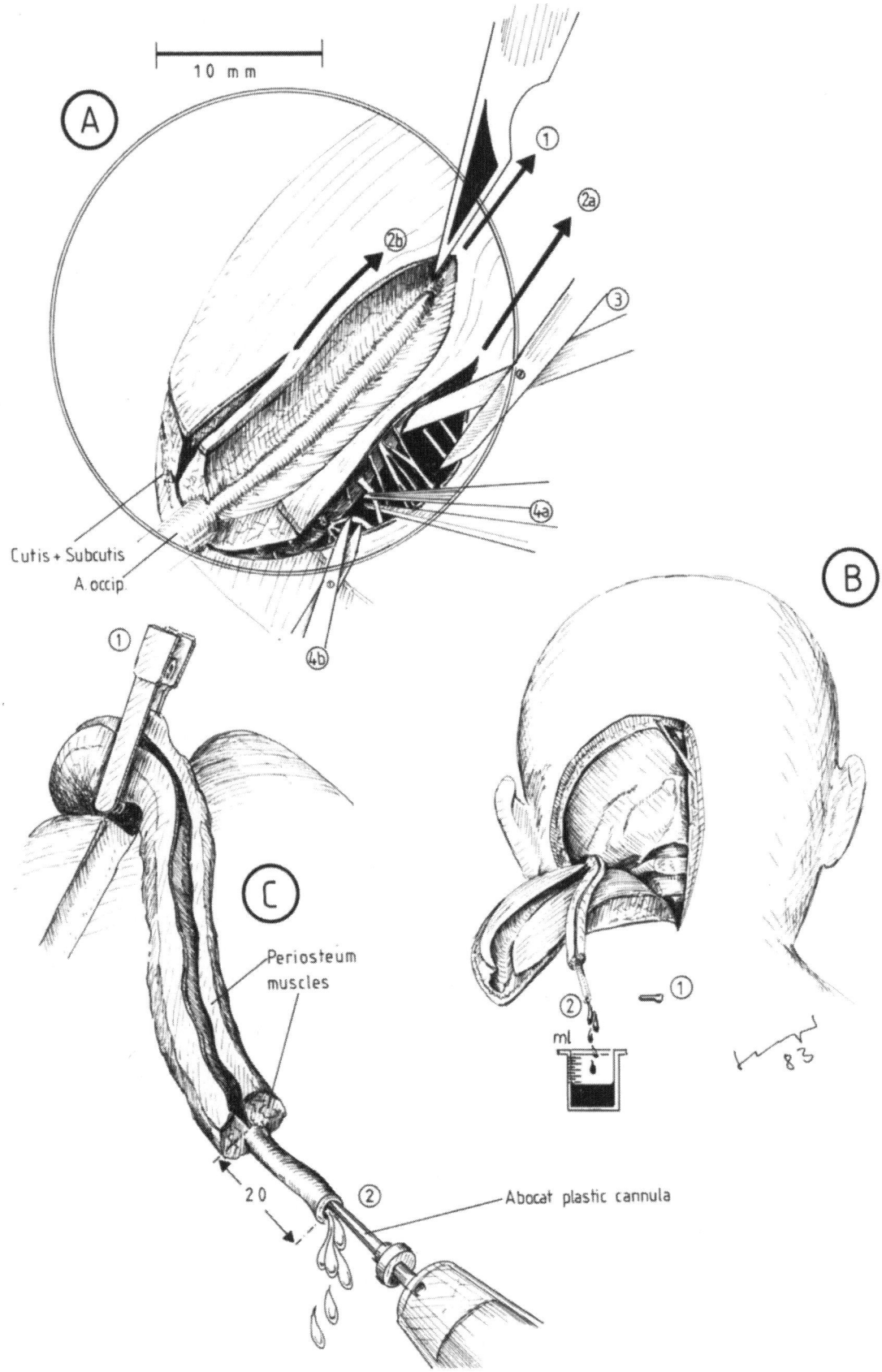
10 mm
A
1
2a
2b
3
4a
4b
Cutis + Subcutis
A. occip.
B
1
2
ml
83
C
1
Periosteum
muscles
20
2
Abocat plastic cannula

Fig. 163. Extra-intracranial bypass
Infratentorial: bypass from A. occipitalis and A. cerebelli inf. post.
Operation

A **1** Trepanation
2 Localization of dura incision

B Microsurgical site, detail from **A.** Dura and arachnoidea are opened up
1 Detachment of arachnoidea from Tonsilla cerebelli and medial Lobulus biventer portions
2a + 2b Lifting Tonsilla cerebelli off Medulla oblongata; cutting of adhesions
3a + 3b Lifting Tonsilla cerebelli and medial Lobulus biventer portions off basal dura; cutting of adhesions

C **1** Lifting of Tonsilla cerebelli and adjoining Lobulus biventer portions by spatula. A. cerebelli inf. post. –"PICA"– and N.XI become recognizable.
For anastomosis, trunk of A. cerebelli inf. post. –"PICA"– is used, not the lateral branch

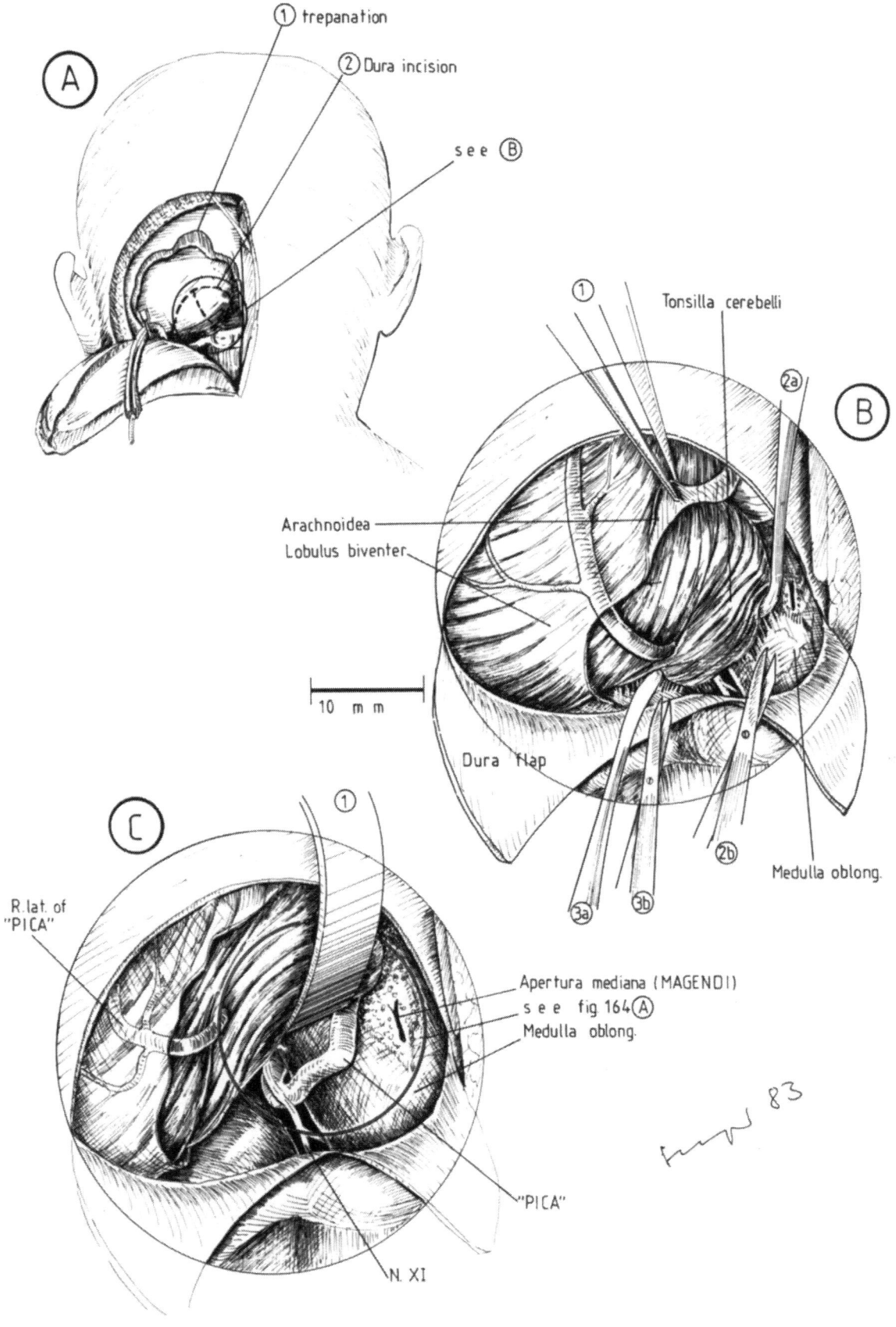
A
1 trepanation
2 Dura incision
see B
B
1
Tonsilla cerebelli
2a
Arachnoidea
Lobulus biventer
10 mm
Dura flap
2b
Medulla oblong.
3a
3b
C
1
R.lat. of "PICA"
Apertura mediana (MAGENDI)
see fig. 164 A
Medulla oblong.
"PICA"
N. XI

Fig. 164. Extra-intracranial bypass
Infratentorial: bypass from A. occipitalis and A. cerebelli inf. post.
Operation

A Deeper insertion of spatula, after separation of additional adhesions between Medulla oblongata and cerebellum
- **1** Retraction of cerebellum
- **2** A piece of rubber foil is placed under A. cerebelli inf. post., after careful freeing of artery from Medulla oblongata
- **3a + 3b** Temporary clipping of A. cerebelli inf. post.
- **4** Incision of A. cerebelli inf. post.

A' Anatomical topographical sketch of Medulla oblongata and A. cerebelli inf. post., corresponding to **A**

B Site, overview. Microsurgical site of Fig. 165 drawn in

C **1** Oblique transection of A. occipitalis

C' Situation after extended incision of A. occipitalis

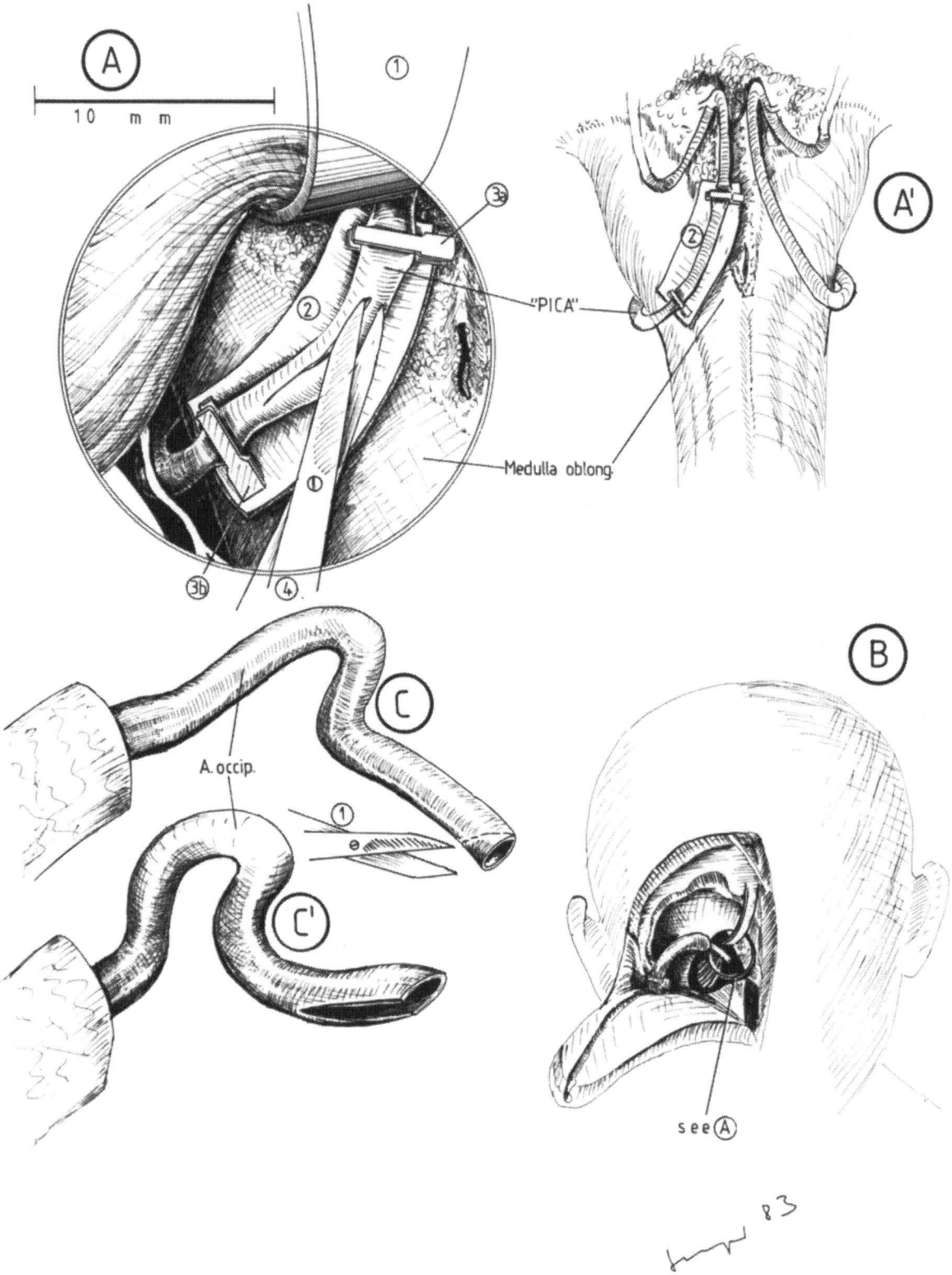
A
10 mm
1
3a
2
"PICA"
Medulla oblong.
1
3b
4
A'
2
C
A. occip.
1
C'
B
see A

Fig. 165. Extra-intracranial bypass
Infratentorial: bypass from A. occipitalis and A. cerebelli inf. post.
Operation

A Microsurgical site. Localization, see overview sketch 164 **B.** Donor vessel – A. occipitalis – is directed in flow direction of receiver vessel – light arrow –. Because suturing is technically difficult in this deep area, placement of donor vessel with or against flow direction depends on the technical possibilities. Application of first stitch

B Second stitch applied

C Initial suturing is done on the side most difficult to reach. For that purpose A. occipitalis is dislocated upwards

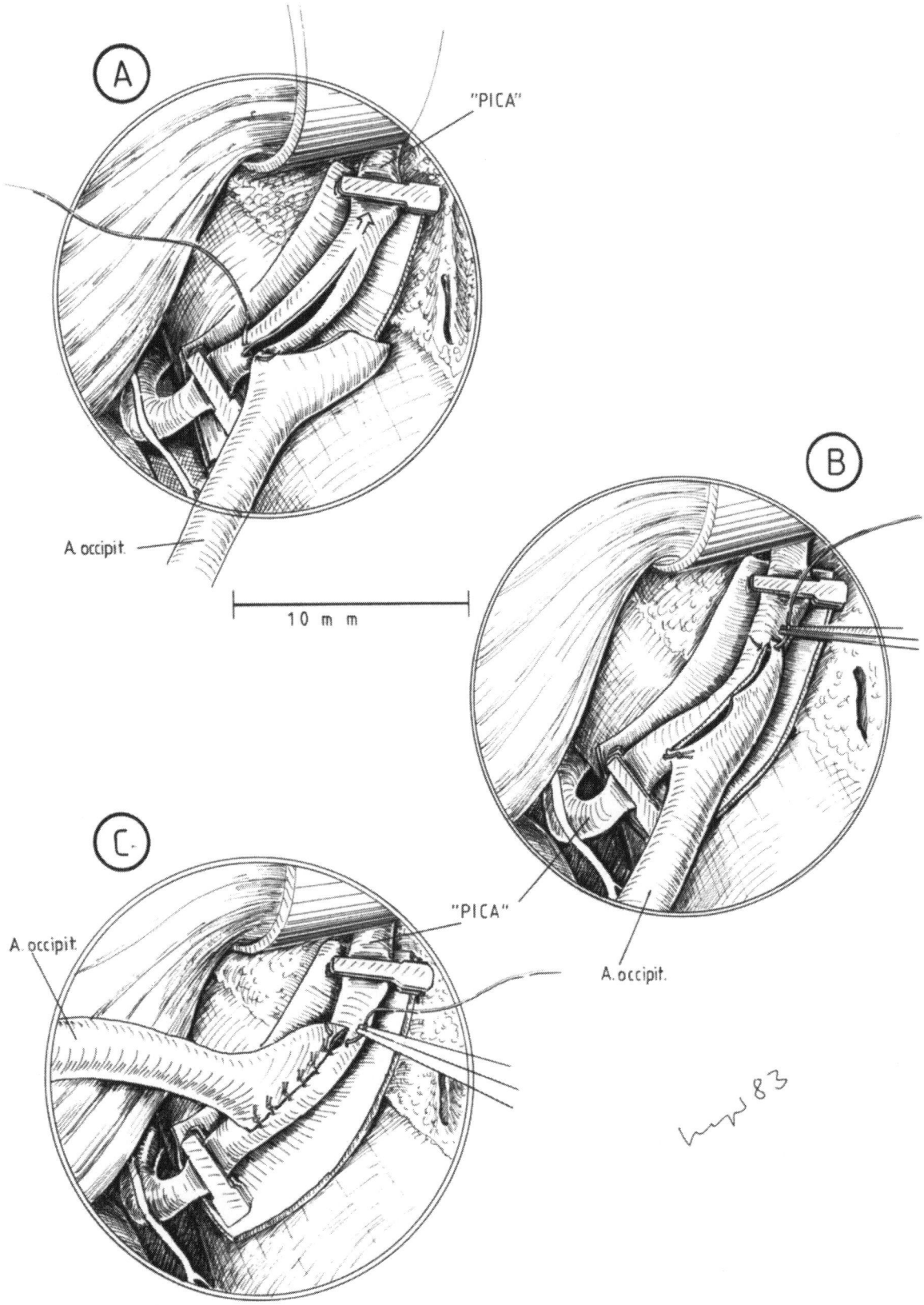
A
"PICA"
A. occipit.
10 m m
B
"PICA"
A. occipit.
C
A. occipit.

Fig. 166. Extra-intracranial bypass
Infratentorial: bypass from A. occipitalis and A. cerebelli inf. post.
Operation

A Application of suture on more easily accessible side of vessel
  1 First, lumen of opened vessel is inspected, to see if contralateral sutures lie correctly
  2 First stitch on the more easily accessible side of vessel

B **1** Finishing of sutures
  2 A. occipitalis is positioned upwards, so that later it may be led through dura gap (light arrow)

C Removal of temporary clip and rubber foil (arrows)

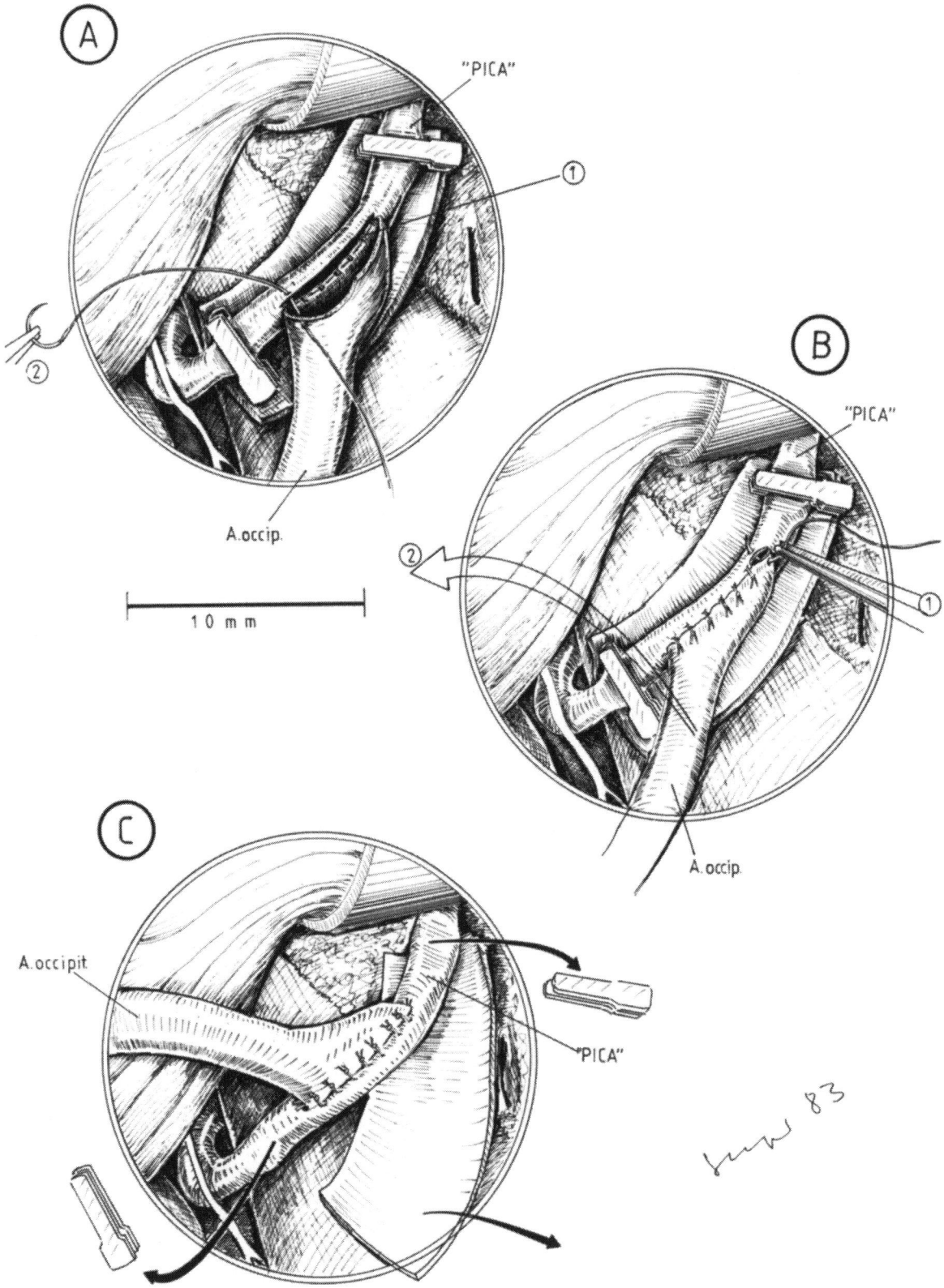
A
"PICA"
1
2
A.occip.
10 mm
B
"PICA"
2
1
A.occip.
C
A.occipit.
"PICA"

Fig. 167. Extra-intracranial bypass
Infratentorial: bypass from A. occipitalis and A. cerebelli inf. post.
Operation

A **1** Removal of temporary clip from A. occipitalis
2 Doppler sonographic check of blood flow in A. occipitalis

A' Microsurgical site
3a **Doppler sonographic check of anastomosis at point where danger of stenosis is greatest**
3b Doppler sonographic check of anastomosis at point where there is less danger of stenosis

B **1** Doppler sonographic check of A. occipitalis after dura closure in order to exclude stenosis at dura penetration point, overview

B' Microsurgical site for **B**
1 As in **B.**
Wound closure

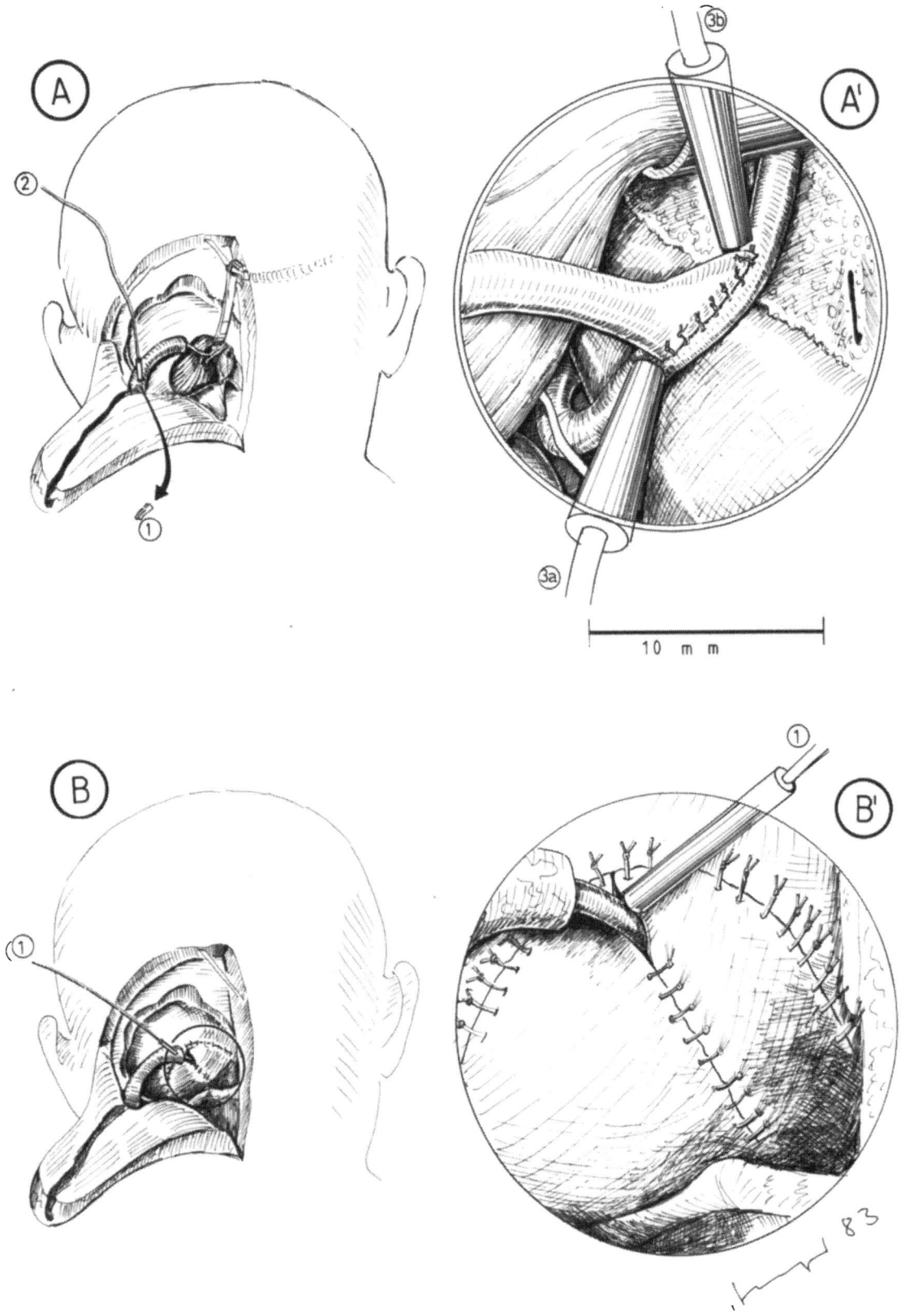
A
2
1
A'
3b
3a
10 mm
B
1
B'
1
83

Chapter 5

Operative Decompressions of N. V and N. VII in the Cerebellopontine Angle (Figs. 168 to 184)

Fig. 168. Decompression of N. V and N. VII in cerebello-pontine angle.
Anatomy of operative approach (arrows)

A Dura gap, through which N. trigeminus leaves liquor space, directly adjoins edge of Lobulus quadrangularis cerebelli. Dura penetration point of N. VII and VIII (= Porus and Meatus acusticus int.) adjoins Flocculus, Brachium pontis and edge of Lobulus quadrangularis.

B Sketch of a portion of skull base showing Sulcus petrosus sup. which surrounds Sinus petrosus sup. Note their adjoining relationships to Porus acusticus int. *–pa–* and to Impressio trigemini *–it–*

C Planum nuchae, through which Sinus transversus, Sinus sigmoideus, Sinus knee *–(k)–* and exit of N. V to N. VIII show translucently. Sulcus petrosus sup. of Os petrosum with Sinus petrosus sup. within tentorial insertion, and edge of Lobulus quadrangularis cerebelli adjoin and run parallel to each other. **Between Sinus petrosus sup. and Lobulus quadrangularis cerebelli lies operative approach.** Starting point of operative approach is Sinus knee (juncture Sinus transversus/sigmoideus and entrance of Sinus petrosus sup. into Sinus transversus/sigmoideus)

Abbreviations:

it	Impressio trigemini of Os petrosum
(k)	Knee of Sinus transversus/sigmoideus (projection)
pa	Porus acusticus int.
pV	Penetration point of N. V at Tentorium
pVII/VIII	Penetration point of N. VII/VIII = Porus acusticus int.
te	Edge of Tentorium

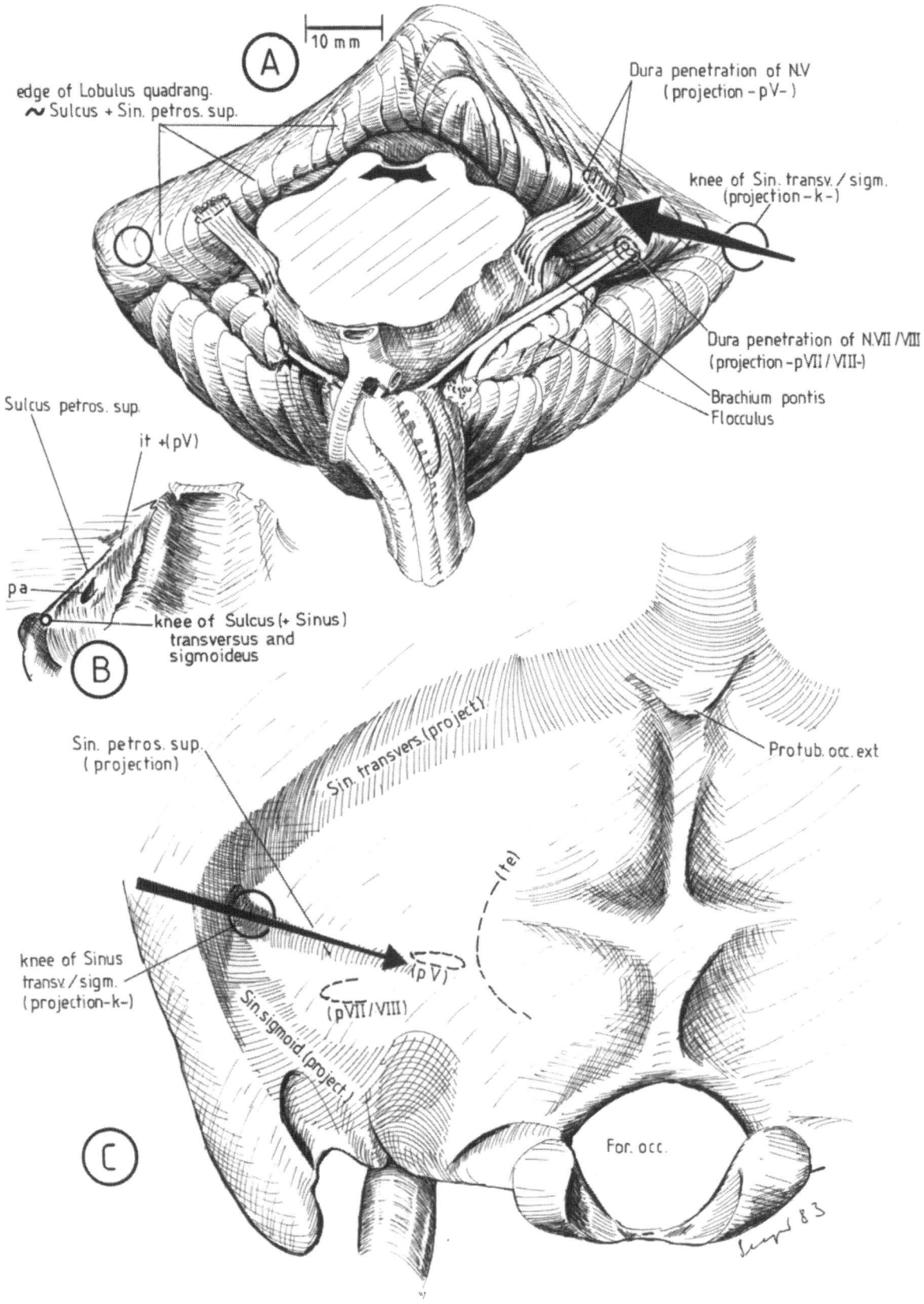
A
10 mm
edge of Lobulus quadrang.
~ Sulcus + Sin. petros. sup.
Dura penetration of N.V
(projection - pV-)
knee of Sin. transv. / sigm.
(projection - k -)
Dura penetration of N.VII / VIII
(projection - pVII / VIII-)
Brachium pontis
Flocculus
Sulcus petros. sup.
it +(pV)
pa
knee of Sulcus (+ Sinus)
transversus and
sigmoideus
B
Sin. petros. sup.
(projection)
Sin. transvers. (project.)
Protub. occ. ext
(te)
knee of Sinus
transv. / sigm.
(projection-k-)
(p V)
(pVII / VIII)
Sin. sigmoid. (project.)
C
For. occ.

Fig. 169. Decompression of N. V and N. VII in cerebello-pontine angle.
Anatomical schematic sketches of operative approach (black arrows)

A Schematic reclination of Lobulus quadrangularis and Pons (double arrows), in order to show position of N.V, which in this sketch is cut through. Note position of Sinus petrosus sup. to the adjoining Tentorium and Os petrosum

B Anatomical sketch of duraclad skull base, detail view, showing arterial loops at N.V and N.VII/VIII

Abbreviations:

k	Knee of Sinus transversus/sigmoideus
pV	Dura penetration point of N.V
pVII/VIII	Penetration point of N.VII/VIII = Porus acusticus int.
VP	V. petrosa sup.

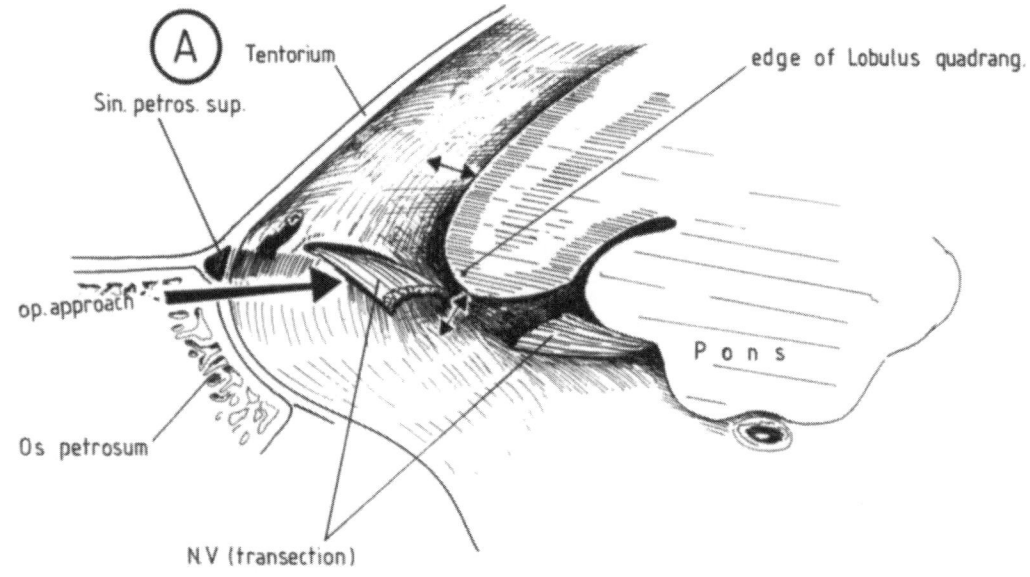
A
Tentorium
Sin. petros. sup.
edge of Lobulus quadrang.
op. approach
Pons
Os petrosum
N.V (transection)

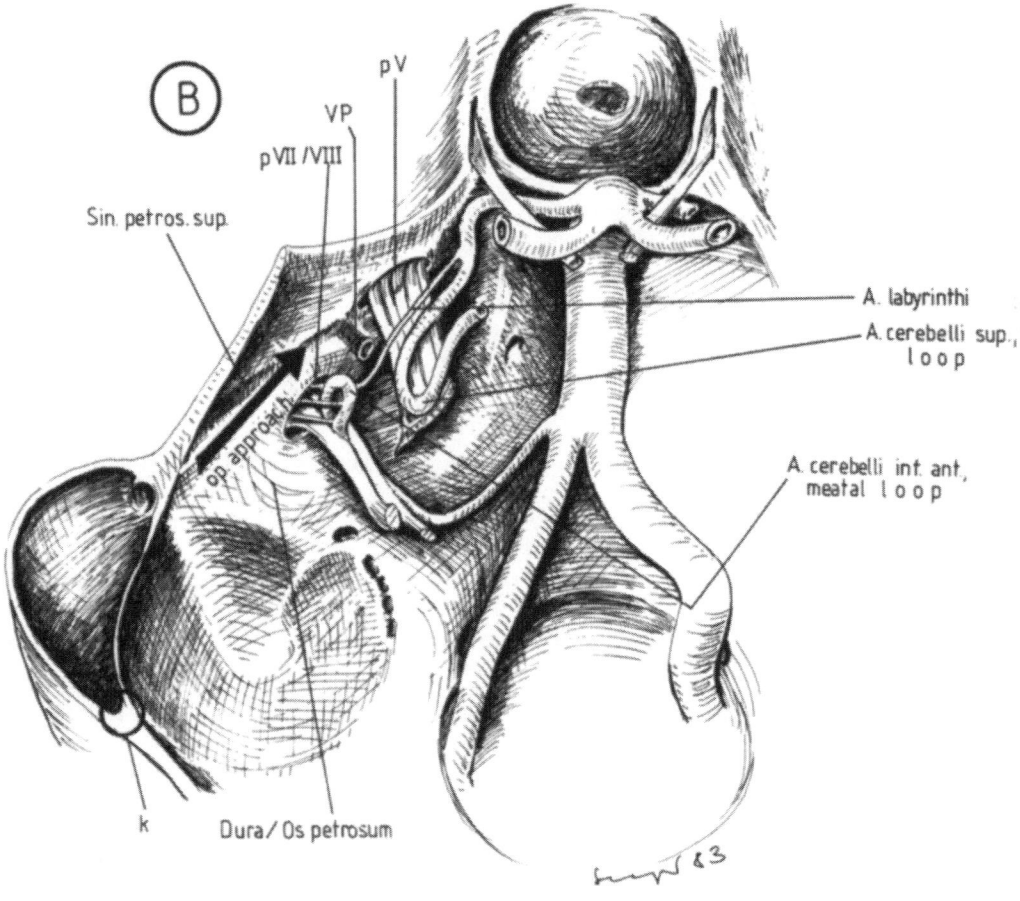
B
pV
VP
pVII /VIII
Sin. petros. sup.
A. labyrinthi
A. cerebelli sup., loop
op. approach
A. cerebelli inf. ant, meatal loop
k
Dura/ Os petrosum

Fig. 170. Decompression of N. V and N. VII in cerebello-pontine angle.
Possibilities of vascularly-induced compression of N.V. and N.VII

A Lower brainstem region, left lateral view, with vessels.
Leptomeningeal structures omitted
a1 – a4 Compression of N. trigeminus by arteries:
a1 by A. cerebelli sup.
a2 A. basilaris
a3 A. vertebralis
a4 A. cerebelli inf. ant. –"AICA"–
b1 – b3 Compression of N. facialis
b1 by meatal loop of "AICA"
b2 A. vertebralis
b3 A. cerebelli inf. post. –"PICA"–
Arrows: Enlargements of arterial loops in the direction of N. trigeminus exit from Pons and near Porus acust. int.

B Typical compression points on N. V. Nomenclature **a1 – a4**

C Typical compression points on N. VII. Nomenclature **b1 – b3** see **A**

Every artery of the posterior fossa may lead to a compression of N. V as well as N. VII (also VIII); most common compressions are: N. V by A. cerebelli sup. (a1), and N. VII by "AICA" b1 *

---

* One also speaks of compressions of other basal cranial nerves such as Nn. IX to XI; however, they are not discussed in this book, since author has not experienced them, and therefore he cannot evaluate them.

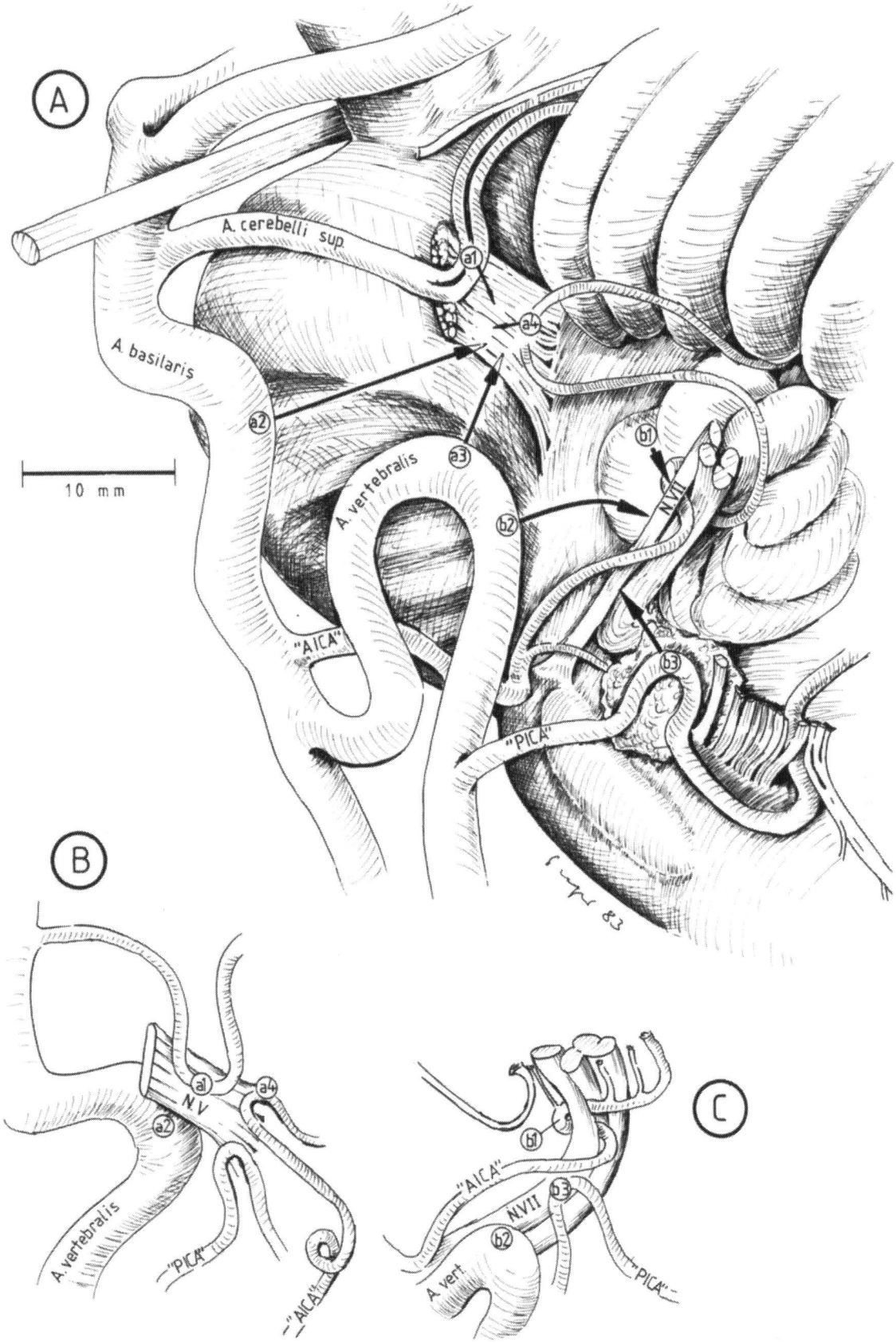
A
A. cerebelli sup.
a1
a4
A. basilaris
a2
a3
10 mm
A. vertebralis
b1
NVII
b2
"AICA"
b3
"PICA"
B
a1
a4
NV
a2
A. vertebralis
"PICA"
"AICA"
C
b1
"AICA"
b3
NVII
b2
A. vert.
"PICA"

Fig. 171. Decompression of N. V and N. VII in cerebello-pontine angle.

A Anatomical sketch, normal finding

B Compression of N. V by A. cerebelli sup. This is the most common cause of trigeminal neuralgia

B' Enlarged detail from **B.**
Light arrows: artery shown compressing N. V, Brachium pontis *–bp–* and Pons *–p–* at exit point of N. V from Pons

Abbreviations:

bi Lobulus biventer
bp Brachium pontis
bl A. basilaris
k Knee of Sinus transversus/sigmoideus (projection)
lss Lobulus semilunaris sup.
p Pons
pl A. cerebri post.
qu Lobulus quadrangularis
si Lobulus semilunaris inf.

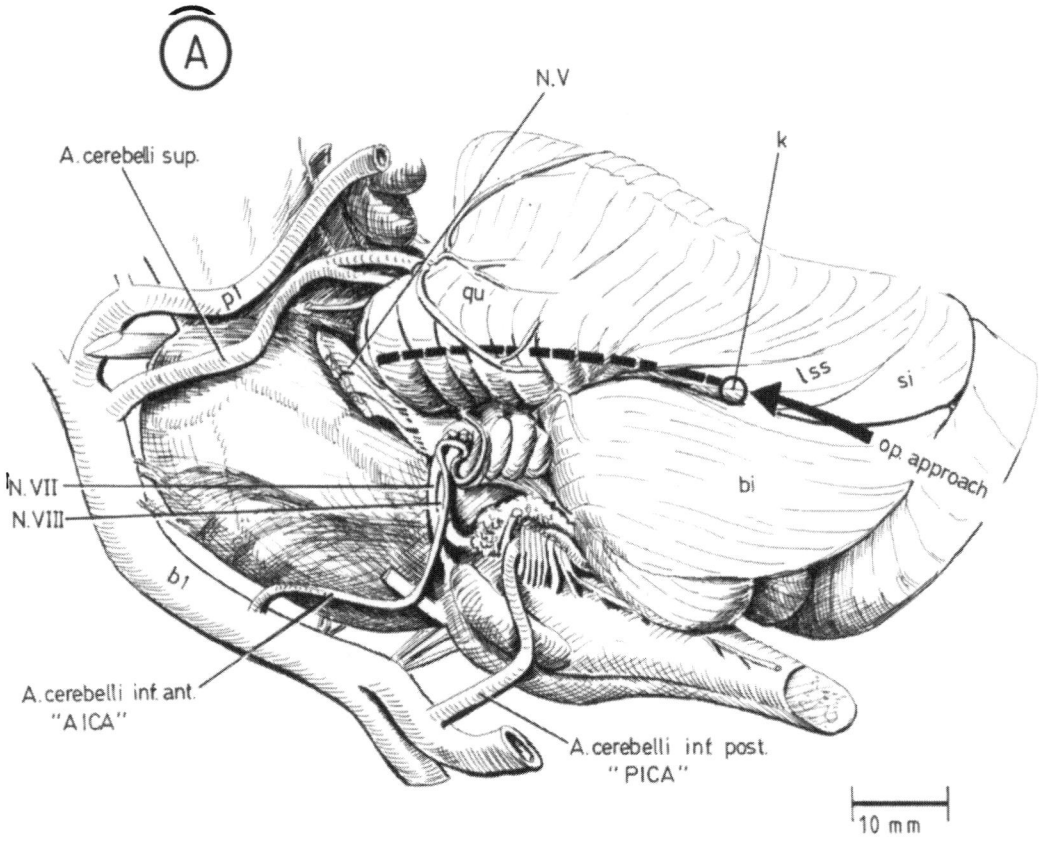
A
N.V
A. cerebelli sup.
k
pl
qu
lss
si
op. approach
bi
N. VII
N. VIII
b1
A. cerebelli inf. ant.
"AICA"
A. cerebelli inf. post.
"PICA"
10 mm

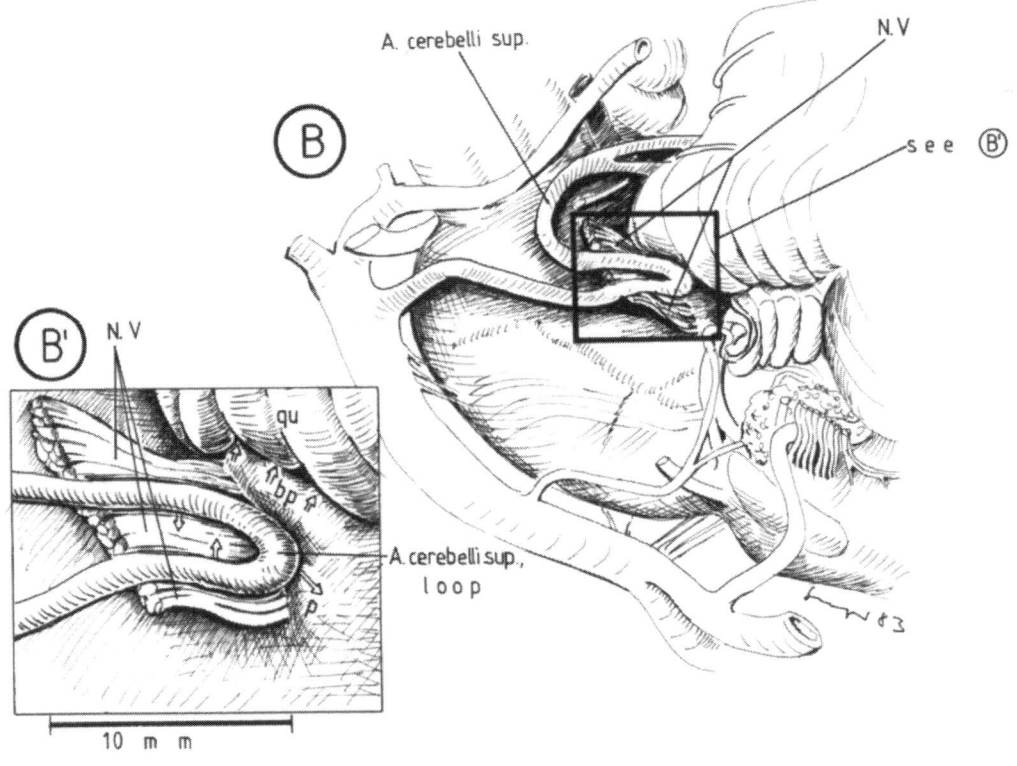
A. cerebelli sup.
N.V
B
see B'
B'
N.V
qu
bp
A. cerebelli sup.,
loop
p
10 mm

Fig. 172. Decompression of N. V and N. VII in cerebello-pontine angle.
Less frequent compression possibilities of N. V
Anatomical sketches

A Compression of N. V by circular looping of A. cerebelli sup. or one of its branches

B Compression by veins, i. e. by lateral pontine vein (or V. petrosa sup.)

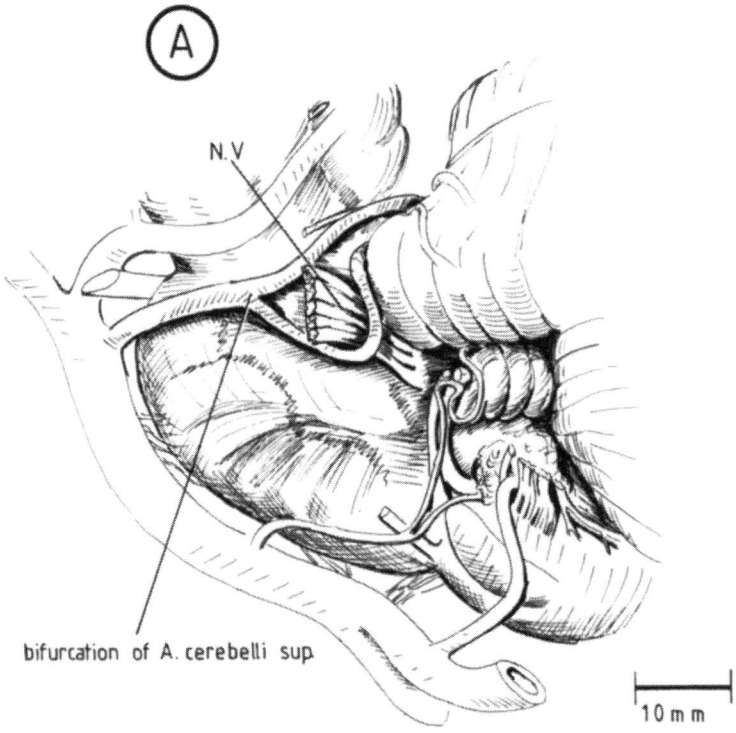
A
N.V
bifurcation of A. cerebelli sup.
10 mm

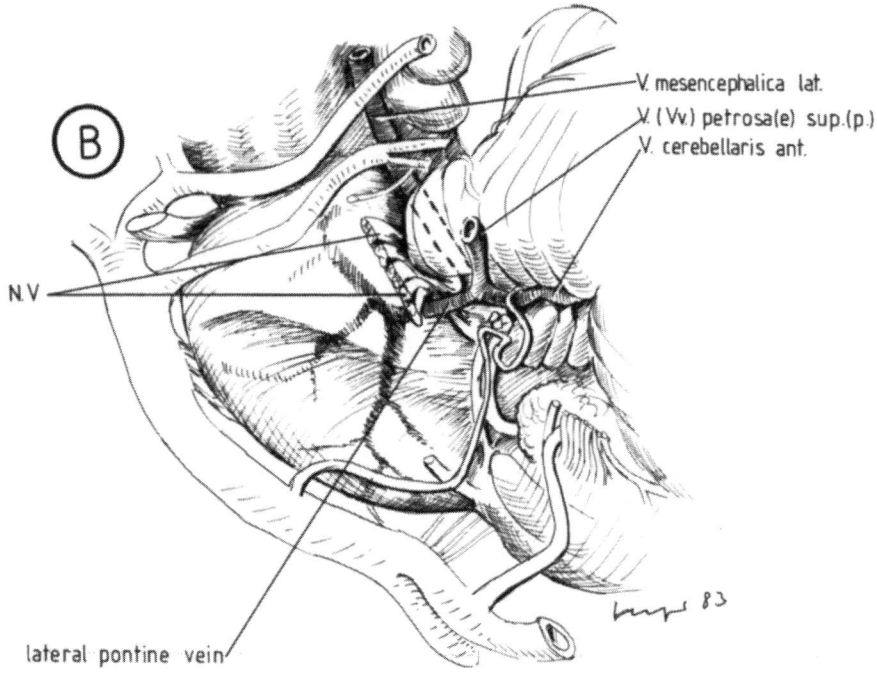
B
V. mesencephalica lat.
V. (Vv.) petrosa(e) sup.(p.)
V. cerebellaris ant.
N.V
lateral pontine vein

Fig. 173. Decompression of N. V and N. VII in cerebello-pontine angle.

Operation

A Localization of skin incision drawn in (broken line). Condition after skin incision and pushing back of muscles. Processus mastoideus exposed. Sinus transversus/sigmoideus drawn in (broken lines)

B Trepanation, anatomical sketch. Burr hole **a** lies above Sinus transversus in order to permit upward view unobstructed by protruding bone structures*. Burr hole **b** lies medial to Sinus sigmoideus, to prevent injury to thin Sinus sigmoideus wall

C Operation site after cutting of skin, fascias and musculature

1 + 2 Further preparation of musculature, periosteum pushed away from Planum nuchae. Note topographical relation between skin incision and Sinus transversus/sigmoideus (skin incision – heavy broken lines – lies just medial of medial Sinus sigmoideus wall – light broken line –)

3 Control of retractor position

Abbreviations:

(ss) Sinus sigmoideus (projection)
(sss) Sinus sagittalis sup. (projection)
(st) Sinus transversus (projection)

---

* Indication from Prof. Dr. G. Yaşargil, Neurosurgical Clinic, University of Zürich.

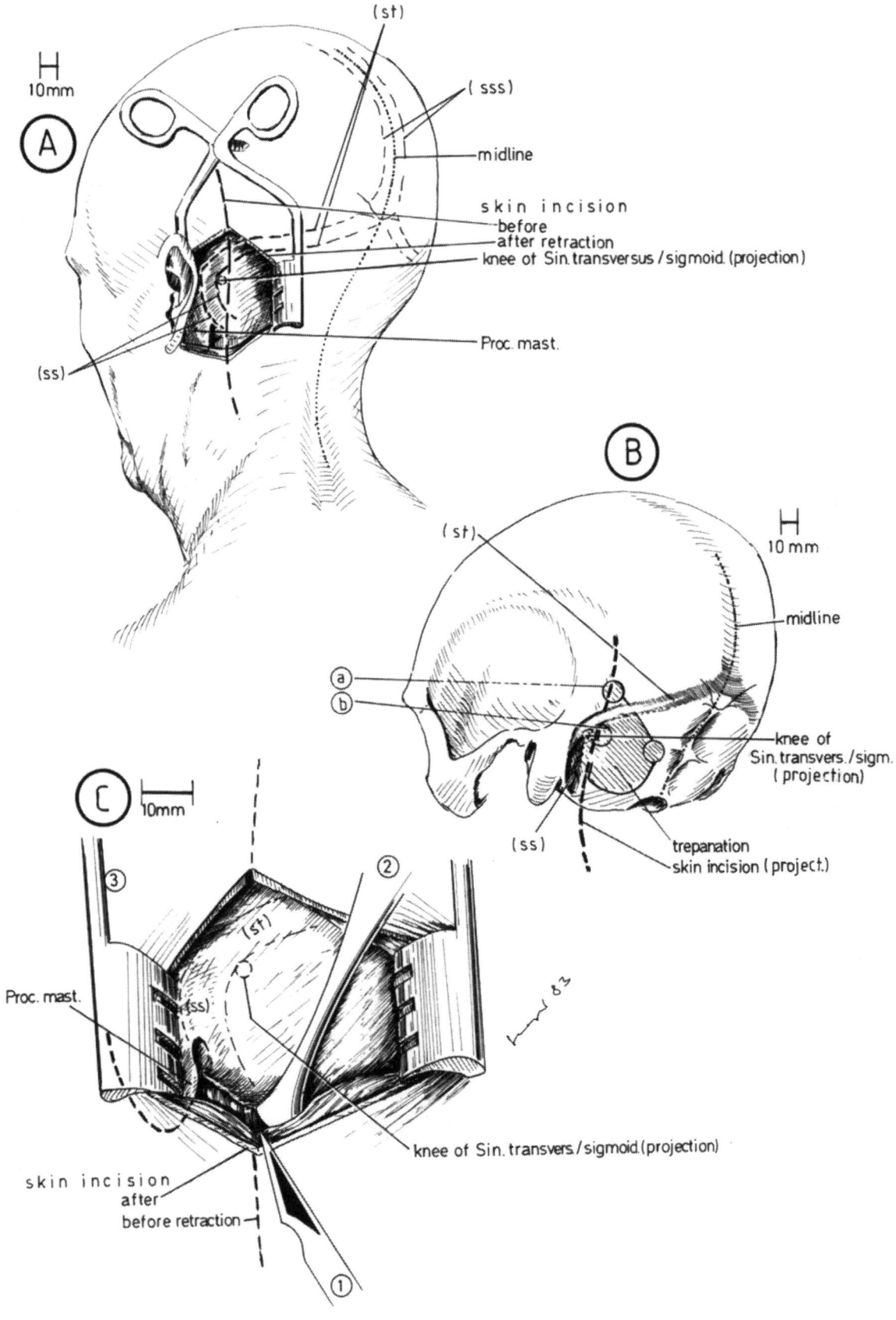
10mm
A
(st)
(sss)
midline
skin incision
before
after retraction
knee of Sin. transversus / sigmoid. (projection)
Proc. mast.
(ss)
B
10 mm
(st)
midline
a
b
knee of
Sin. transvers. / sigm.
(projection)
(ss)
treparation
skin incision (project.)
C
10mm
3
2
(st)
Proc. mast.
(ss)
knee of Sin. transvers. / sigmoid. (projection)
skin incision
after
before retraction
1

Fig. 174. Decompression of N. V and N. VII in cerebello-pontine angle.
Operation

A **1** Wider opening of wound spreader, after drilling burr holes (light arrow)
2 Continuation of craniotomy

B **1** Loosening of dura from Sinus transversus as far as Sinus knee *–(k)–*
2 Loosening on dura from bone medial to Os mastoideum
3a + 3b Cautious bone resection over Sinus sigmoideus (projection) *–(ss)–* as far as Processus mastoideus

C Edges of Sinus transversus and Sinus sigmoideus are exposed

Arrows: Especially endangered are Sinus sigmoideus edges (projection *–(ss)–*)

Abbreviations:

k Knee of Sinus transversus/Sinus sigmoideus
(k) Knee of Sinus transversus/Sinus sigmoideus (projection)
(ss) Sinus sigmoideus (projection)
st Sinus transversus
(st) Sinus transversus (projection)

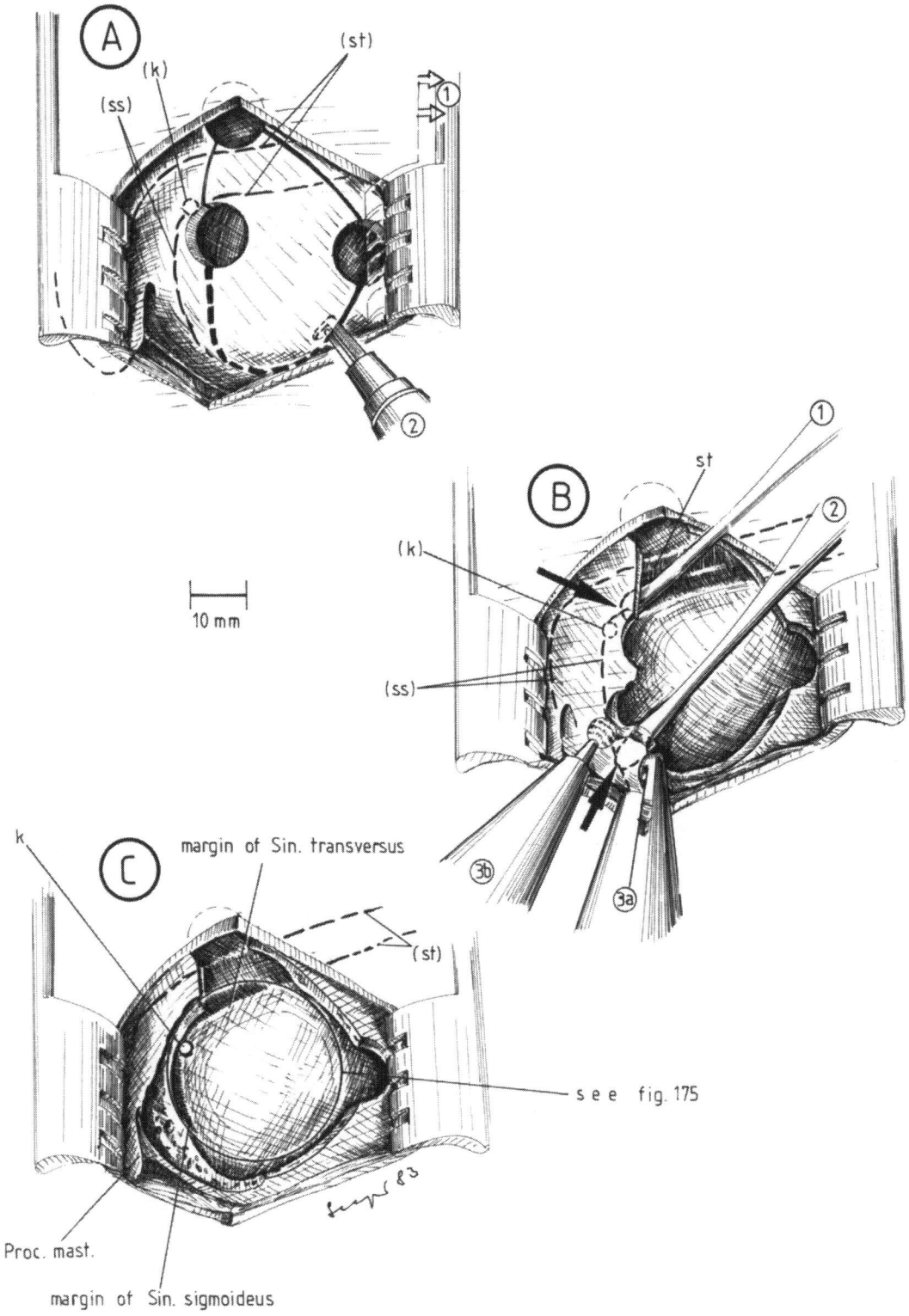
A
(st)
(k)
(ss)
1
2
B
st
1
2
(k)
10 mm
(ss)
3b
3a
C
k
margin of Sin. transversus
(st)
see fig. 175
Proc. mast.
margin of Sin. sigmoideus

Fig. 175. Decompression of N. V and N. VII in cerebello-pontine angle.
Microsurgical operation. Dura opening

A **1** Dura incision
2 Suture of Lacuna near sinus

B Cerebellar surface after folding back of dura flaps

C Anatomical sketch of microsurgical site **B;** dorsal view of cerebellum, not dorso-lateral view, as during operation

Abbreviations:

bi Lobulus biventer cerebelli
fh Fissura horizontalis cerebelli
k Knee of sinus
lq Lobulus quadrangularis
si Lobulus semilunaris inf.
ss Lobulus semilunaris sup.

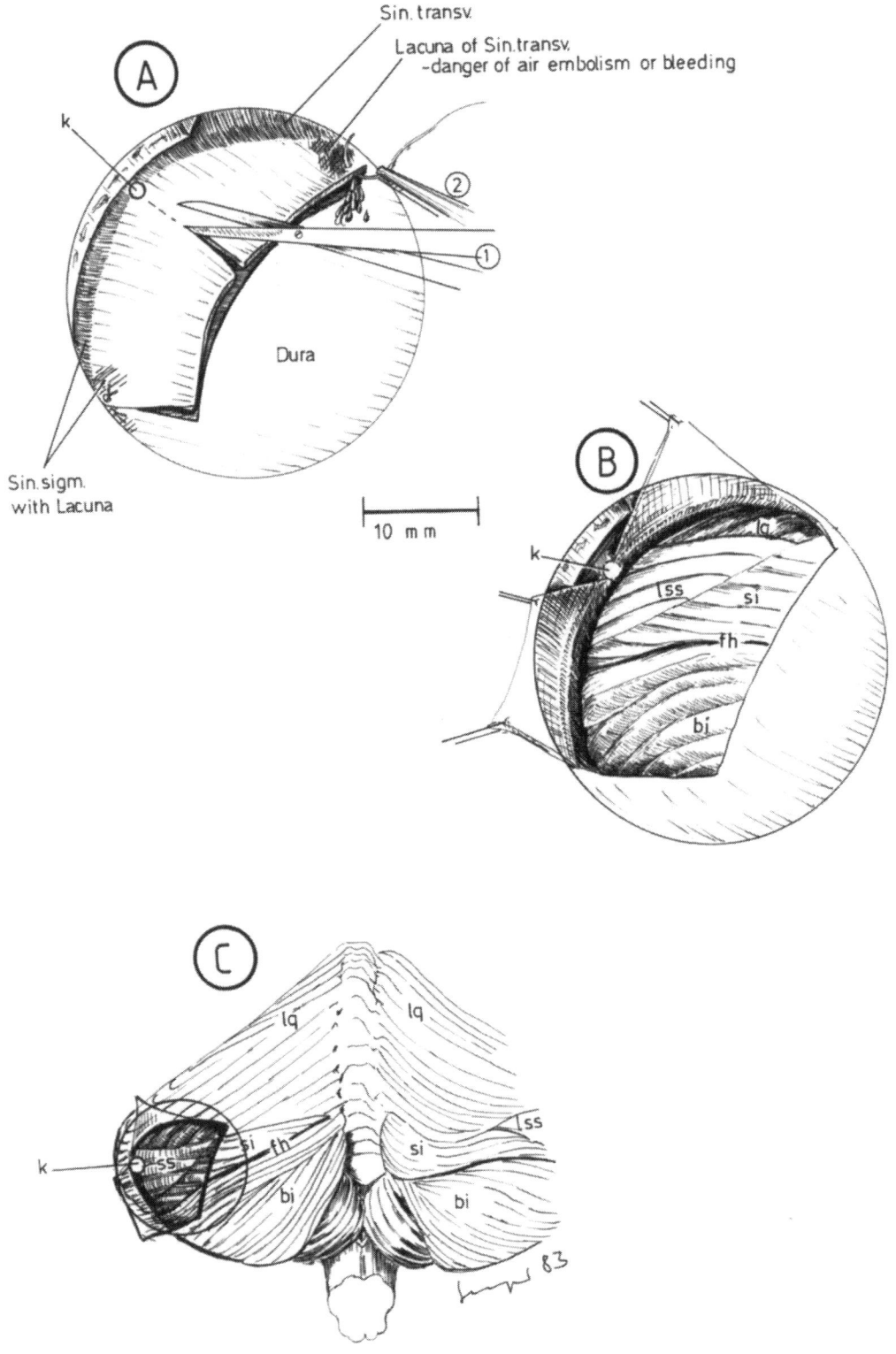
A
Sin. transv.
Lacuna of Sin.transv.
-danger of air embolism or bleeding
k
2
1
Dura
Sin.sigm.
with Lacuna
10 mm
B
k
lq
lss
si
fh
bi
C
lq
lq
lss
si
fh
si
ss
k
bi
bi
83

Fig. 176. Decompression of N. V and N. VII in cerebello-pontine angle.
Microsurgical operation. Reclination of cerebellum

A Insertion of spatula

A' Anatomical sketch for microsurgical site **A.** Arrow: view as in **A**

B After separation of slight adhesions, spatula is inserted more deeply

B' Anatomical sketch for microsurgical site **B**

C Enlarged detail from **B.** Separation of adhesions in the area of N. VII/VIII, Flocculus, V. petrosa sup. and N. V

Abbreviations:

bi Lobulus biventer
fh Fissura horizontalis cerebelli
k Knee of Sinus transversus/sigmoideus
lss Lobulus semilunaris sup.
qu Lobulus quadrangularis
si Lobulus semilunaris inf.
PS V. petrosa sup.

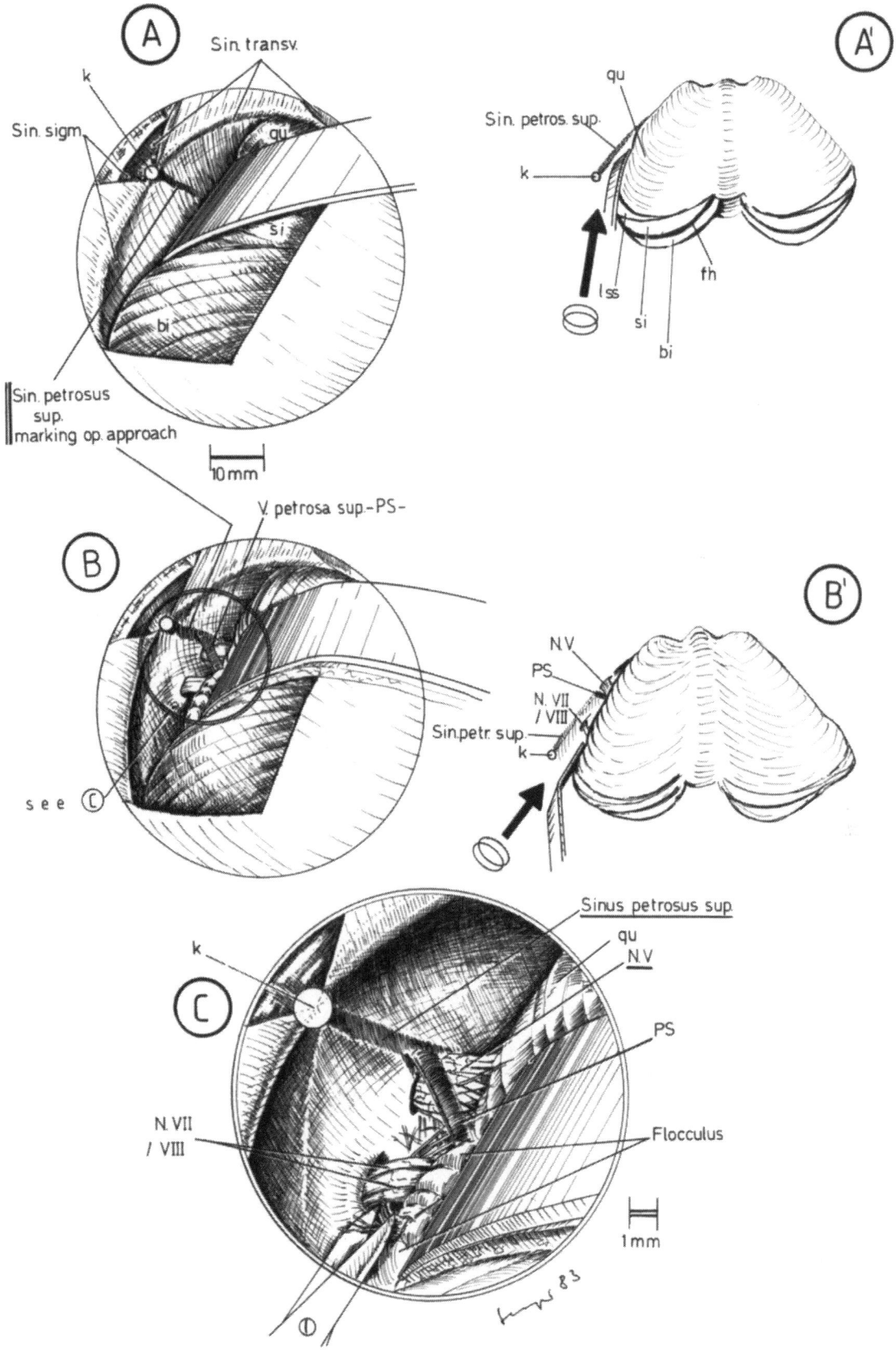
A
Sin. transv.
k
Sin. sigm.
qu
si
bi
Sin. petrosus sup. marking op. approach
10 mm
A'
qu
Sin. petros. sup.
k
lss
si
bi
th
V. petrosa sup.-PS-
B
see C
B'
N.V.
PS
N. VII / VIII
Sin.petr. sup.
k
Sinus petrosus sup.
qu
N.V
k
C
PS
N. VII / VIII
Flocculus
1 mm
D

Fig. 177. Decompression of N. V and N. VII in cerebello-pontine angle.
Microsurgical operation

A **1** Separation of adhesions between Flocculus *–fl–* and V. petrosa sup. *–PS–*

2 Separation of arachnoidal adhesions of N. V., A. cerebelli sup. and Lobulus quadrangularis *–qu–*. Further reclination of cerebellum by changing spatula position (light arrows)

A' Anatomical transection sketch of microsurgical site **A.** Anatomical topographical relation of loop of A. cerebelli sup., to N. V. and Pons

B **1** Separation of arachnoidal adhesions near A. cerebelli sup. loop

2 Reclination of deeper lying cerebellar structures over N. V (structures close to surface can be reclined over N. V 5 to 10 mm, but deeper structures not more than 5 mm)

B' Anatomical topographical sketch for **B.** Section plane **A'** drawn in (broken line)

Abbreviations:

bp Brachium pontis
fl Flocculus
k Knee of Sinus transversus/sigmoideus
qu Lobulus quadrangularis
PS V. petrosa sup.

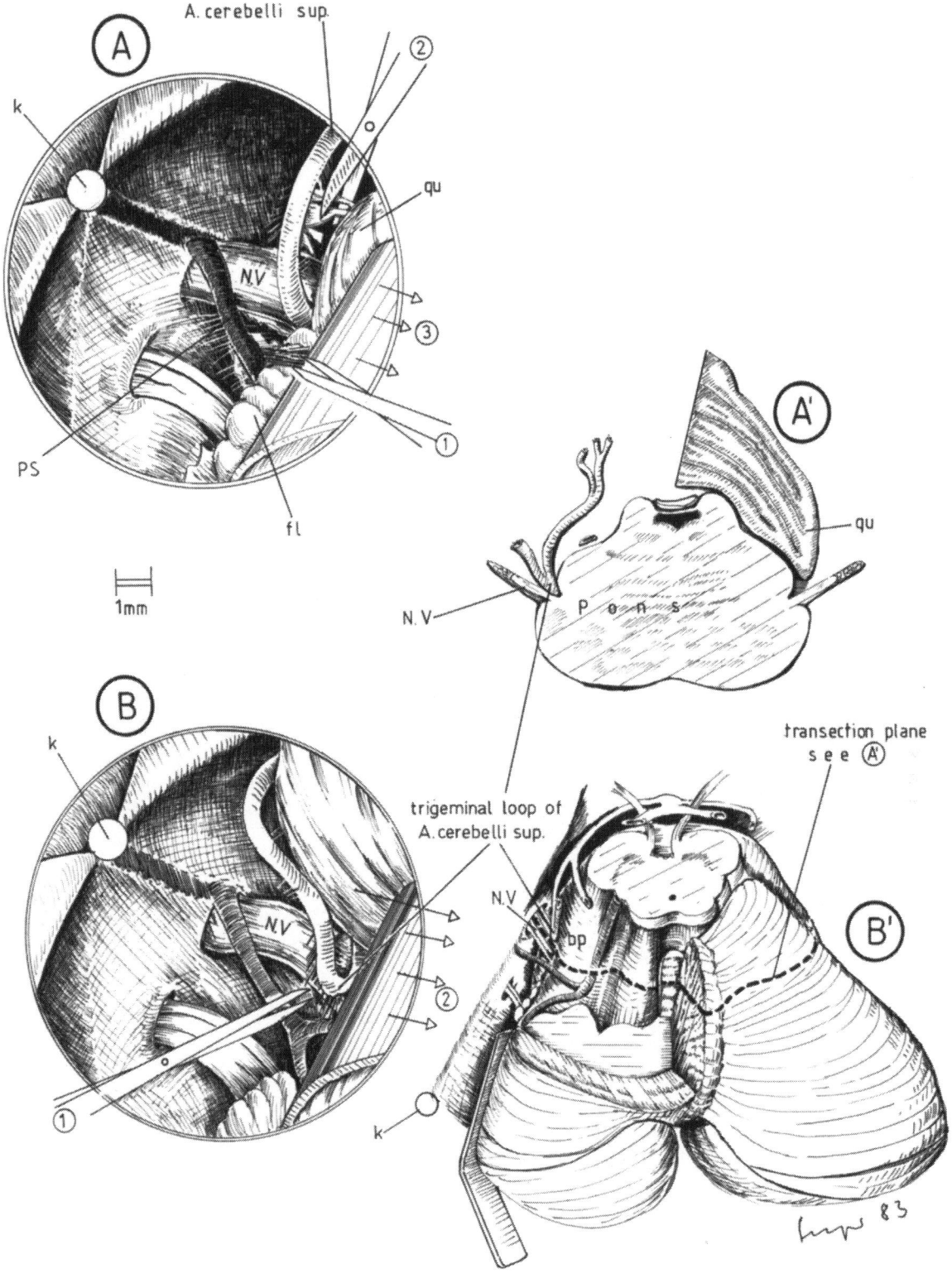
A
A. cerebelli sup.
k
qu
N.V
PS
fl
1mm
A'
qu
N.V
P o n s
B
k
N.V
trigeminal loop of
A. cerebelli sup.
transection plane
see A'
N.V
bp
B'
k

Fig. 178. Decompression of N. V and N. VII in cerebello-pontine angle.
Microsurgical operation

A **1** Loosening and cutting of remaining adhesions between N. VII/VIII and Flocculus *–fl–*

2 Loosening of remaining adhesions at dura penetration point of N. V

3 Separation of remaining arachnoidal adhesions on A. cerebelli sup. loop

4 Again, slight forward positioning of spatula (light arrows), until the juncture Pons – Brachium pontis can be seen, at pontine N. V exit

B **1** Lifting of A. cerebelli sup. loop from N. V. and Brachium pontis *–bp–*.
Light arrow: small muscle piece is positioned between dorsal surface of N. V and A. cerebelli sup. loop

B' Operation site, overview

2 Excision of small muscle piece from nape muscles

3 Positioning of muscle piece between N. V. and A. cerebelli sup. loop, see **B**

Abbreviations:

bp Brachium pontis
fl Flocculus
k Knee of Sinus transversus/sigmoideus
p Pons

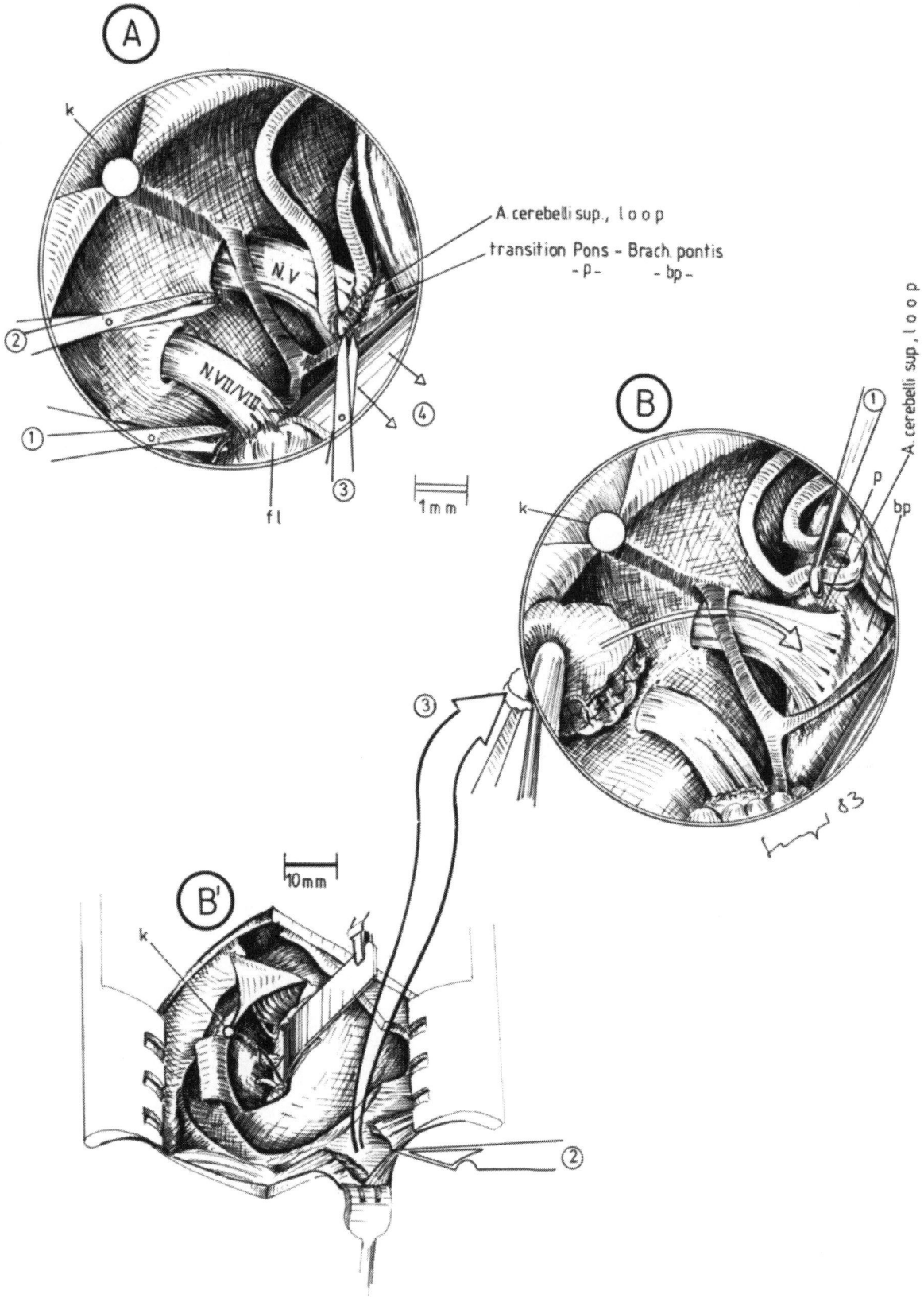
A
k
A. cerebelli sup., l o o p
transition Pons - Brach. pontis
- p - - bp -
N. V
N. VII/VIII
fl
1mm
B
k
A. cerebelli sup., l o o p
p
bp
B'
10mm
k

Fig. 179. Decompression of N. V and N. VII in cerebello-pontine angle.
Microsurgical operation

A **1** Insertion of muscle piece under V. petrosa sup. –*PS*–. Fascia and muscle are soaked with thrombin-calcium-solution*

2 Injection of fibrogen concentrate* beneath muscle (between muscle and N. V)

3 Attachment of A. cerebelli sup. loop to fascia by means of tissue glue*, similar to **2**

A' Anatomical transection sketch for **A.** Muscle positioning between artery and nerve

B Dura suture, wound closure

Abbreviation:

PS V. petrosa sup.

* Immuno.

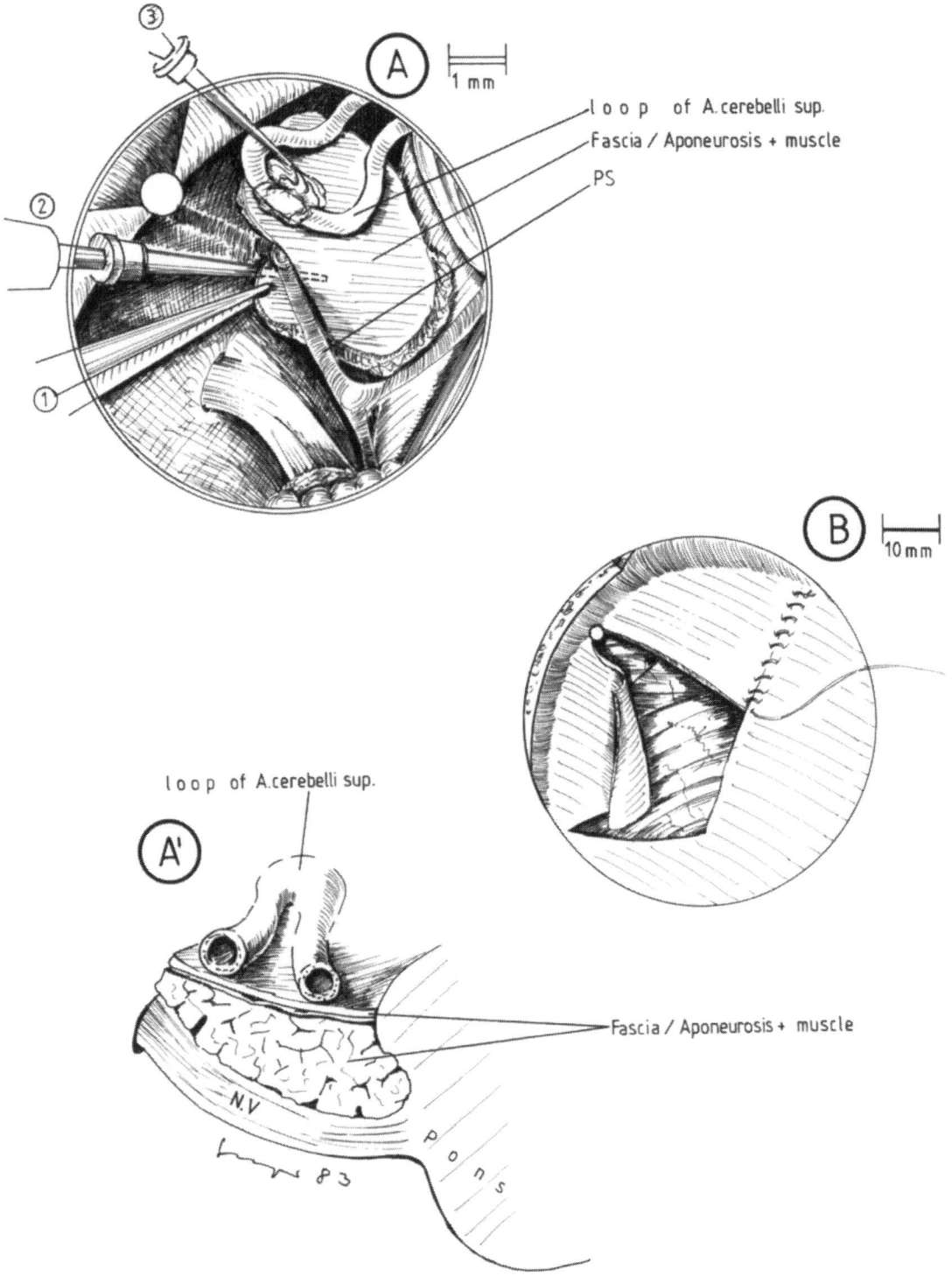
A
1 mm
loop of A.cerebelli sup.
Fascia / Aponeurosis + muscle
PS
B
10 mm
loop of A.cerebelli sup.
A'
Fascia / Aponeurosis + muscle
N.V
Pons
83

Fig. 180. Decompression of N. V and N. VII in cerebello-pontine angle.
Microsurgical operation
Clinical example of trigeminal neuralgia with facial tic on left side caused by A. basilaris loop compression of N. V and N. VII. After operation trigeminal neuralgia and facial tic have disappeared

A Angiogram shows A. basilaris loop, pointing toward the right side

A' Loop is not only pointing to the right side, but also dorsally

B In ap-angiogram (right sided A. cubitalis) one recognizes hypoplasia of right A. vertebralis

B' As **B,** lateral view

C Position sketch of A. basilaris and brain stem with hypoplastic right A. vertebralis based on angiogram

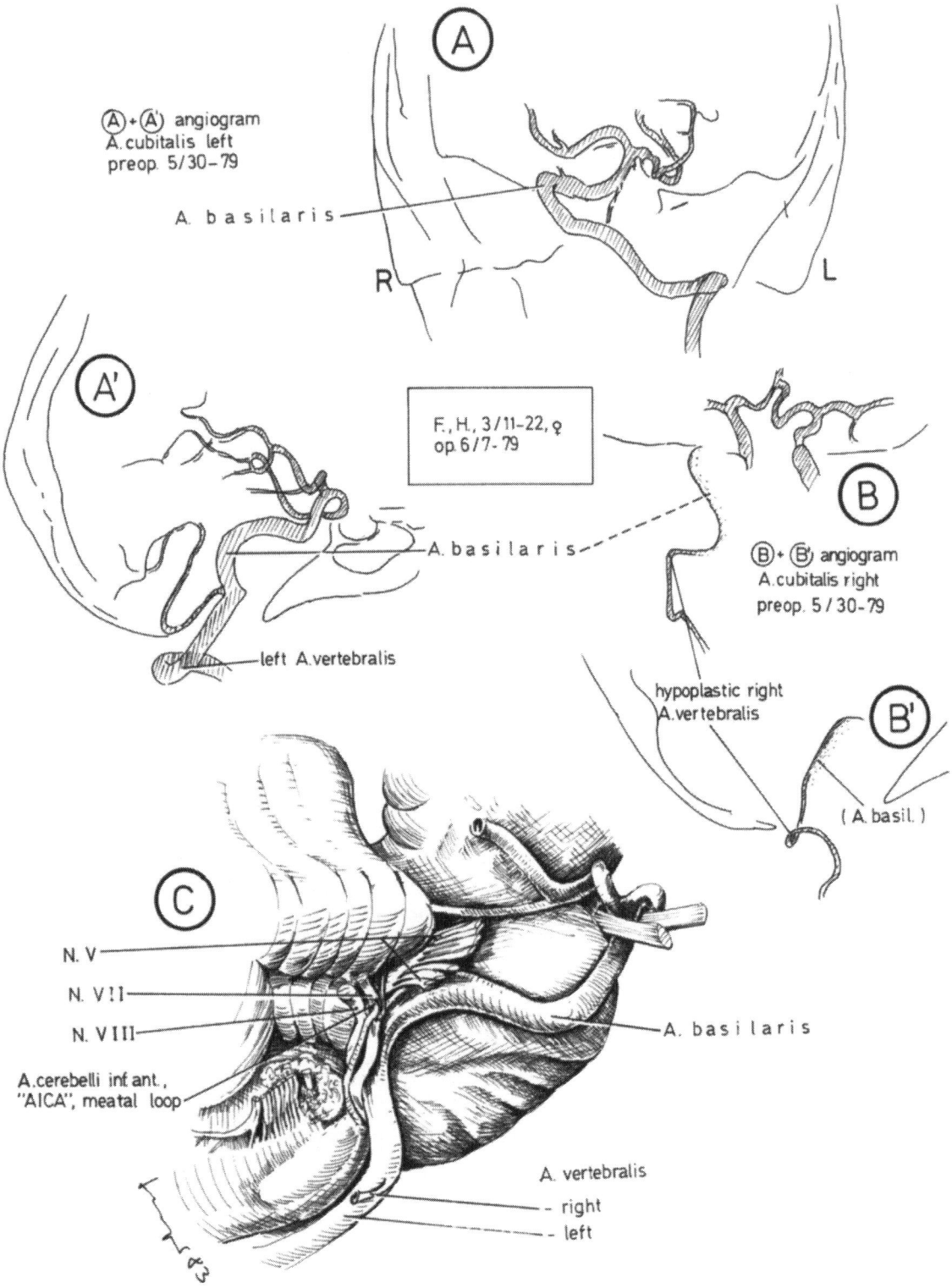
A
Ⓐ+Ⓐ' angiogram
A.cubitalis left
preop. 5/30-79
A. basilaris
R
L
A'
F., H., 3/11-22, ♀
op. 6/7-79
A. basilaris
left A.vertebralis
B
Ⓑ+Ⓑ' angiogram
A.cubitalis right
preop. 5/30-79
hypoplastic right
A.vertebralis
B'
(A. basil.)
C
N. V
N. VII
N. VIII
A.cerebelli inf.ant.,
"AICA", meatal loop
A. basilaris
A. vertebralis
- right
- left

Fig. 181. Decompression of N. V and N. VII in cerebello-pontine angle.
Microsurgical operation

A Microsurgical site. For teaching purposes, reclination of cerebellum between spatula and Porus acusticus int. is drawn approx. 2 cm wide. This site constitutes a combination of several microsurgical sites where, each time, reclination amounted to only 0,5 cm (repeated repositioning of spatula). One recognizes the close topographical relation of A. basilaris to N. V, VII and VIII

A' Anatomical sketch of cerebellum and lower brain stem, corresponding to microsurgical site **A**

B Cerebellum and lower brain stem, view from right sided dorsobasal direction. The drawn-in right cerebellum-pontine angle is deformed, corresponding to deformation caused by the atypical path of A. basilaris. Broken lines: projection of A. basilaris upon brain stem.

Arrows: **I** Operative approach to N. VII
II Operative approach to N. V

Abbreviations:

fl Flocculus
(k) Knee of Sinus transversus/sigmoideus (projection)
pch Plexus chorioideus
sp Sinus petrosus sup.
te Tentorium
PS V. petrosa sup.

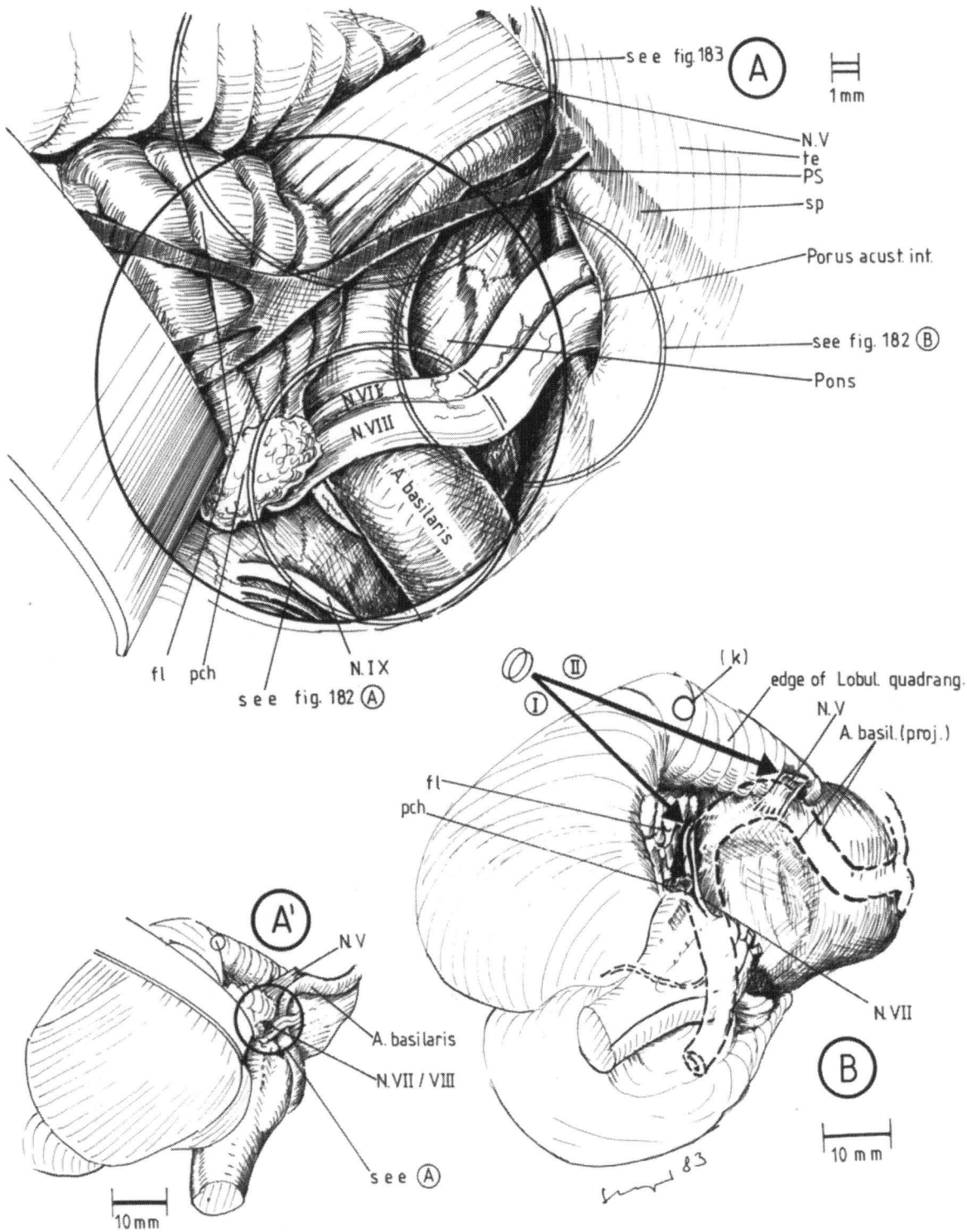
see fig. 183
A
1 mm
N.V
te
PS
sp
Porus acust. int.
see fig. 182 B
Pons
N.VII
N.VIII
A. basilaris
fl
pch
N.IX
see fig. 182 A
II
I
(k)
edge of Lobul. quadrang.
N.V
A. basil. (proj.)
fl
pch
N.VII
B
10 mm
A'
N.V
A. basilaris
N.VII / VIII
see A
10 mm

Fig. 182. Decompression of N. V and N. VII in cerebello-pontine angle.
Microsurgical operation

A Medial preparation
- **1** **Slight** reclination of A. basilaris by sucker
- **2** Separation of adhesions between A. basilaris and N. VII at its exit from Fossa supraolivaris
- **3** Separation of adhesions between N. VII and A. basilaris at the middle portion of nerve path
- **4** Repositioning of sucker, to check whether further adhesions must be separated
- **5** Interposition of a muscle piece taken from nape muscles (with remnants of fibrous tissue)

B Lateral preparation at Porus acusticus int.
- **1** Repositioning of sucker (during all preparations in the cerebello-pontine angle, minimal suction and cotton wool layer beneath sucker should be used)
- **2** Separation of adhesions between N. VII and N. VIII. A. labyrinthi with branches is preserved
- **3** + **4** Separation of further adhesions of A. basilaris, N. VII and N. VIII

Abbreviations:

fl Flocculus
obl Medulla oblongata
pch Plexus chorioideus

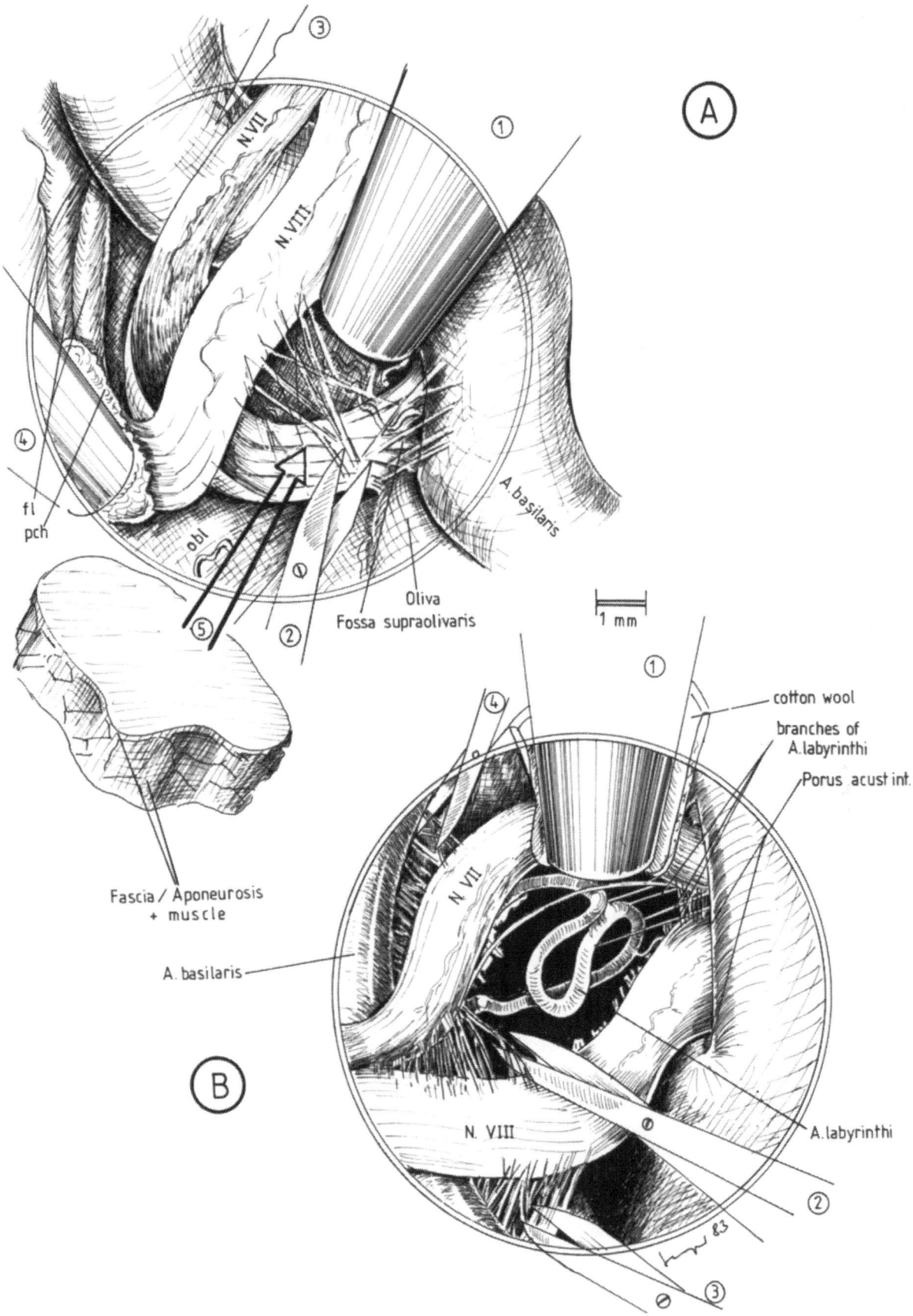
A
B
N. VII
N. VIII
A. basilaris
Oliva
Fossa supraolivaris
fl
pch
obl
1 mm
cotton wool
branches of
A. labyrinthi
Porus acust. int.
Fascia / Aponeurosis
+ muscle
A. basilaris
A. labyrinthi

Fig. 183. Decompression of N. V and N. VII in cerebello-pontine angle.
Microsurgical operation

A Microsurgical site of N. V. As in Fig. 181, this presentation constitutes a combination of several microsurgical sites

- **1** Separation of adhesions between N. V. and Pons *–p–*, as well as Lobulus quadrangularis *–qu–*
- **2** Repositioning of spatula, after separation of adhesions
- **3** Separation of adhesions between Tentorium *–tc–* and N. V
- **4** Separation of adhesions between A. basilaris and N. V
- **5a + 5b** Preparation and separation of adhesions of N. V, Brachium pontis/Pons *–bp/p–*, as well as Flocculus. Note: V. petrosa sup. *–PS–* is hypoplastic

B Supplement to **A**

- **2** Normally, Lobulus quadrangularis covers exit point of N. V from Brachium pontis/pons area *–bp/p–*. Only after preparation of Lobulus quadrangularis with separation of arachnoidal adhesions between Lobulus quadrangularis, brain stem and N. V., can reclination – as in **2** – be carried out, arrow

Abbreviations:

bp	Brachium pontis
bp/p	Brachium pontis/pons transition area
f	Flocculus
p	Pons
qu	Lobulus quadrangularis
te	Tentorium
PS	V. petrosa sup.

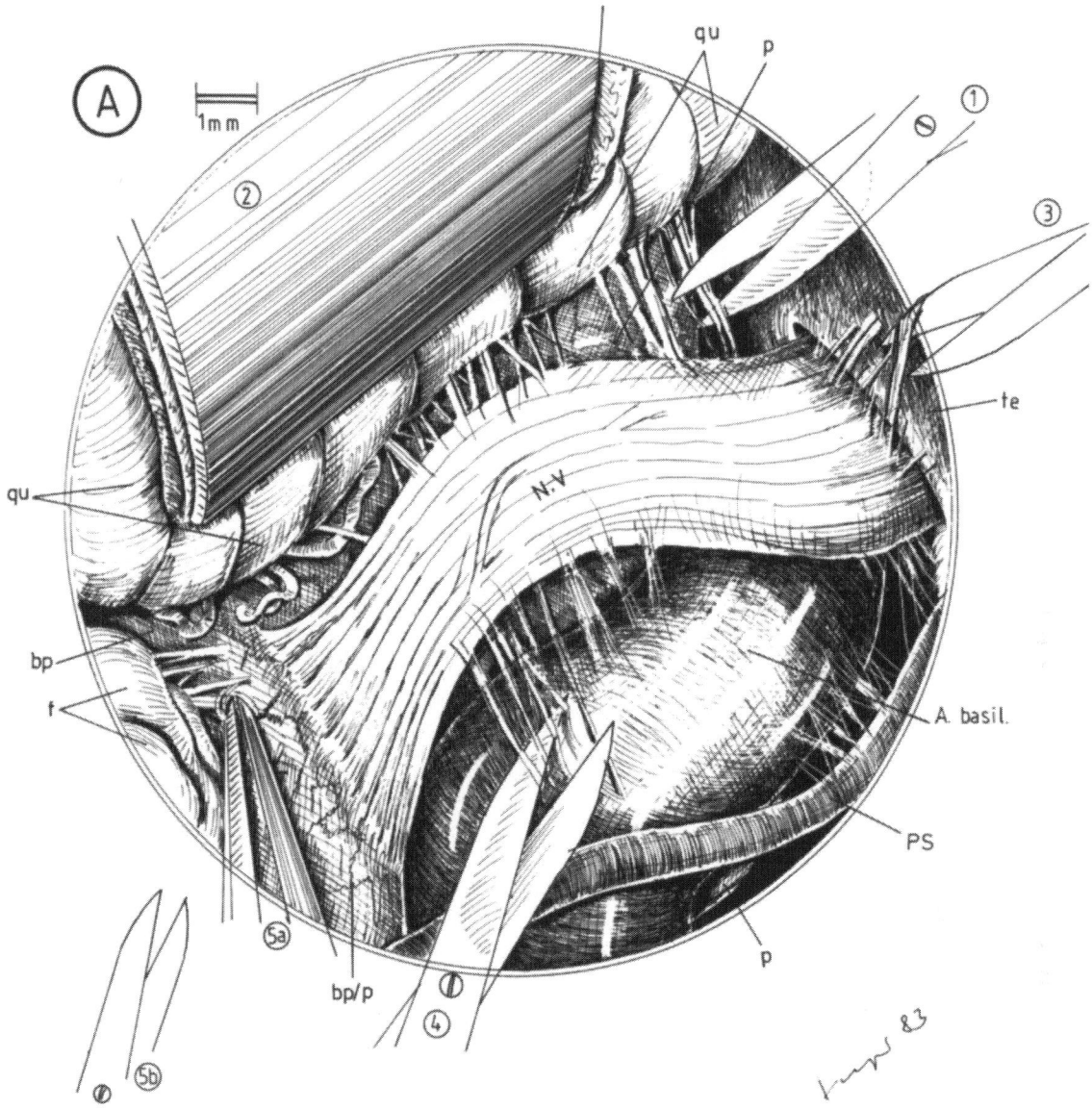
A
1mm
qu
p
1
2
3
te
N.V
qu
bp
f
A. basil.
PS
p
5a
bp/p
4
5b

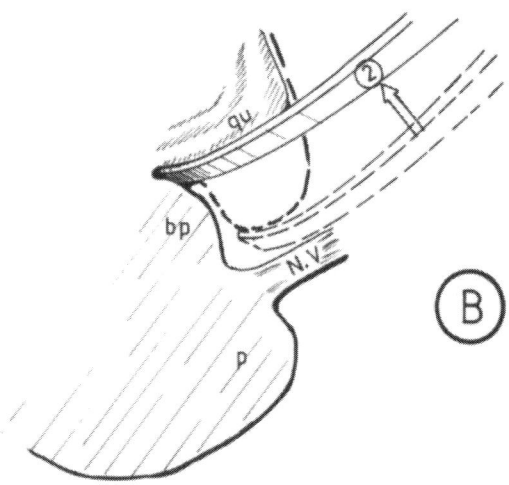
2
qu
bp
N.V
B
p

Fig. 184. Decompression of N. V and N. VII in cerebello-pontine angle.
Microsurgical operation

A Microsurgical site. Muscle piece taken from nape muscles (with connective tissue) was inserted between N. V, VII and VIII and A. basilaris

1 Muscle piece, soaked with thrombin/calcium solution, is squirted with fibrinogen concentrate*, in order to attach to A. basilaris

2 Pressing of muscle piece against A. basilaris. **The thinner the fibrin film, the more reliable is the gluing**

B + B' Brain stem transections of mid-Pons and upper Medulla oblongata

B Positioning of muscle between A. basilaris and N. V. Light arrow: Pushing A. basilaris away from N. V

B' Positioning of muscle between A. basilaris and N. VII. Light arrow: Pushing A. basilaris from N. VII.
Wound closure

Abbreviations:

fl Flocculus
pch Plexus chorioideus
qu Lobulus quadrangularis
PS V. petrosa sup.

* Immuno.

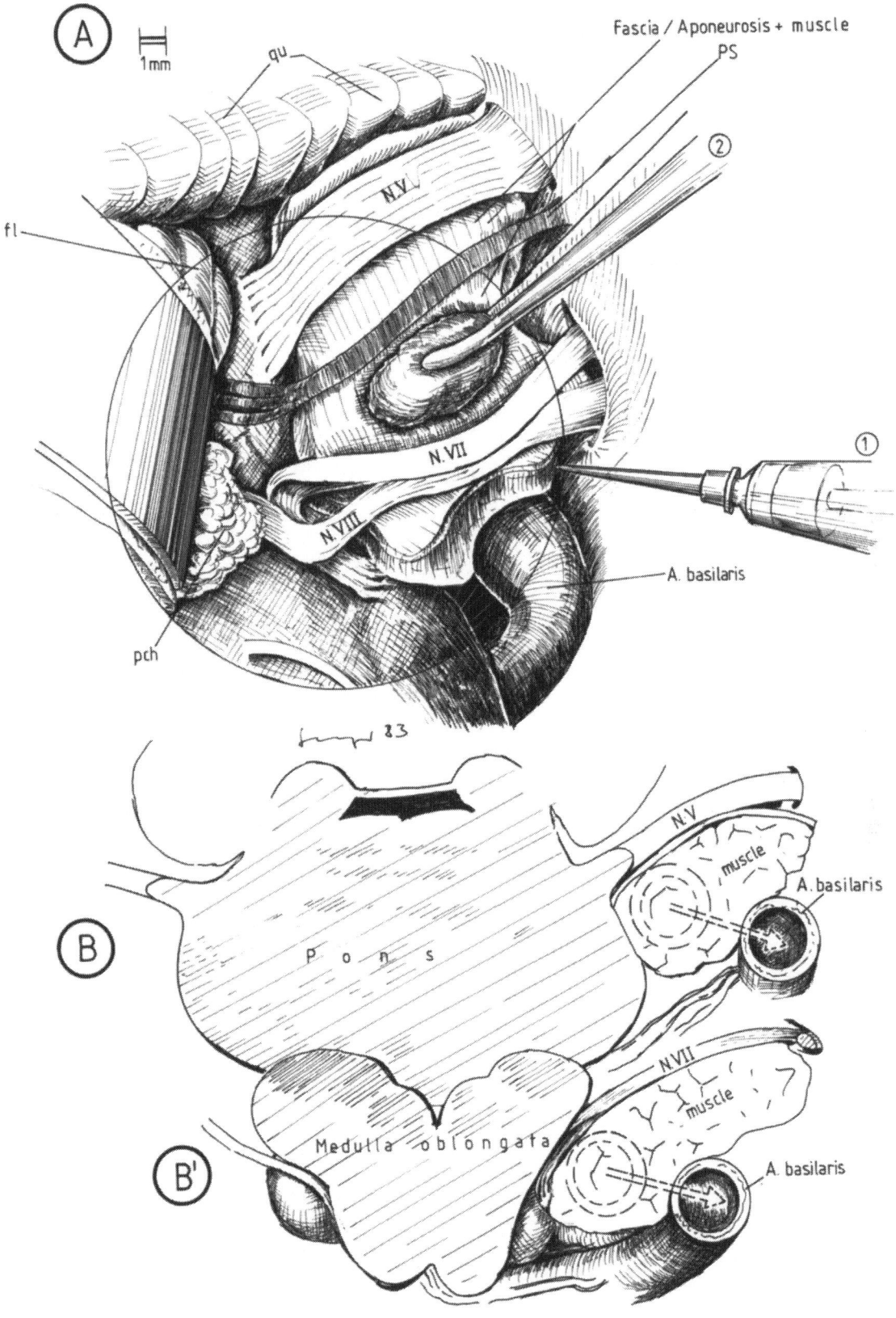
A
1mm
qu
Fascia / Aponeurosis + muscle
PS
②
N.V.
fl
N.VII
①
N.VIII
A. basilaris
pch
B
N.V
muscle
A. basilaris
P o n s
N.VII
muscle
Medulla oblongata
B'
A. basilaris

Chapter 6

Operations at the Base of Fossa cranii post. (Figs. 185 to 200)

Epidermoid, pre- and paramedullary (Figs. 185 to 194)

Fig. 185. Basal tumors of posterior Fossa.
Clinical example of epidermoid: pre- and paramedullary, pre- and parapontine, pre- and paramesencephalic; no pre- or postoperative neurological deficits.
Diagnostic procedures

A Premedullary tumor between Clivus and Medulla oblongata, extending to the right

B Pre- and parapontine tumor portion. Beyond Tentorium temporomedially –*x*– a tumor portion is seen which expanded from Cisterna ambiens, beneath parahippocampal area, into supratentorial space

C Tumor lies in front of and alongside Mesencephalon and widens Cisterna ambiens irregularly

A' – C' Postoperative findings: no tumor remnant can be recognized; supratentorial temporomedial portion –*x*– is removed also

Abbreviations:

m Mesencephalon
o Medulla oblongata
p Pons
p-m Ponto-mesencephalic transition
x Temporo-medialy tumor portion

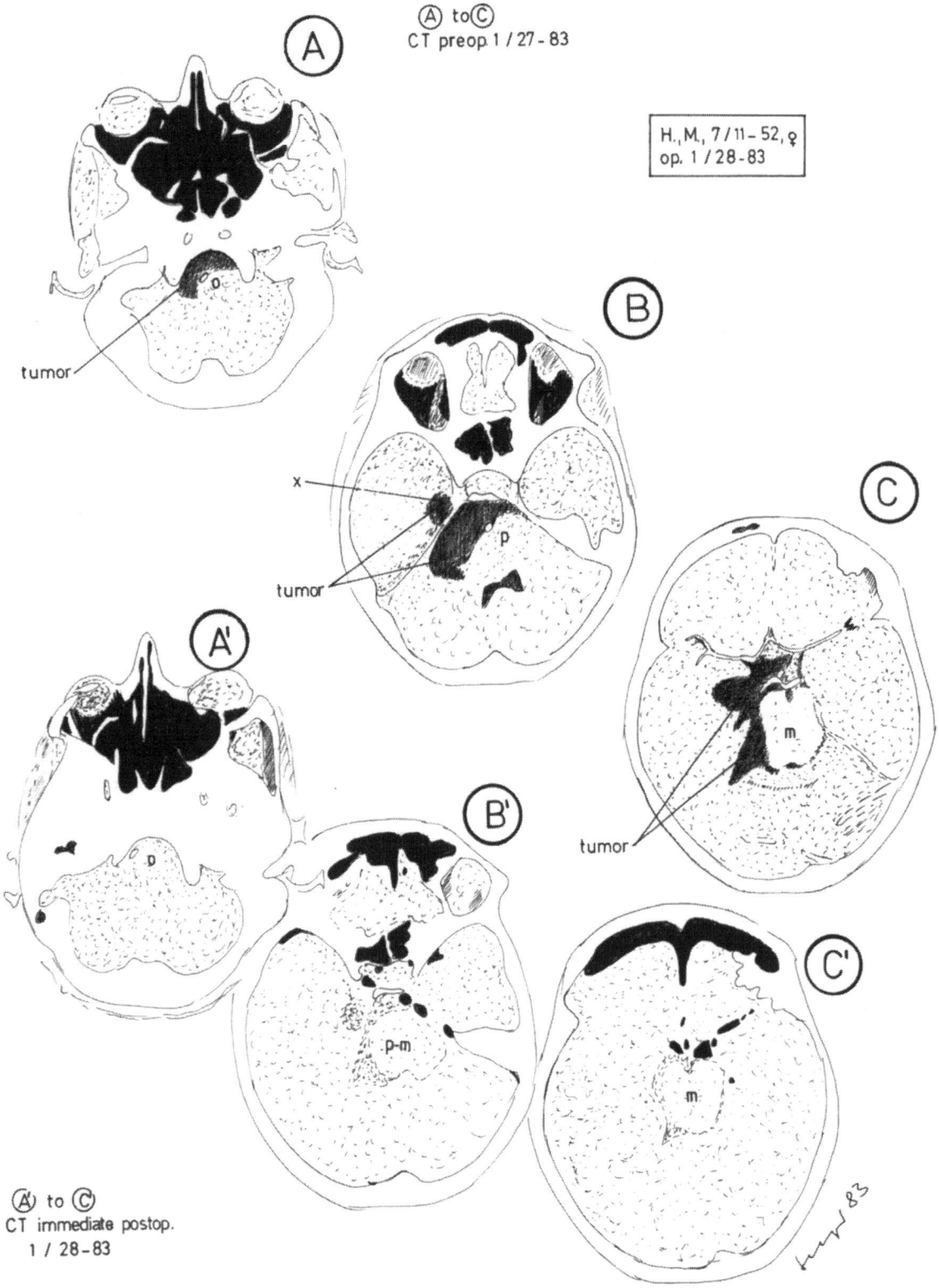
Ⓐ to Ⓒ
CT preop. 1 / 27 - 83
H., M., 7 / 11 - 52, ♀
op. 1 / 28 - 83
A
tumor
B
x
tumor
C
tumor
A'
B'
p-m
C'
Ⓐ' to Ⓒ'
CT immediate postop.
1 / 28 - 83

Fig. 186. Basal tumors of posterior Fossa.
Operation of an epidermoid.
Microsurgical operation

A Anatomical sketch corresponding to Fig. 185 CTs.
Anatomical section planes lie transverse to brain stem axis, and thus lie in a different plane than that of CTs Fig. 185 **A – C**

B Anatomical section sketch, section planes see **A.** Tumor displaced Medulla oblongata and expanded within several cisterns

C Anatomical section sketch, section plane see **A.** Pons is compressed and displaced

D Anatomical section sketch, section plane see **A.** Tumor reaches from Corpora quadrigemina area to N. oculomotorius, surrounding it.
(x): temporo-medial portion, projection on Tentorium undersurface

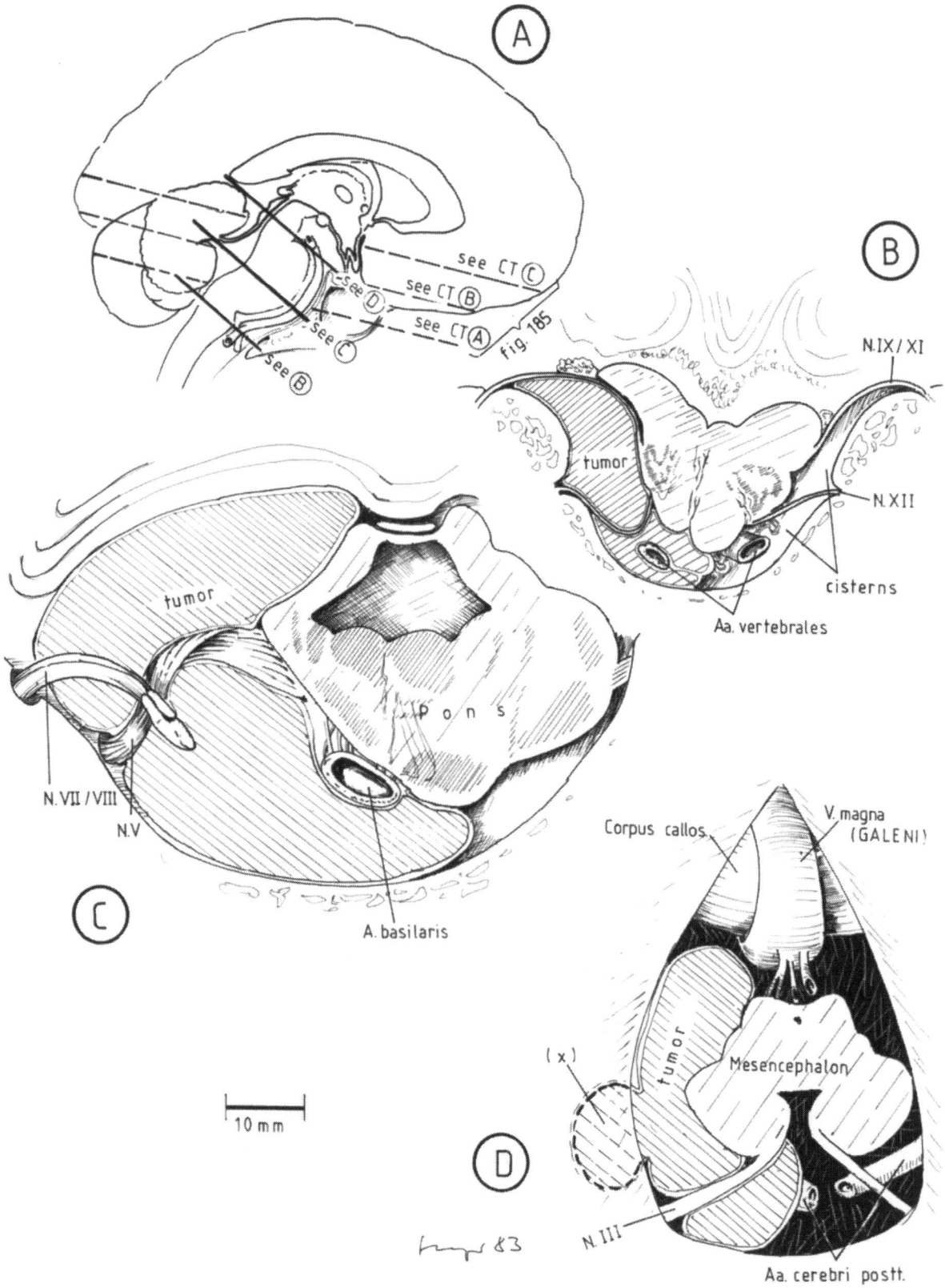
A
see CT C
see CT B
see CT A
see D
see C
see B
fig. 185
B
N.IX/XI
tumor
N.XII
cisterns
Aa. vertebrales
tumor
pons
N.VII/VIII
N.V
A. basilaris
C
Corpus callos.
V. magna (GALENI)
tumor
Mesencephalon
(x)
10 mm
D
N.III
Aa. cerebri postt.

Fig. 187. Basal tumors of posterior Fossa.
Operation of an epidermoid.
Microsurgical operation

A Position of trepanation and dura incision, indicated on skull sketch. Position of skull corresponds to head position during operation

A' Sketch of skull base, view from above, trepanation sketched in, supplement to **A.** Arrow: initial direction of operative approach

B Operative site after trepanation and dura opening

C Reclination of cerebellum using spatula. Arrow: microsurgical view for Fig. 188

Abbreviations:

fo Edge of Foramen occipitale
pm Processus mastoideus
ss Sinus sigmoideus
st Sinus transversus

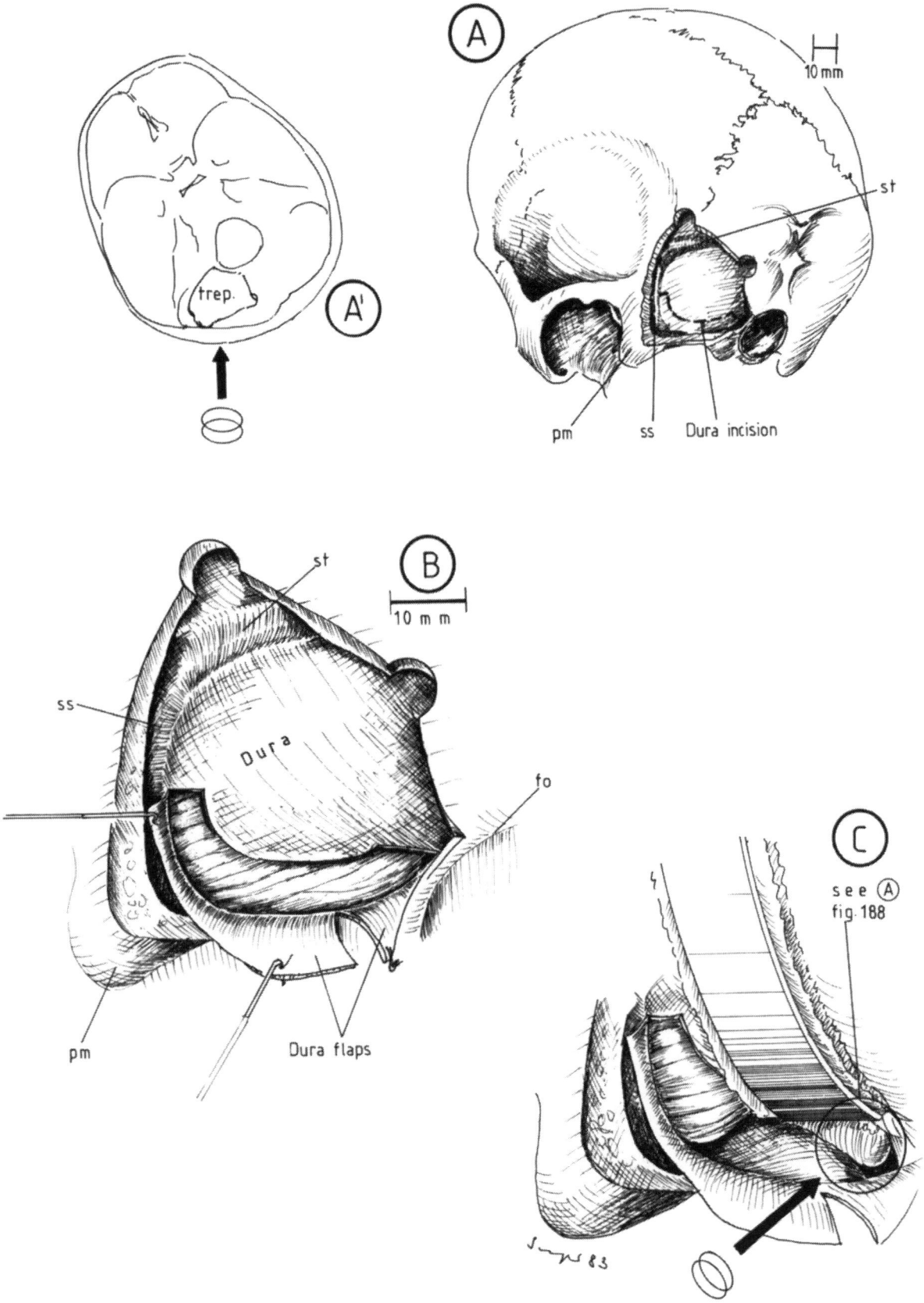
A
10 mm
st
pm
ss
Dura incision
trep.
A'
B
st
10 m m
ss
Dura
fo
pm
Dura flaps
C
see A
fig. 188

Fig. 188. Basal tumors of posterior Fossa.
Operation of an epidermoid.
Microsurgical operation

A Microsurgical site. Continuation of Fig. 187
- **1** Reclination of Tonsilla cerebelli
- **2** Pulling away an artery (branch or hypoplastic trunk of A. cerebelli inf. post. –PICA–)
- **3a + 3b** Opening and pulling away arachnoidea lying over lower tumor end

B **1a** Holding tumor with sucker
- **1b** Hollowing tumor with curette
- **2a + 2b** The same procedure as in **1a + 1b** applied to a medial tumor lump in a second cistern chamber, in front of Medulla oblongata and A. vertebralis

C Anatomical position of tumor portions shown in **A + B;** posterior view, not lateral inferior view as microsurgical site

Abbreviations:

pch Plexus chorioideus
tj Tuberculum jugulare

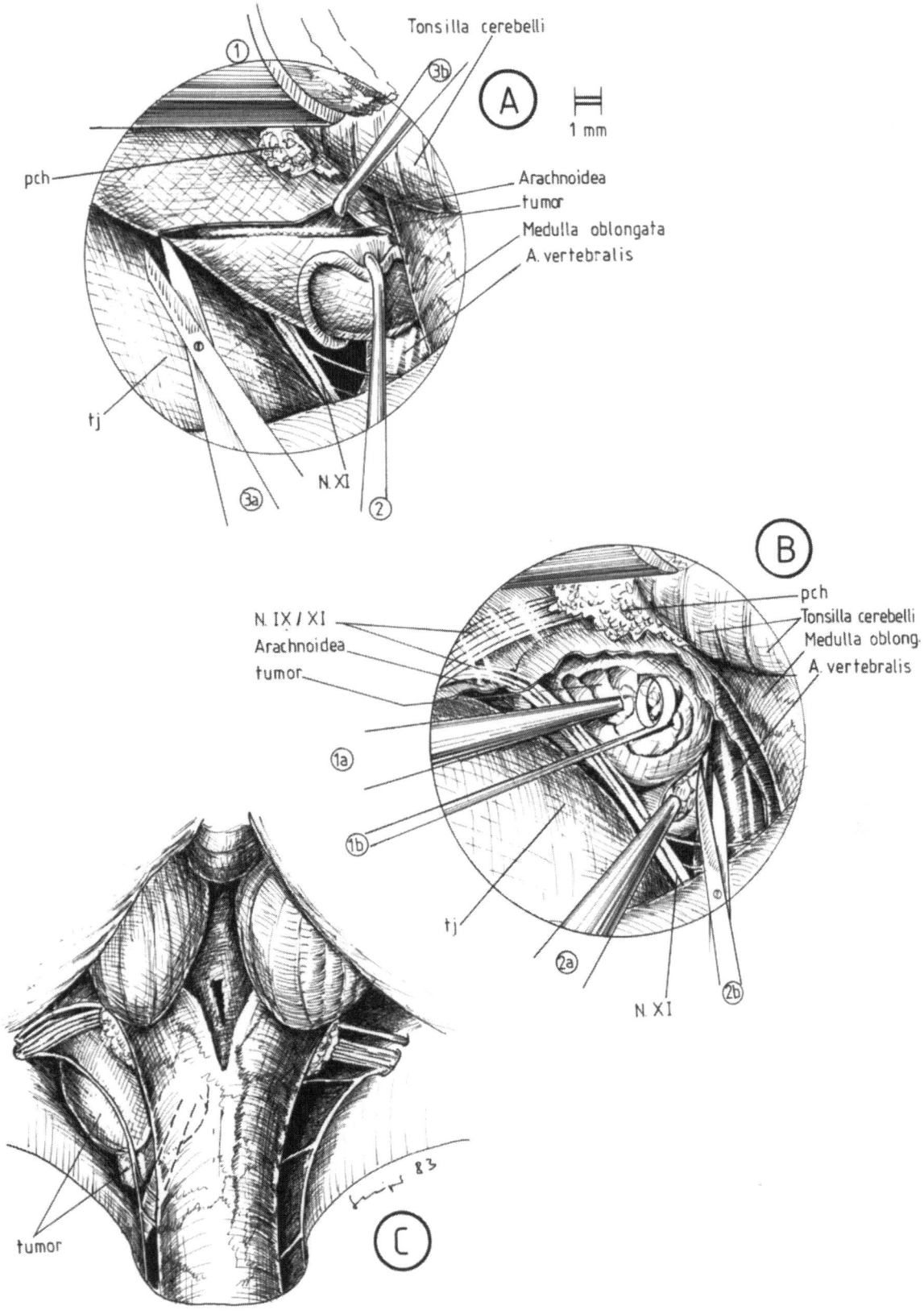
Tonsilla cerebelli
1
3b
A
1 mm
pch
Arachnoidea
tumor
Medulla oblongata
A. vertebralis
tj
N. XI
3a
2
B
pch
N. IX / XI
Tonsilla cerebelli
Arachnoidea
Medulla oblong.
tumor
A. vertebralis
1a
1b
tj
2a
N. XI
2b
tumor
C

Fig. 189. Basal tumors of posterior Fossa.
Operation of an epidermoid.
Microsurgical operation

A Topographical relation after removal of lower tumor portions

B **1** Spatula placed farther laterally
2 Change of microsurgical approach (arrow)

C Microsurgical site, enlargement from **B**
1 Preparation and incision of arachnoidea and tumor (broken line), corresponding to **D** –*x*–. Microsurgical preparation corresponding to this sketch is presented in Fig. 190

D Anatomical sketch showing caudal tumor portion removed as far as hatched zone –*x*–

Abbreviations:

df Dura flap
fl Flocculus
mo Medulla oblongata
pch Plexus chorioideus
tj Tuberculum jugulare
to Tonsilla cerebelli
vl A. vertebralis
x Tumor resection surface (broken line in **C**)
PS V. petrosa sup.

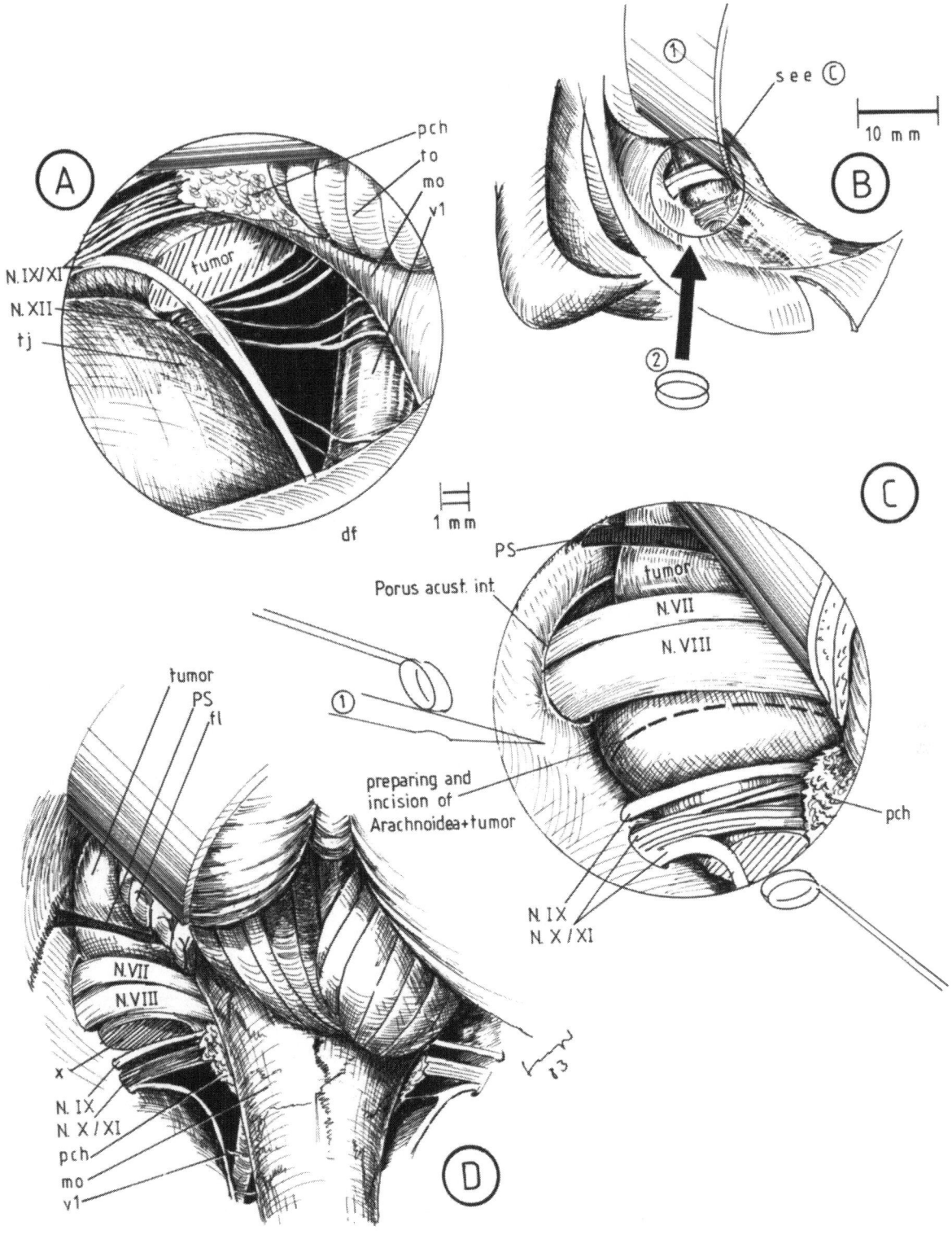
A
pch
to
mo
v1
tumor
N. IX/XI
N. XII
tj
df
1 mm
B
see C
10 mm
1
2
C
PS
tumor
Porus acust. int.
N. VII
N. VIII
1
preparing and
incision of
Arachnoidea+tumor
pch
N. IX
N. X / XI
D
tumor
PS
fl
N. VII
N. VIII
x
N. IX
N. X / XI
pch
mo
v1

Fig. 190. Basal tumors of posterior Fossa.
Operation of an epidermoid.
Microsurgical operation

A **1a** Holding (and removal by suction) of tumor portion beneath N. IX to XI

1b Hollowing tumor with curette

2a + 2b The same procedure as in **1a + 1b** beneath N. VII and VIII

3 Arachnoidea preparation and tumor incision as in Fig. 188 **A + B,** here between V. petrosa sup. *–PS–* and N. VII

B Loosening of tumor from undersurface of N. VII and N. VIII. Arachnoidal layer *–a–* covering tumor is left on undersurface of N. VII and N. VIII. Tumor shell can be separated from thickened arachnoidea in a single piece *

2 + 3 Examination of arachnoidal niches for tumor remnents. Arrow: Change of view direction for **C**

C Loosening of tumor-enclosed N. V. Nerve fascicles are held together by arachnoidal layer, which is saved. In the meantime V. petrosa sup. *–PS–*, solitary and grossly hypoplastic, was interrupted

Abbreviations:

a Membranous cisternal arachnoidea
fl Flocculus
sp Sinus petrosus sup.
PS V. petrosa sup. (After ligation)
VP V. petrosa sup. (before Ligation)

---

* Tumor was completely enveloped by greatly thickened membranous cisternal arachnoidea (which here faciliated preparation and particularly protected cranial nerves sheathed by cisternal membranes).

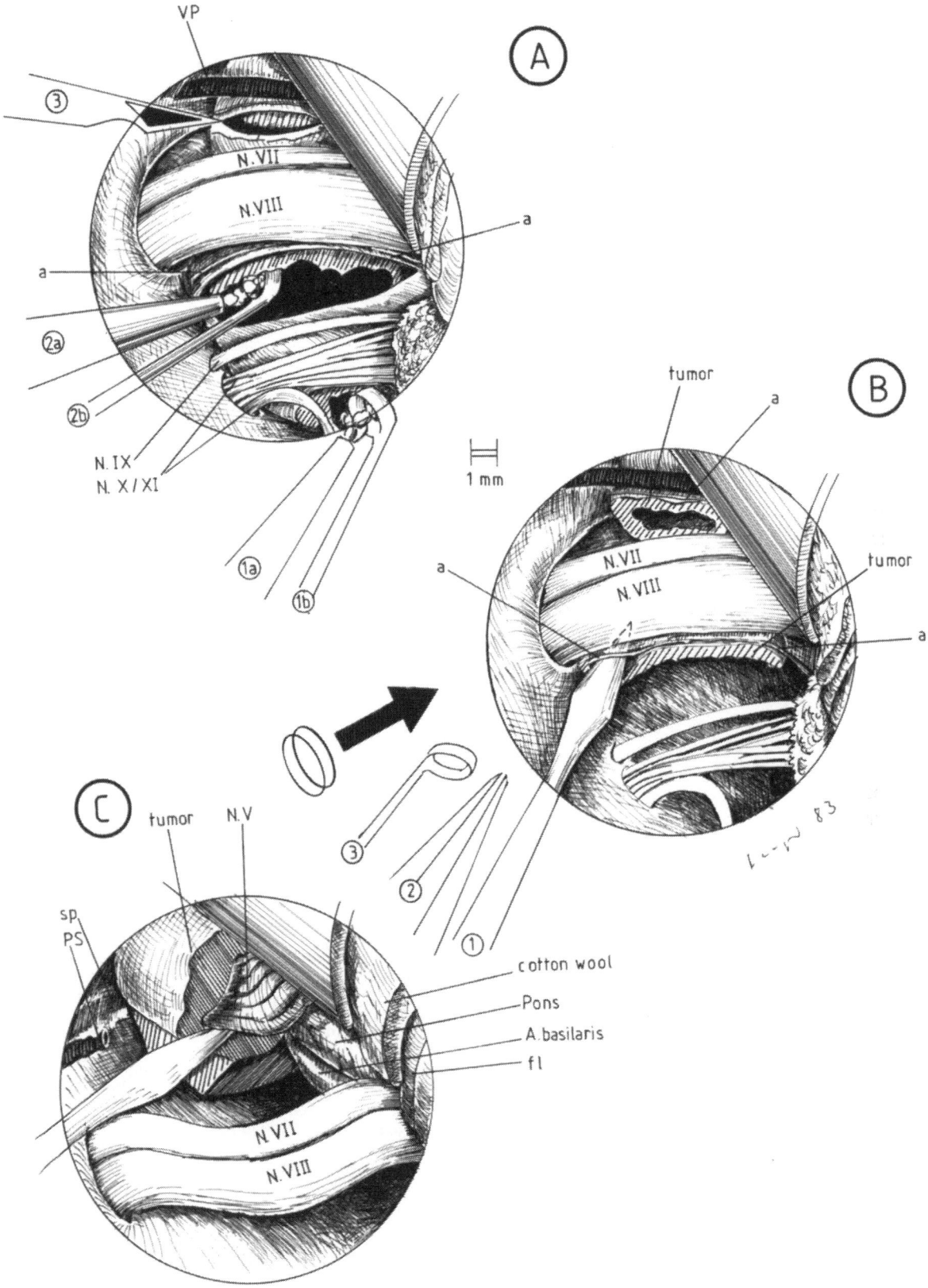
A
VP
3
N.VII
N.VIII
a
a
2a
2b
N. IX
N. X / XI
1a
1b
B
tumor
a
1 mm
N.VII
N.VIII
a
tumor
a
3
2
1
C
tumor
N.V
sp
PS
cotton wool
Pons
A.basilaris
fl
N.VII
N.VIII

Fig. 191. Basal tumors of posterior Fossa.
Operation of an epidermoid.
Microsurgical operation

A Microsurgical site. Tumor loosened from N. V on all sides, however, tumor portions crowd rostrally and displace trigeminal fibers downwards.

B Site after removal of additional tumor portions

C Anatomical sketch of cerebellar and brain stem preparation, dura structures drawn in. Arrows: **A – C:** operative approaches for Figs. 192–194

- **a** Preparation in the direction of prepontine cistern and Cisterna interpeduncularis
- **b** Preparation in Fissura horizontalis cerebelli as far as Corpora quadrigemina region
- **c** Preparation in Cisterna ambiens as far as base of parahippocampus region

Trigonum lemnisci at lateral mesencephalon wall is, because of rich vascularization, specifically designated

Abbreviations:

bc Brachium conjunctivum
bp Brachium pontis
fl Flocculus
sp Sinus petrosus sup.
PS V. petrosa sup. (remnant)

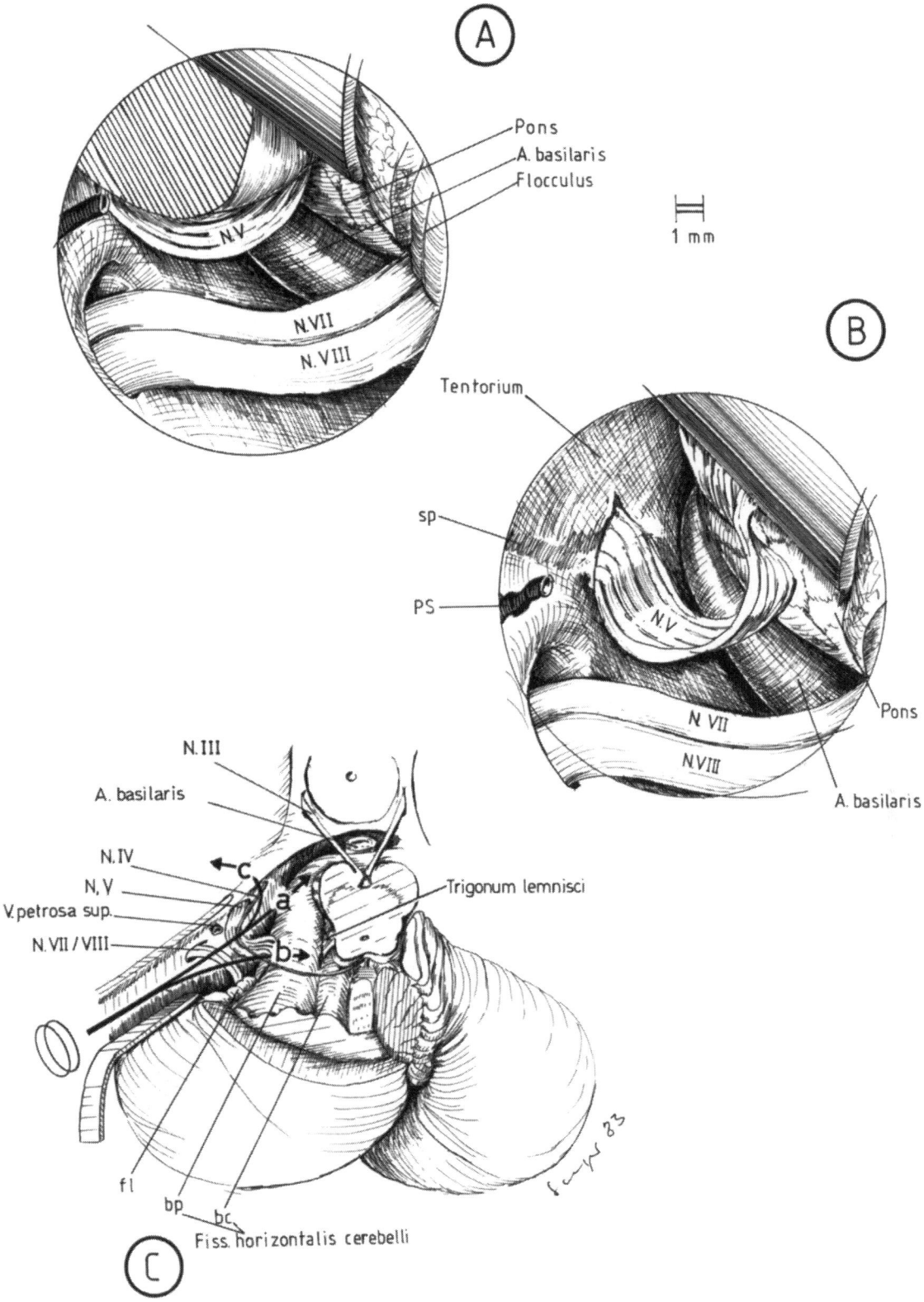
A
Pons
A. basilaris
Flocculus
N.V
N.VII
N.VIII
1 mm
B
Tentorium
sp
PS
N.V
N. VII
N.VIII
Pons
A. basilaris
N.III
A. basilaris
N.IV
N, V
V.petrosa sup.
N.VII / VIII
c
a
b
Trigonum lemnisci
fl
bp
bc
Fiss. horizontalis cerebelli
C

Fig. 192. Basal tumors of posterior Fossa.
Operation of an epidermoid.
Microsurgical operation.
Microsurgical preparation **a + b** from Fig. 191 **C**

A **1** Further insertion of spatula and pulling back Lobulus quadrangularis *–qu–*. Brachium pontis *–bp–* becomes visible

2a + 2b Arachnoidea preparation and opening of tumor as before. During tumor hollowing, A. cerebri post., N. IV and Crus cerebri *–cc–* gradually become visible

B **1** Spatula lying on Lobulus quadrangularis *–qu–*, is moved farther rostrally on Lobulus quadrangularis

2 Light arrows: reclination of rostral Lobulus quadrangularis portions *–qu–*

C Enlarged detail from **B**

1 New spatula position

2 Arachnoidea preparation, tumor incision, and tumor hollowing as before.
Arrow **b:** operative approach in direction of Fissura horizontalis cerebelli and Cisterna quadrangularis

Abbreviations:

a Arachnoidea
bp Brach. pontis
cc Crus cerebri
qu Lobulus quadrangularis
te Tentorium

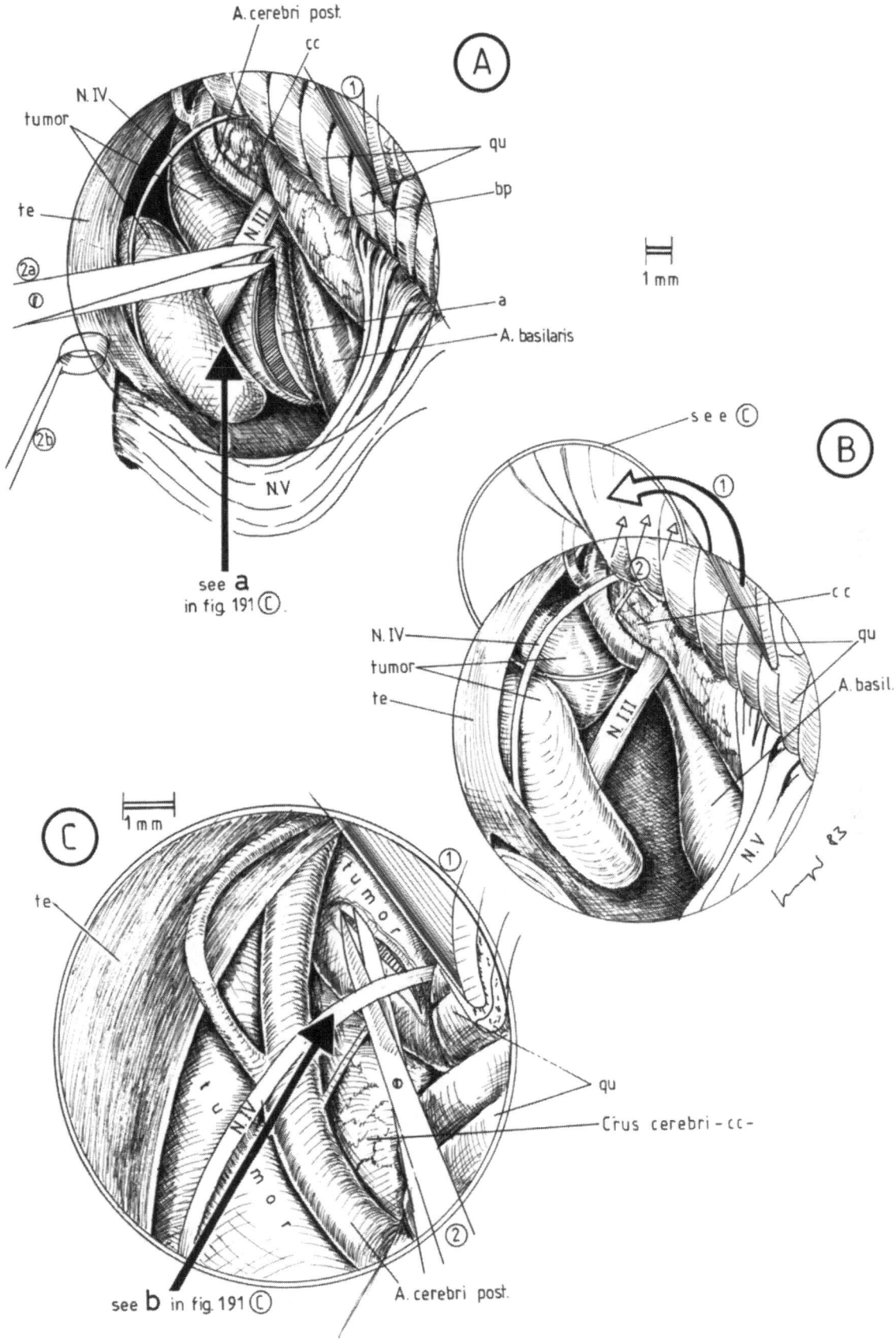
A
A. cerebri post.
cc
N. IV
tumor
te
qu
bp
N. III
2a
a
A. basilaris
2b
N. V
1 mm
see a
in fig. 191 C.
B
see C
cc
N. IV
tumor
te
qu
A. basil.
N. III
N. V
C
1 mm
te
tumor
qu
Crus cerebri - cc -
N. III
tumor
see b in fig. 191 C
A. cerebri post.

Fig. 193. Basal tumors of posterior Fossa.
Operation of an epidermoid
Microsurgical operation. Continuation of Fig. 192

A **1** Adjustment of spatula. One sees that Cisterna quadrigemina is free of tumor

2 Posterior and inferior to Corpora quadrigemina, in Fissura horizontalis cerebelli, there are still tumor remnants. (Arrow: approach **b** of Fig. 191 **C**)

3 Preparation of lateral tumor portions at Tentorium edge

B Removal of tumor remnants at Tentorium edge. Vessels and nerves are still sheathed by arachnoidal layer which is to be preserved. Arrows: varying approaches

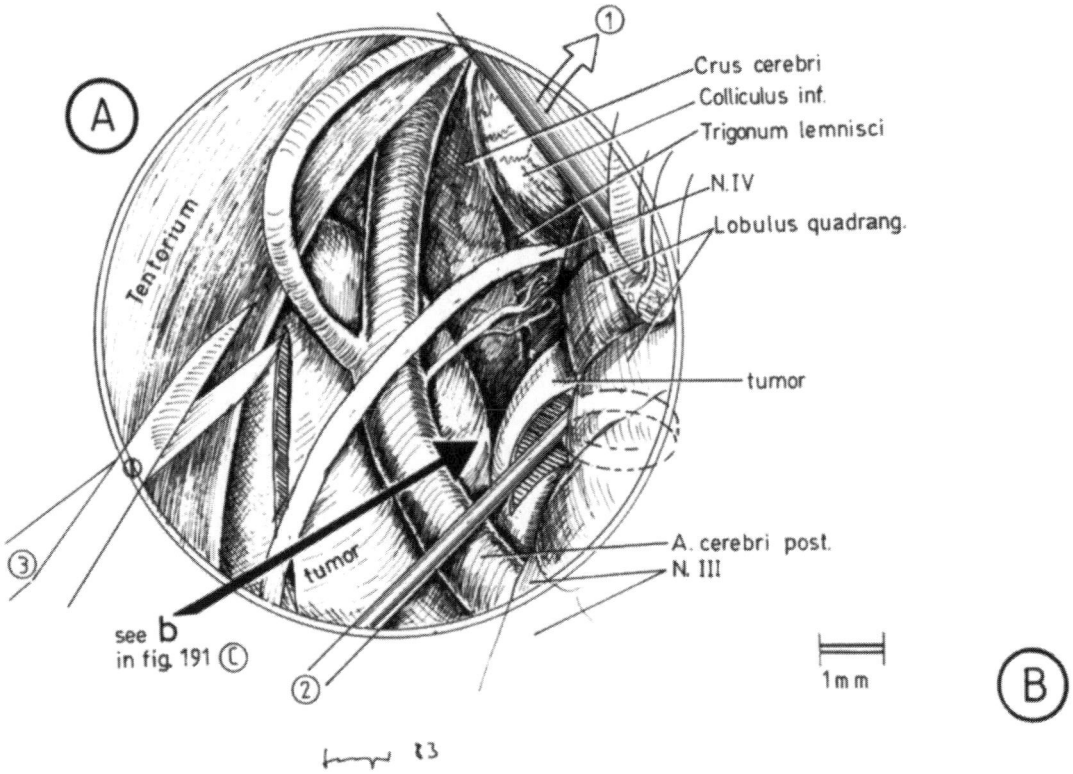
A
Tentorium
Crus cerebri
Colliculus inf.
Trigonum lemnisci
N.IV
Lobulus quadrang.
tumor
A. cerebri post.
N. III
tumor
see b
in fig. 191 C
1mm
B

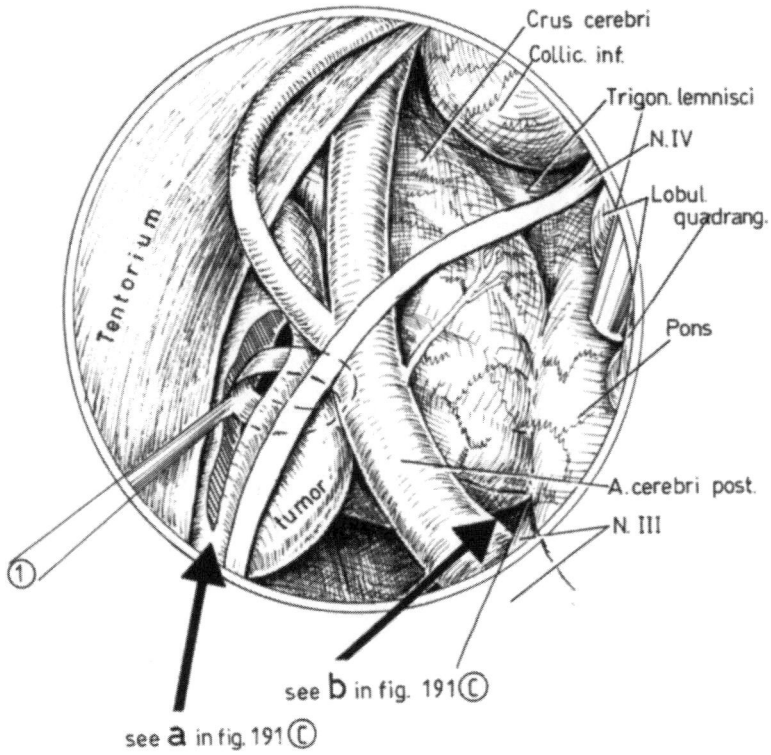
Crus cerebri
Collic. inf.
Trigon. lemnisci
N.IV
Lobul.
quadrang.
Pons
Tentorium
tumor
A.cerebri post.
N. III
see b in fig. 191 C
see a in fig. 191 C

Fig. 194. Basal tumors of posterior Fossa.
Operation of an epidermoid
Microsurgical operation

A **1** Cautious bipolar coagulation close to Trigonum lemnisci with minimal amperage

2 After pushing N. IV aside, temporo-basal tumor portion is removed, which also lies in an arachnoidal chamber. Arrow: approach to Cisterna ambiens and temporo-basal region

A' Site after tumor removal. **a, b, c** (arrows): approach directions (**a:** to Cisterna ambiens, **b:** to Fissura horizontalis cerebelli, **c:** to Cisterna ambiens and temporobasal region)
See also Fig. 191 **C.** Check shows no further tumor. Wound closure

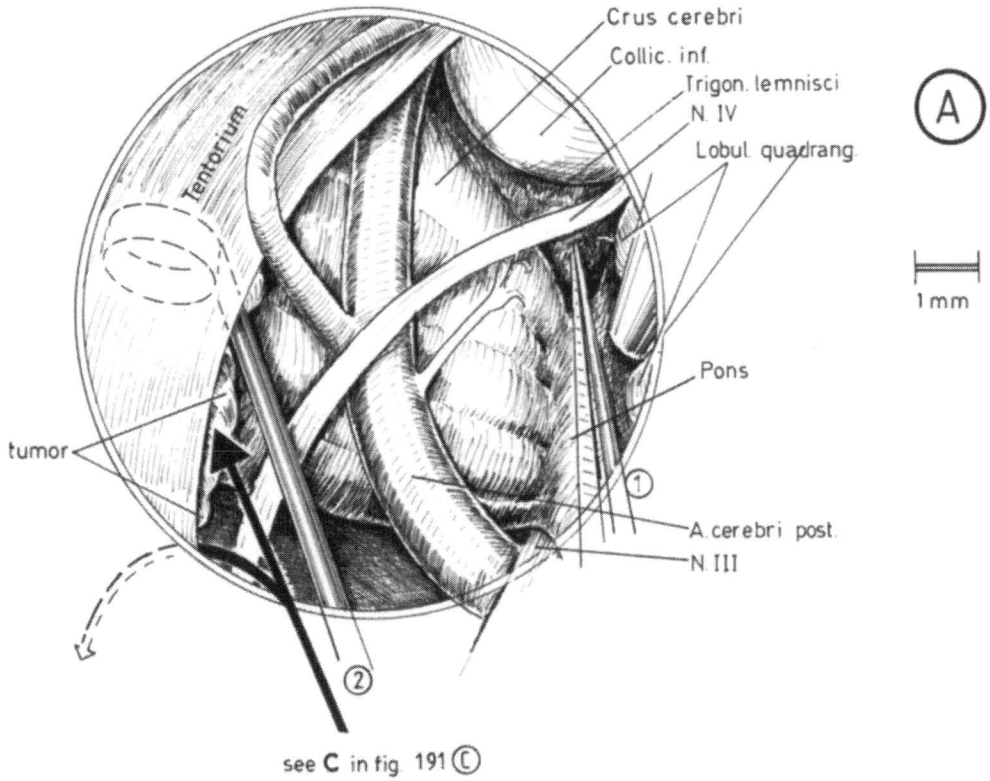
Crus cerebri
Collic. inf.
Trigon. lemnisci
N. IV
Lobul. quadrang.
Tentorium
A
1 mm
Pons
tumor
1
A. cerebri post.
N. III
2
see C in fig. 191 C

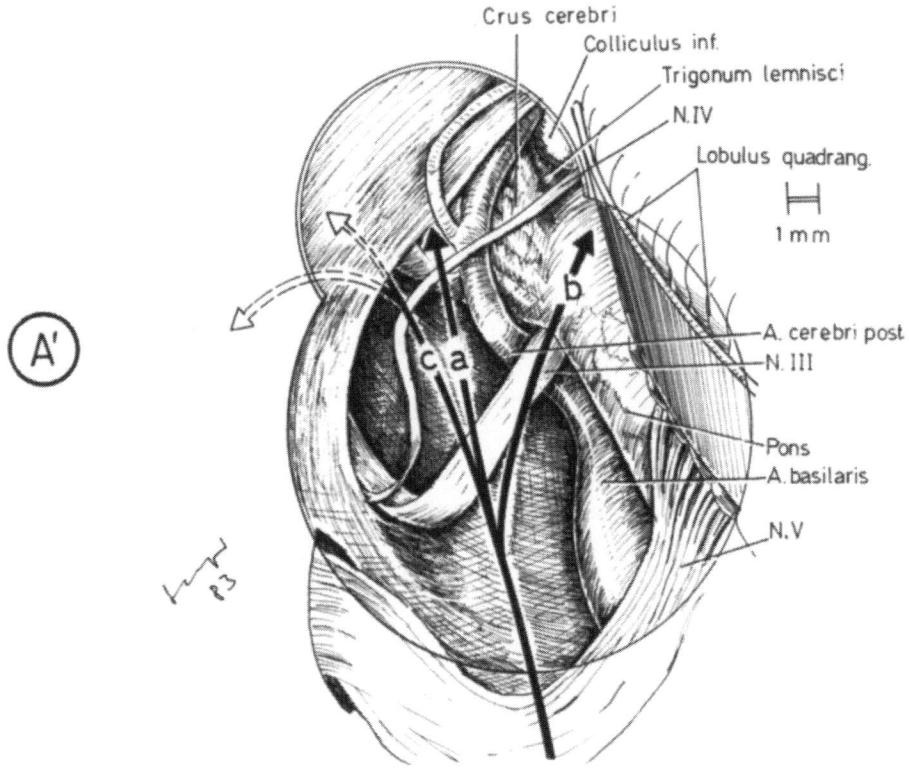
Crus cerebri
Colliculus inf.
Trigonum lemnisci
N.IV
Lobulus quadrang.
1 mm
A'
b
c
a
A. cerebri post.
N. III
Pons
A. basilaris
N.V

Extradural tumor with shift of Sinus sigmoideus (Figs. 195 to 200)

Fig. 195. Basal tumors of posterior Fossa.
Operation of richly vascularized extradural tumor, with **Sinus sigmoideus displacement**
Clinical example of aneurysmatic bone cyst in left cerebellopontine angle. One year ago hoarseness, noises in left ear, dizziness and vomiting. Neurological findings attributable to left caudal cranial nerves. Due to dangerous bleeding, biopsy attempt by outside hospital had to be terminated. Histological: aneurysmatic bone cyst. Two months later, partial embolization and renewed operative attempt, again terminated due to bleeding. One year later patient refered to our hospital. Additional peripheral VII paresis, postoperatively. After radical tumor removal*, diagnosis was verified
Diagnostic procedures

A	Old trepanation area *–t–* in preoperative X-ray
B – B''	CT: broad tumor surface connecting to Os petrosum, which shows gross asymmetry as compared to the other side. In addition, tumor reaches skull surface in previous trepanation area *–t–*
C + C'	Carotis angiogram shows tumor contrast medium uptake from A. carotis externa branches
D	Lateral enlarged detail from **C**
E	Poor showing of left Sinus sigmoideus in phlebogram, probably indicating medial displacement

Abbreviations:

ao A. occipitalis
t Trepanation

---

* N. VII graft reconstruction carried out later on by Prof. Helms, Director, Hals-Nasen-Ohren-Klinik (ENT-Department), University of Mainz.

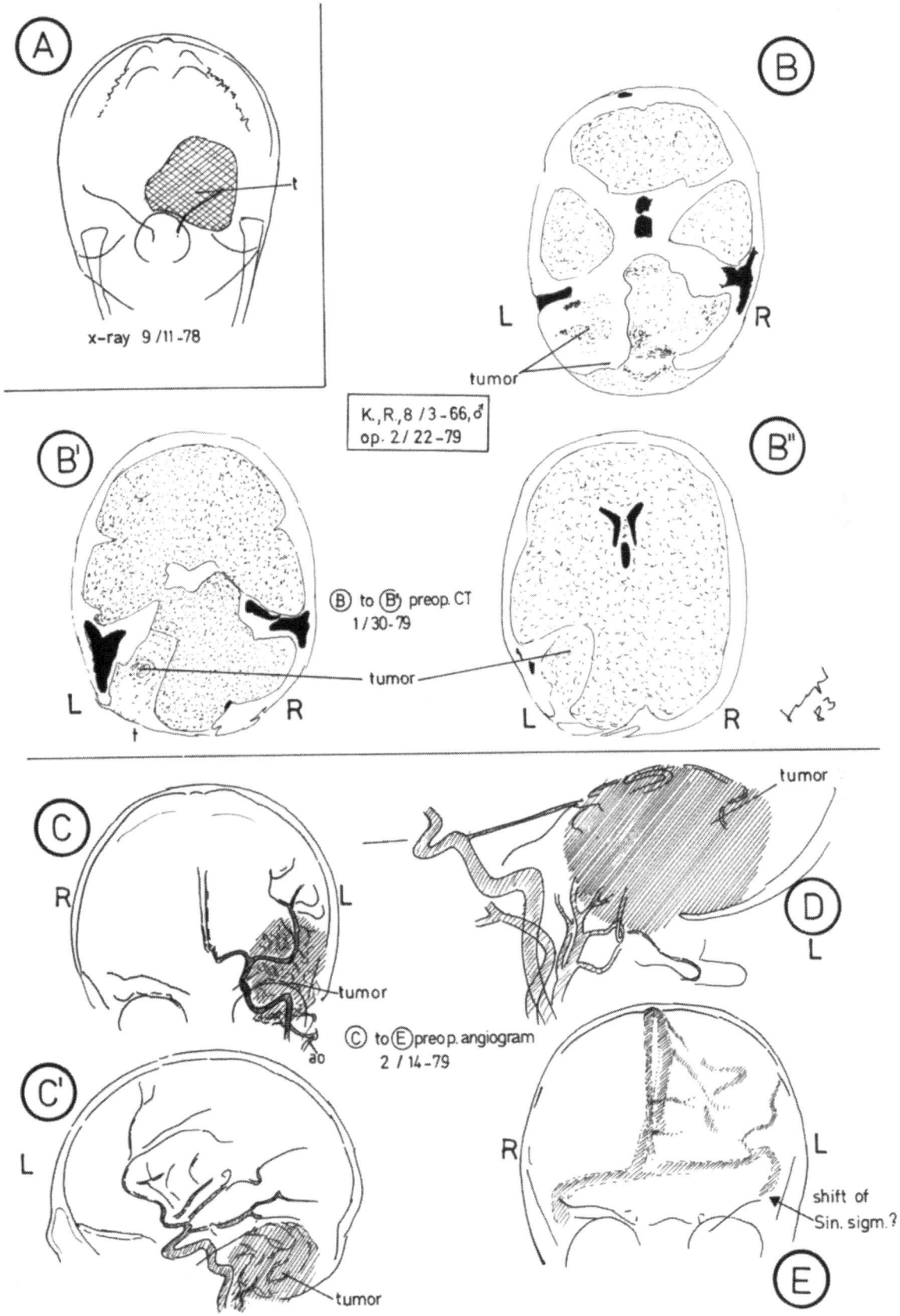
A
t
x-ray 9/11-78
B
L
R
tumor
K., R., 8/3-66, ♂
op. 2/22-79
B'
B''
Ⓑ to Ⓑ' preop. CT
1/30-79
tumor
L
R
t
L
R
C
R
L
tumor
ao
tumor
D
L
Ⓒ to Ⓔ preop. angiogram
2/14-79
C'
L
tumor
R
L
shift of
Sin. sigm.?
E

Fig. 196. Basal tumors of posterior Fossa.
Operation of richly vascularized extradural tumor, with Sinus sigmoideus displacement
Anatomical sketches

A Schematic horizontal section based on CT **B'** of Fig. 195. Sinus sigmoideus is luxated medially out of Sulcus sigmoideus

B Skull drawing, with Sinus sigmoideus displacement (projection), superior view.
Arrows: displacement direction of Sinus sigmoideus – broken line –

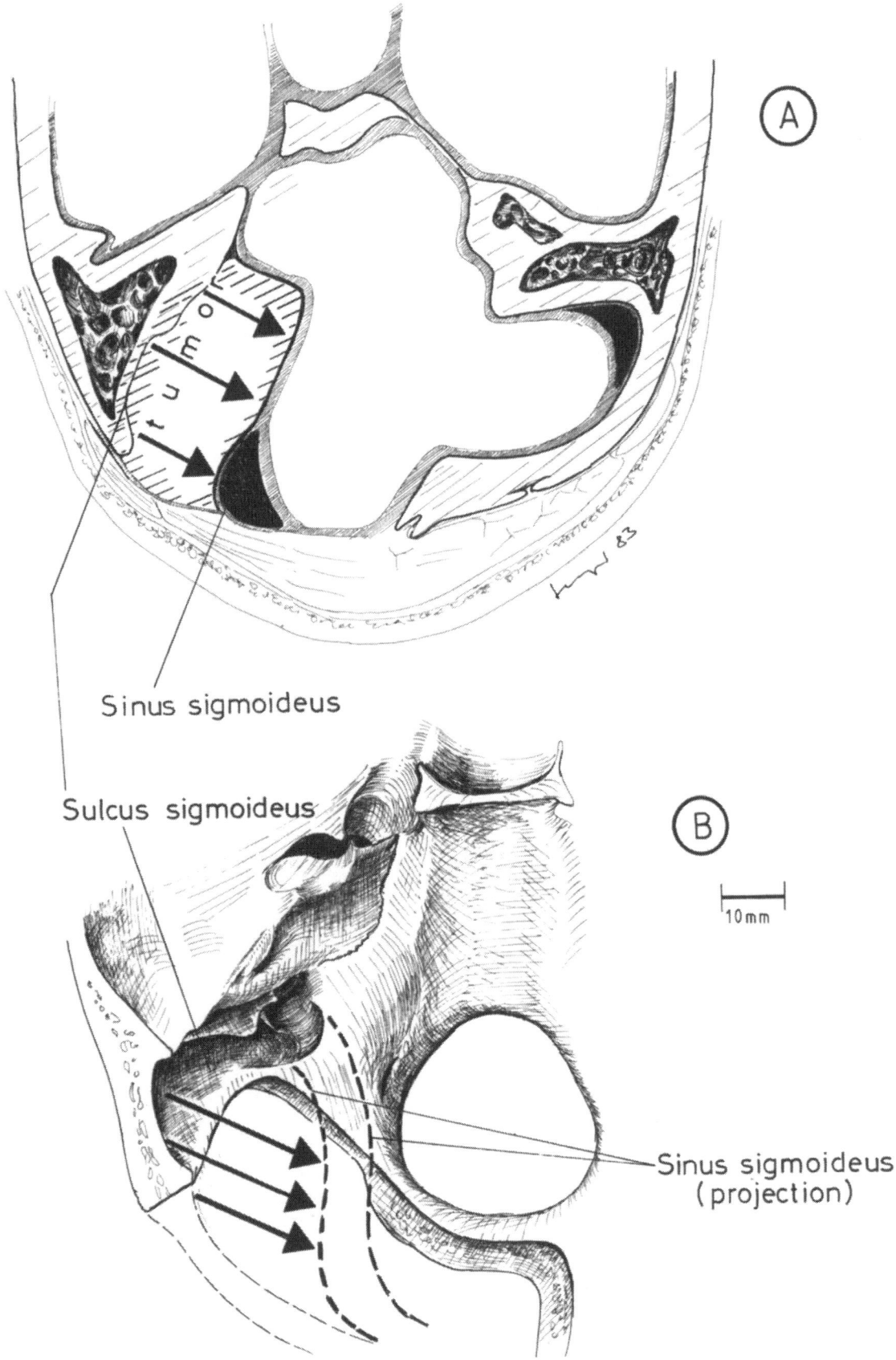
A
O
E
U
t
Sinus sigmoideus
Sulcus sigmoideus
B
10 mm
Sinus sigmoideus
(projection)

Fig. 197. Basal tumors of posterior Fossa.
Operation of richly vascularized extradural tumor, with Sinus sigmoideus displacement
Anatomical model presentation. Continuation of Fig. 195

A Superior view of skull base, dura and displaced Sinus sigmoideus drawn in

B Anatomical model of operation site, posterior view

In **A** + **B** dura sheath of N.VII/VIII not shown

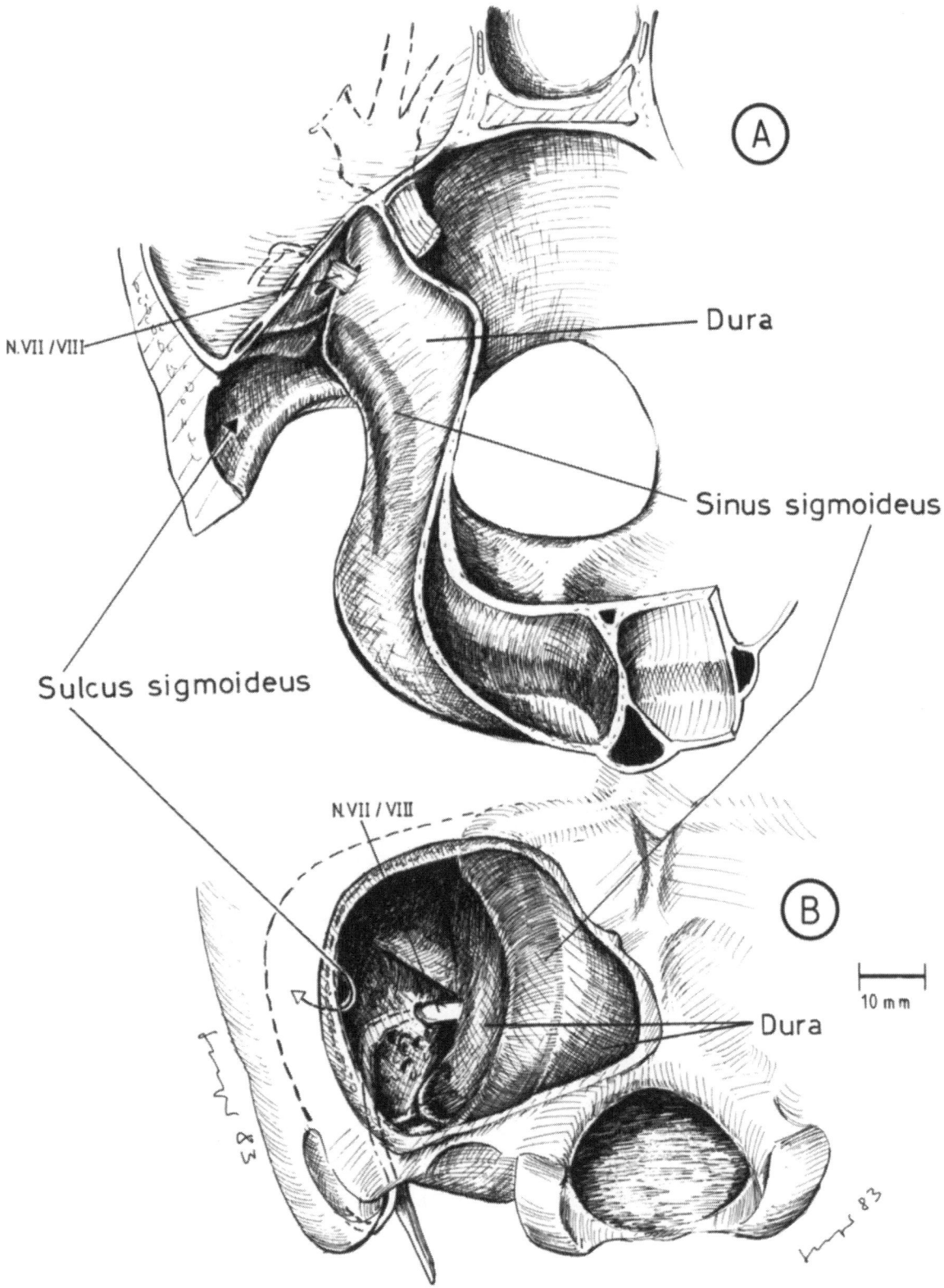
A
N.VII / VIII
Dura
Sinus sigmoideus
Sulcus sigmoideus
N.VII / VIII
B
10 mm
Dura

Fig. 198. Basal tumors of posterior Fossa.
Operation of richly vascularized extradural tumor, with Sinus sigmoideus displacement
Operative tumor exposure

A Skin incision, posterior view (correct position on operation table see **B'**)
- **1** Skin incision
- **2** Monopolar coagulation of subcutis and fascia

B Situation after skin and muscle incision
- **1** Incision of scarred periosteum at trepanation edge
- **2** Pulling back periosteum, exposure of trepanation edge.
  Arrow: operative approach when patient is positioned on operative table, corresponding to anatomical sketch **B'**

B' During operation patient's head is turned sideways, in this example to the left – the side of tumor – as for acoustic neurinoma operation.
Arrow: operative approach

C Removal of external tumor capsule scarred by previous operation. At first, relief of Sinus sigmoideus could not be identified within scar tissue. Previous operative approach had been partially carried out through Sinus sigmoideus
- **1a** Drilling of Os mastoideum, similar to acoustic neurinoma operation
- **1b** Incision of scarred tumor capsule
- **2** Preparation of capsule back from tumor surface by forceps
- **3** As **2**, carried out by dissector

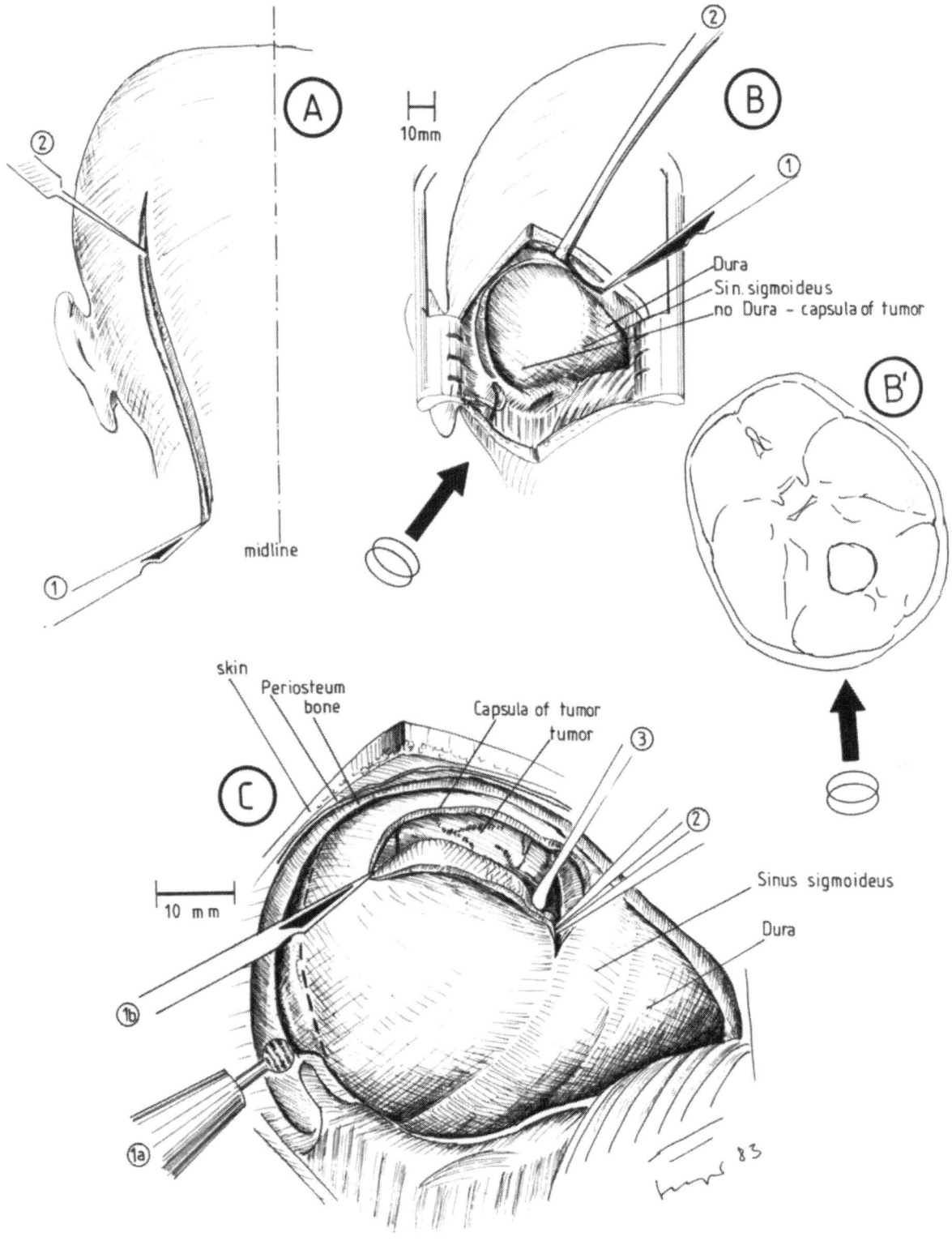
A
B
B'
C
10mm
midline
Dura
Sin. sigmoideus
no Dura - capsula of tumor
skin
Periosteum
bone
Capsula of tumor
tumor
10 mm
Sinus sigmoideus
Dura

Fig. 199. Basal tumors of posterior Fossa.
Operation of richly vascularized extradural tumor, with Sinus sigmoideus displacement
Isolation of richly vascularized tumor

A **1** Incision of tumor capsule portions
2 Pulling back flaps
3 Loosening of smooth tumor surface from dura (originally lying on posterior surface of Os petrosum)
4 Application of gelfoam to bleeding Sinus sigmoideus gaps after removal of scars from previous operative approach. Gelfoam is soaked with Calcium/Thrombin
5 Fibrinogen concentrate* is squirted under gelfoam. Bleeding stops immediately

B **1** Application of cotton wool to Sinus sigmoideus, for protection against heat
2 Extensive irrigation and suction
3 Cautious, thorough, time-consuming bipolar coagulation of tumor surface

---

* Immuno.

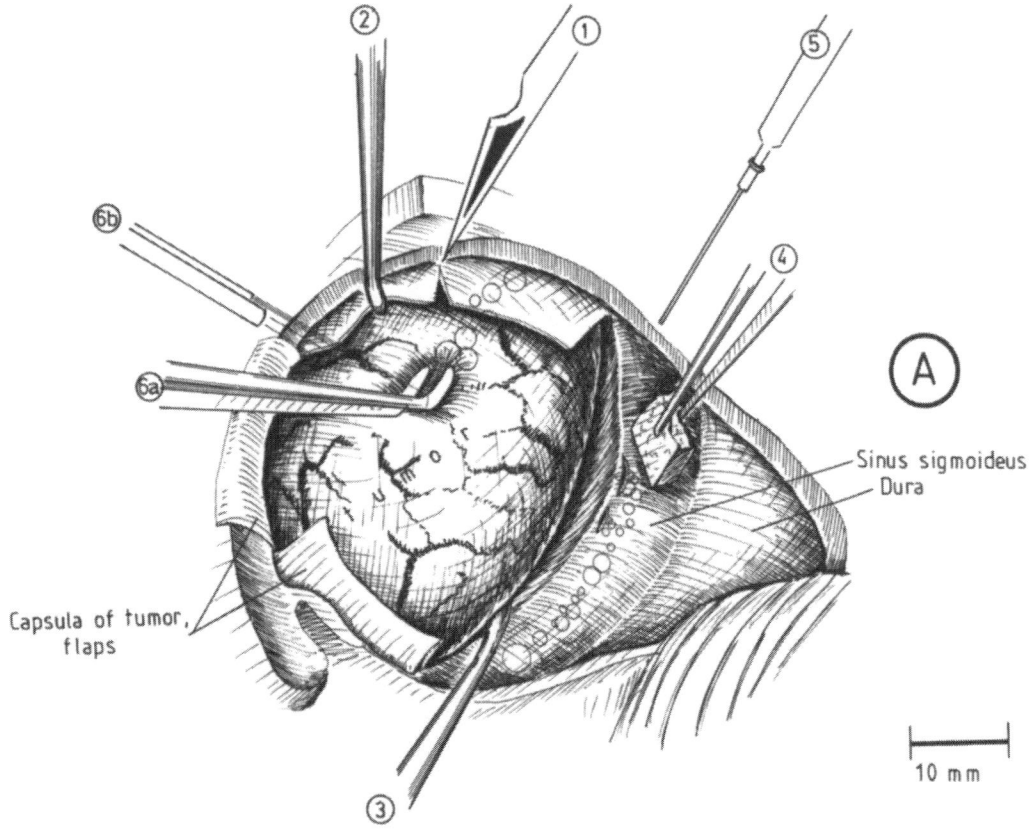
2
1
5
6b
4
6a
A
Sinus sigmoideus
Dura
Capsula of tumor, flaps
10 mm
3

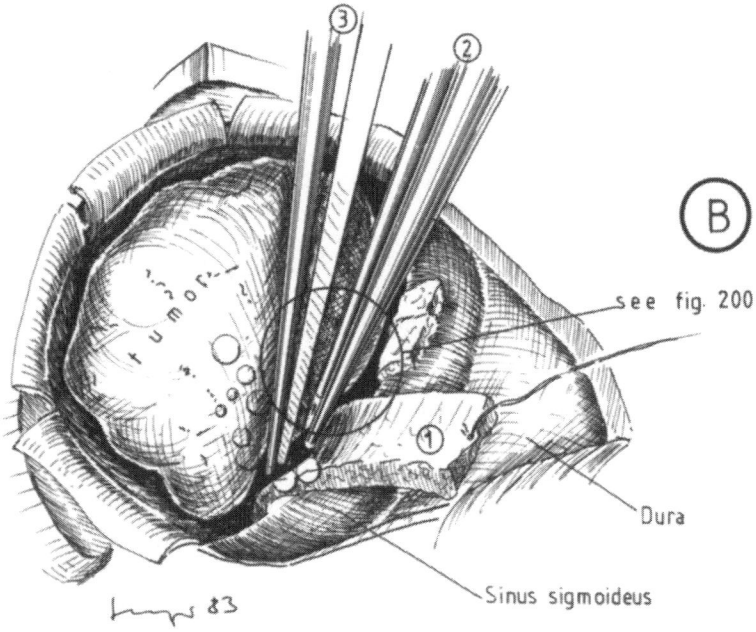
3
2
B
see fig. 200
1
Dura
Sinus sigmoideus

Fig. 200. Basal tumors of posterior Fossa.
Operation of richly vascularized extradural tumor, with Sinus sigmoideus displacement

A Situation after tumor removal

1 Scraping of tumor remnants from posterior surface of Os petrosum partially destroyed by tumor

2a + 2b Coagulation of bleeding tumor residuals

B **1a + 1b** Removal of tumor-infiltrated bone portions from posterior surface of Os petrosum

2a + 2b Hemostasis

Wound closure

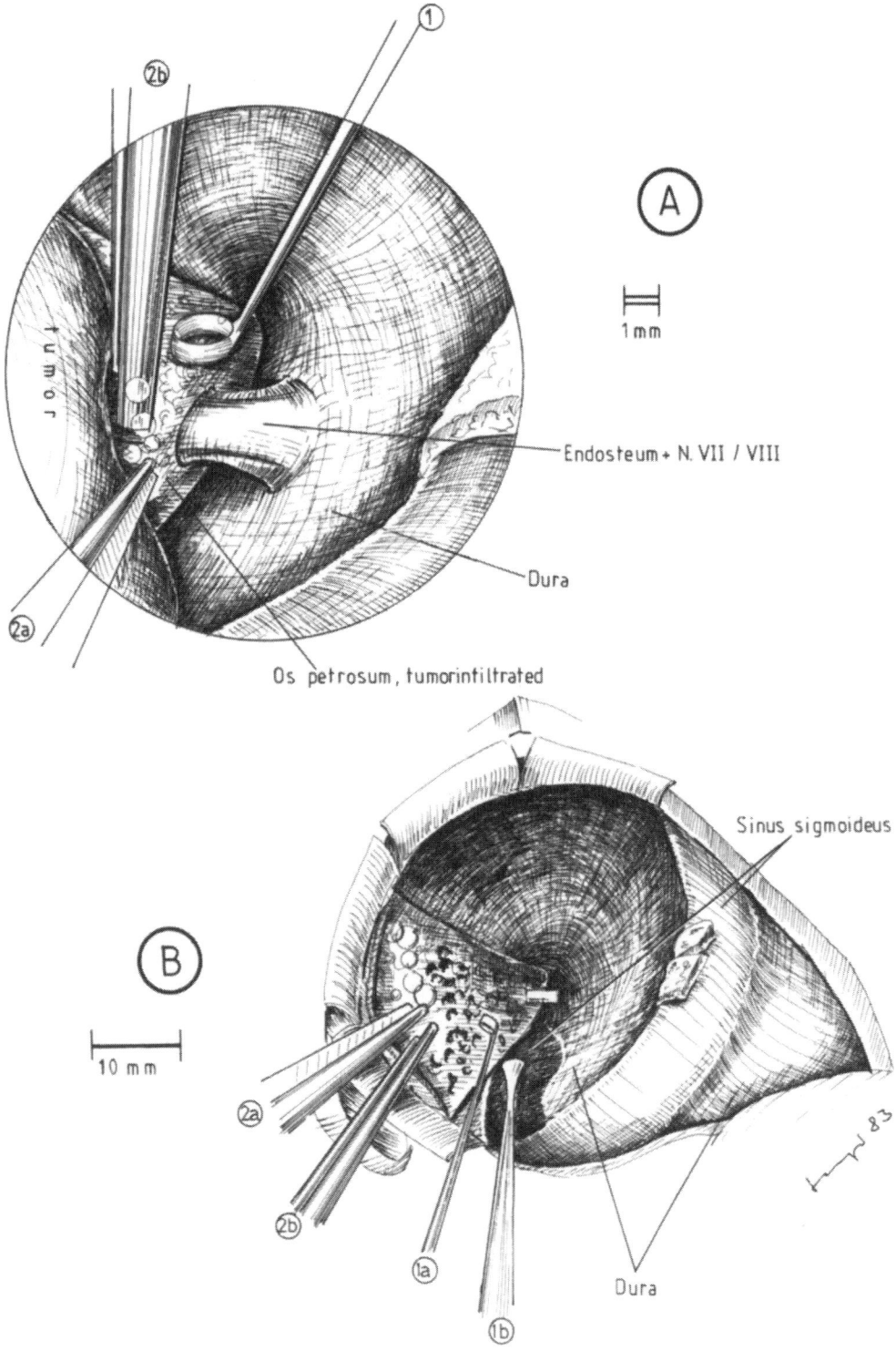
1
2b
A
1mm
tumor
Endosteum + N. VII / VIII
Dura
2a
Os petrosum, tumorinfiltrated
Sinus sigmoideus
B
10 mm
2a
2b
1a
1b
Dura
83

References

Chapter 1

Van Alyea, O. E.: Sphenoid sinus. Anatomic study, with consideration of the clinical significance of the structural characteristics of the sphenoid sinus. Arch. Otolaryng. **34,** 225–253 (1941).

Bailey, P.: Tumors of the hypophysis cerebri. In: Cytology and Cellular Pathology of the Nervous System (Penfield, W., ed.), pp. 905–951. New York: Hoeber (1932).

Bailey, P., Cushing, H.: Studies in acromegaly. VII. The microscopical structure of the adenomas in acromegalic dyspituitarism (fugitiative acromegaly). Amer. J. Path. **4,** 545–563 (1928).

Bakay, L.: The results of 300 pituitary adenoma operations. J. Neurosurg. **7,** 240–255 (1950).

Bateman, G. H.: Trans-sphenoidal hypophysectomy. A review of 70 cases treated in the past two years. Trans. Amer. Acad. Ophthal. Otolaryng. **66,** 103–110 (1962).

Benda, C.: Pathologische Anatomie der Hypophysis. In: Handbuch der pathologischen Anatomie des Nervensystems (Flatau, E., Jacobsohn, L., Minor, L., eds.), Bd. 2, pp. 1418–1438. Berlin: S. Karger (1904).

Bergland, R. M., Ray, B. S., Torack, M.: Anatomical variations in the pituitary gland and adjacent structures in 225 human autopsy cases. J. Neurosurg. **28,** 93–99 (1968).

Borchardt, H.: Diskussion zum Vortrag Hochenegg. Verhandl. Ges. Chir. **37,** 85 (1908).

Borchardt, H.: The operative cure of acromegaly by removal of a hypophysial tumor. Ann. Surg. **48,** 783 (1908).

Broeckaert, J.: A contribution to the surgery of the hypophysis. J. Laryngol. **28,** 340–352 (1913).

Broeckaert, J.: Contribution à la chirugie de l'hypophyse. Presse Otolaryngolog. Belge **11,** 297–315 (1912).

Busch, W.: Die Morphologie der Sella turcica und ihre Beziehungen zur Hypophyse. Virchow's Arch. **320,** 437–458 (1951).

Calcaterra, T. C., Rand, R. W.: Current adjuncts for surgery of the sphenoid sinus and pituitary gland. Laryngoscope **86,** 1692–1698 (1976).

Chiari, O.: Ueber eine Modifikation der Schloffer'schen Operation von Tumoren der Hypophyse. Wien. Klin. Wschr. **25,** 5–6 (1912).

Collins, W. F., jr.: Transsphenoidal surgery in pituitary adenomas. In: The Pituitary – a Current Review (Allen, M. B., Mahesh, V. B., eds.), pp. 431–442. New York–San Francisco–London: Academic Press (1977).

Cope, V. Z.: Surgery of the pituitary fossa. Brit. J. Surg. **4,** 107–144 (1916).

Cummings, C. W., Johnson, J.: Transethmoidal approach to the pituitary adenomas. In: Current Techniques in Operative Neurosurgery (Schmidek, H. H., Sweet, W. H., eds.), pp. 173–180. New York: Grune & Stratton (1977).

Cushing, H.: Surgical experiences with pituitary disorders. J. A. M. A. **63,** 1515–1525 (1914).

Cushing, H.: Intracranial tumours. Notes upon a series of two thousand verified cases with surgical-mortality percentages pertaining thereto. Springfield, Ill.: Ch. C Thomas (1932).

Cushing, H.: Dyspituitarism: twenty years later. With special consideration of pituitary adenomas. Arch. Int. Med. **51,** 487–557 (1933).

Denker, A.: Hypophysentumoren. Int. Centralbl. Laryngol. Rhinol. **37,** 225 (1922).

Derome, P. J., Jedynak, C. P., Peillon, F.: Pituitary Adenomas; Biology, Physiopathology and Treatment. Paris: Asclepios (1980).

Dostoiewsky, A.: Ueber den Bau der Vorderlappen des Hirnanhanges. Arch. Mikr. Anat. **26,** 592–598 (1886).

Eiselsberg, A.: The operative cure of acromegaly by removal of a hypophysial tumor. Ann. Surg. **48,** 783–784 (1908).

Eiselsberg, A.: Operations upon the hypophysis. Ann. Surg. **52,** 1–14 (1910).

Eiselsberg, A., Frankl-Hochwart, L.: Über operative Behandlung der Tumoren der Hypophysengegend. Neurol. Zbl. **26,** 994–1001 (1907).

Erdheim, J.: Ueber Hypophysenganggeschwülste und Hirncholesteatome. S. Ber. Akad. Wiss. Wien, Math.-Naturw. Kl. Abt. III, **113,** 537–726 (1904).

Erdheim, J.: Über das eosinophile und basophile Hypophysenadenom. Frankf. Z. Path. **4,** 70–86 (1910).

Escher, F.: Hypophysektomie. Fortschr. Hals-Nasen-Ohrenheilk. **12,** 1–225 (1965).

Fahlbusch, R., Rjosk, H. K., v. Werder, K.: Operative treatment of prolactinproducing adenomas. In: Treatment of Pituitary Adenomas (Fahlbusch, R., Werder, K. v., eds.). Stuttgart: G. Thieme (1978).

Fein, J.: Zur Operation der Hypophyse. Wien. Klin. Wschr. **23,** 1035 (1910).

Ferner, H.: Die Hypophysenzisterne des Menschen und ihre Beziehung zum Entstehungsmechanismus der sekundären Sellaerweiterung. Z. Anat. Entwgesch. **121,** 407–416 (1960).

Fujii, K., Chambers, S. M., Rhoton, A. L.: Neurovascular relationships of the sphenoid sinus. A microsurgical study. J. Neurosurg. **50,** 31–39 (1979).

Guiot, G.: Transsphenoidal approach in surgical treatment of pituitary adenomas: general principles and indications in non-functioning adenomas. In: Diagnosis and Treatment of Pituitary Tumors (Kohler, P. O., Ross, G. T., eds.), pp. 159–178. Amsterdam: Excerpta Medica (1973).

Guiot, G.: Considerations on the surgical treatment of pituitary adenomas. In: Treatment of Pituitary Adenomas (Fahlbusch, R., Werder, K. v., eds.), pp. 202–218. Stuttgart: G. Thieme (1978).

Guiot, G., Derome, P.: Surgical problems of pituitary adenomas. In: Advances and Technical Standards in Neurosurgery (Krayenbühl, H., et al., eds.), Vol. 3, pp. 3–35. Wien–New York: Springer (1976).

Guleke, N.: Die Eingriffe am Gehirnschädel, Gehirn, an der Wirbelsäule und am Rückenmark. In: Allgemeine und spezielle Operationslehre (Guleke, N., Zenker, R., eds.), Vol. 2, 2nd ed., pp. 335–343. Berlin–Göttingen–Heidelberg: Springer (1950).

Halstead, A. E.: Remarks on the operative treatment of tumors of the hypophysis. With the report of two cases operated by an oro-nasal method. Trans. Amer. Surg. Assoc. **28,** 73–93 (1910).

Hamberger, C. A., Hammer, G.: Der transnasale Weg der Hypophysektomie. In: Hals-Nasen-Ohren-Heilkunde (Berendes, J., Link, R., Zöllner, F., eds.), Vol. 1, pp. 795–818. Stuttgart: G. Thieme (1964).

Hamberger, C. A., Hammer, G., Norlén, G., Sjogren, B.: Transantrosphenoidal hypophysectomy. Arch. Otolaryngol. **74,** 22–28 (1961).

Hammer, G., Rådberg, C.: The sphenoidal sinus. – An anatomical and roentgenologic study with reference to transsphenoid hypophysectomy. Acta Radiol. **56,** 401–422 (1961).

Hardy, J.: L'exérèse des adénomas hypophysaires par voie transsphénoidale. Un. Med. Can. **91,** 933–945 (1962).

Hardy, J.: La chirugie de l'hypophyse par voie transsphénoidale ouverte. Etude comparative de deux modalités techniques. Ann. Chir. (Paris) **21,** 1011–1022 (1967).

Hardy, J.: Transsphenoidal microsurgery of the normal and pathological pituitary. Clin. Neurosurg. **16,** 185–216 (1969).

Hardy, J.: Transsphenoidal hypophysectomy. J. Neurosurg. **34,** 582–594 (1971).

Hardy, J.: Transsphenoidal surgery of hypersecreting pituitary tumors. In: Diagnosis and Treatment of Pituitary Tumors (Kohler, P. O., Ross, G. T., eds.), pp. 179–194. Amsterdam: Excerpta Medica (1973).

Hardy, J.: Subnasal trans-sphenoidal approach to the pituitary. In: Microneurosurgery (Rand, R. W., ed.), ed. 2., pp. 105–130. St. Louis: Mosby (1978).

Hardy, J., Townsend, P. R., Gerundulo, D. G.: Forces applied by nasal speculums during transsphenoidal operations. Surg. Neurol. **10,** 361–363 (1978).

Hardy, J., Wigser, S. M.: Transsphenoidal surgery of pituitary fossa tumors with televised radiofluoroscopic control. J. Neurosurg. **23,** 612–620 (1965).

Henderson, W. R.: The pituitary adenomata. A follow-up study of the surgical results in 338 cases (Dr. Harvey Cushing's series). Brit. J. Surg. **26,** 811–921 (1939).

Heimbach, S. B.: Follow-up studies on 105 cases of verified chromophobe and acidophilic pituitary adenomata after treatment by transfrontal operation and x-ray irradiation. Acta Neurochir. (Wien) **7,** 101–155 (1959).

Heuer, G. J.: The surgical approach and the treatment of tumors and other lesions about the optic chiasm. Surg. Gynec. Obstet. **53,** 489–518 (1931).

Hirsch, O.: Eine neue Methode der endonasalen Operation von Hypophysentumoren. Wien. Med. Wschr. **59,** 636–637 (1909).

Hirsch, O.: Zur endonasalen Operation von Hypophysentumoren. Wien. Med. Wschr. **60,** 749–750 (1910).

Hochenegg, J.: Zur Therapie der Hypophysentumoren. Dtsch. Z. Chir. **100,** 317–326 (1909).

Horsley, V.: On the technique of operations on the central nervous system. Brit. Med. J. **2,** 411–423 (1906).

Kahler, O.: Zur Operation der Hypophysentumoren. Z. Ohrenheilk. **75,** 287–308 (1917).

Kanavel, A. B.: The removal of tumors of the pituitary body by an infranasal route. J.A.M.A. **53,** 1704–1707 (1909).

Kanavel, A. B., Grinker, J.: Removal of tumors of the pituitary body. Surg. Gynec. Obstet. **10,** 414–418 (1910).

Karduck, A., Bock, W. J.: Rhinological findings following transantrosphenoidal surgery of the pituitary gland. Acta Otolaryngol. **85,** 449–452 (1978).

Kern, E. B., Laws, E. R., Randall, R., Westwood, W. B.: A transseptal, transsphenoidal approach to the pituitary: An old technique in the managament of pituitary tumors and related disorders. Trans. Amer. Acad. Ophthalmol. Otolaryngol. **84,** 997–1010 (1977).

Killian, G.: Die submucöse Fensterresektion der Nasenscheidewand. Arch. Laryngol. Rhinol. **16,** 362–387 (1904).

Kirchner, J. A., Van Gilder, J. C.: Transethmoidal hypophysectomy: Some surgical landmarks. Trans. Amer. Acad. Ophthalmol. Otolaryngol., sect. Otolaryngol. **80,** 391–196 (1975).

Kocher, T.: Ein Fall von Hypophysis-Tumor mit operativer Heilung. Deutsch. Z. Chir. **100,** 13–37 (1909).

Krogius, A.: Neue Methode, den Nasopharyngealraum für die Operation von Basalfibromen und Hypophysengeschwülsten freizulegen. Zbl. Chir. **36,** 1420 (1909).

Landolt, A. M.: Progress in Pituitary Adenoma Biology. Results of Research and Clinical Applications. In: Advances and Technical Standards in Neurosurgery (Krayenbühl, H., et al., eds.), Vol. **5,** pp. 3–49. Wien–New York: Springer (1978).

Landolt, A. M.: Technique of Transsphenoidal Operation for Pituitary Adenomas. In: Advances and Technical Standards in Neurosurgery (Krayenbühl, H., et al., eds.), Vol. **7,** pp. 119–171. Wien–New York: Springer (1980).

Landolt, A. M., Kistler, G. S.: Morphology of chromophobe adenoma. In: Treatment of Pituitary Adenomas (Fahlbusch, R., Werder, K. v., eds.), pp. 154–171. Stuttgart: G. Thieme (1978).

Landolt, A. M., Siegfried, J.: Zur Behandlung maligner, metastasierender Tumoren mit der stereotaktischen transsphenoidalen Elektrokoagulation der Hypophyse. Schweiz. Med. Wschr. **100,** 1297–1306 (1970).

Landolt, A. M., Wilson, C. B.: Tumors of the sella and the parasellar area in adults. In: Neurological Surgery, 2nd ed. (Youmans, J. R., ed.). Philadelphia: Saunders (1980).

Lang, J.: Klinische Anatomie des Kopfes. Berlin–Heidelberg–New York: Springer (1981).

Lanz, T. von, Wachsmuth, W.: Praktische Anatomie, Vol. 1/1B. Berlin–Heidelberg–New York: Springer (1979).

Lautenschläger, A.: Die prämaxilläre Hypophysenoperation. Chirurg **1,** 30–33 (1929).

Laws, E. R.: Transsphenoidal approach to lesions in and about the sella turcica. In: Current Techniques in Operative Neurosurgery (Schmidek, H. H., Sweet, W. H., eds.), pp. 161–172. New York: Grune & Stratton (1977).

Laws, E. R., Kern, E. B.: Complications of trans-sphenoidal surgery. Clin. Neurosurg. **23,** 401–416 (1976).

Laws, E. R., Trautmann, J. C., Hollenhorst, R. W.: Transsphenoidal decompression of the optic nerve and chiasm. Visual results in 62 patients. J. Neurosurg. **46,** 717–722 (1977).

Loewe, L.: Ueber die Freilegung der Sehnervenkreuzung und der Hypophysis und über die Beteiligung des Siebbeinlabyrinthes am Aufbau der Supraorbitalplatte. Z. Augenheilk. **19,** 456–464 (1908).

Macbeth, R. G.: An approach to the pituitary via a nasal osteoplastic flap. J. Laryngol. Otol. **75,** 70–77 (1961).

Macbeth, R. G.: Hypophysectomy by the nasal route in advanced carcinoma of the breast. J. Roy. Coll. Surg. Edinburgh **6,** 199–205 (1961).

Macbeth, R. G., Hall, M.: Hypophysectomy as a rhinological procedure. Arch. Otolaryngol. **75,** 440–450 (1962).

Montgomery, W. W.: Transethmoidosphenoidal hypophysectomy with septal mucosal flap. Arch. Otolaryngol. **78,** 68–77 (1963).

Moszkowicz, L.: Zur Technik der Operation an der Hypophyse. Wien. Klin. Wschr. **20,** 792–795 (1907).

Mundinger, F., Riechert, T.: Hypophysentumoren – Hypophysektomie. Stuttgart: G. Thieme (1967).

Nager, F. R.: The paranasal approach to intrasellar tumors. J. Laryng. **55,** 361–381 (1940).

Netzer, H. R., McCoy, E. G.: Transseptal transsphenoidal hypophysectomy. A new approach. Arch. Otolaryng. **86,** 252–255 (1967).

Nowikoff, W. N.: Ein neuer Weg für Eingriffe an der Hypophyse. Zbl. Chir. **40,** 1000–1003 (1913).

Nurnberger, J. L., Korey, S. R.: Pituitary chromophobe adenomas. A clinical study of the sella syndrome: Neurology, metabolism, therapy. New York: Springer Publishing Comp. (1953).

Oehlecker, F.: Zur Trepanation des Türkensattels bei Tumoren der Hypophyse und der Gehirnbasis. Langenbeck's Arch. Klin. Chir. **121,** 490–511 (1922).

Olivecrona, H.: The surgical treatment of intracranial tumors. VIII. The pituitary adenomas. In: Handbuch der Neurochirurgie (Olivecrona, H., Tönnis, W., eds.), Vol. 4, part 4, pp. 228–301. Berlin–Heidelberg–New York: Springer (1967).

Palacios, E., Fine, M., Haughton, V. M.: Multiplanar anatomy of the head and neck for computed topography. New York: J. Wiley & Sons (1980).

Parkinson, D.: A surgical approach to the cavernous portion of the carotid artery. Anatomical studies and case report. J. Neurosurg. **23,** 474–483 (1965).

Parkinson, D.: Carotid cavernous fistula: direct repair with preservation of the carotid artery. Technical note. J. Neurosurg. **38,** 99–106 (1973).

Preysing, H.: Beiträge zur Operation der Hypophyse. Verh. Dtsch. Laryng. **20,** 51–66 (1913).

Proust, R.: La chirurgie de l'hypophyse. J. Chir. (Paris) **1,** 665–680 (1980).

Rand, R. W., Heuser, G., Adamas, D. A.: Ten-year experience with stereotaxie cryohypophysectomy. Progr. Neurol. Surg. **6,** 252–271 (1975).

Renn, W. H., Rhoton, A. L.: Microsurgical anatomy of the sellar region. J. Neurosurg. **43,** 288–298 (1975).

Romeis, B.: Hypophyse. In: Handbuch der mikroskopischen Anatomie des Menschen (v. Möllendorf, W., ed.), Vol. 6, part 3. Berlin: J. Springer (1940).

Rhoton, A. L., Jr.: Micro-operative techniques. In: Neurological Surgery (Youman, J. R., ed.), ed. 2., Vol. 1, pp. 1160–1194. Philadelphia: Saunders (1982).

Rhoton, A. L., Jr.: Ring curettes for transsphenoidal pituitary operations. Surg. Neurol. **18,** 28–33 (1982).

Rhoton, A. L., Jr., Hardy, D. G., Chambers, S. M.: Microsurgical anatomy and dissection of the sphenoid bone, cavernous sinus and sellar region. Surg. Neurol. **12,** 63–104 (1979).

Rhoton, A. L., Jr., Merz, W.: Suction tubes for conventional and microscopic neurosurgery. Surg. Neurol. **15,** 120–124 (1981).

Rhoton, A. L., Jr., Yamamoto, I., Peaace, D. A.: Microsurgery of the third ventricle: Part II. Operative approaches. Neurosurgery **8,** 357–377 (1981).

Rubinstein, L. J.: Tumors of the central nervous system. In: Atlas of Tumors Pathology. 2nd series, fascicle 6. Washington, D. C.: Armed Forces Institute of Pathology (1972).

Samii, M., Draf, W.: Course on Surgery of the Skull Base. Hannover, West-Germany (1979).

Samii, M., Draf, W.: Course in the Surgery of the Anterior Skull Base. Hannover, West-Germany (1980).

Samii, M., Jannetta, P. J.: Symposium on Cranial Nerves. Hannover, West-Germany (1980).

Schloffer, H.: Zur Frage der Operation an der Hypophyse. Beitr. Klin. Chir. **50,** 767–817 (1906).

Schloffer, H.: Erfolgreiche Operationen eines Hypophysentumors auf nasalem Wege. Wien. Klin. Wschr. **20,** 621–624 (1907).

Schloffer, H.: Weiterer Bericht über den Fall von operiertem Hypophysentumor. (Plötzlicher Exitus letalis 2½ Monate nach der Operation.) Wien. Klin. Wschr. **20,** 1075–1078 (1907).

Seeger, W.: Atlas of Topographical Anatomy of the Brain and Surrounding Structures. Wien–New York: Springer (1978).

Seeger, W.: Microsurgery of the Spinal Cord and Surrounding Structures. Anatomical and Technical Principles. Wien–New York: Springer (1982).

Smoler, F.: Zur Operation der Hypophysentumoren auf nasalem Wege. Wien. Klin. Wschr. **22,** 1488–1489 (1909).

Svien, H. L., Colby, M. Y.: Treatment for chromophobe adenoma. Springfield, Ill.: Ch. C Thomas (1967).

Tiefenthal: Technik der Hypophysenoperation. Münch. Med. Wschr. **67,** 794 (1920).

Tindall, G. T., Collins, W. F., Kirchner, J. A.: Unilateral septal technique for transsphenoidal microsurgical approach to the sella turcica. J. Neurosurg. **49,** 138–142 (1978).

Tönnis, W., Oberdisse, K., Weber, E.: Bericht über 264 operierte Hypophysenadenome. Acta Neurochir. (Wien) **3,** 113–130 (1953).

Tönnis, W.: Diagnostik der intrakraniellen Geschwülste. In: Handbuch der Neurochirurgie (Olivecrona, H., Tönnis, W., eds.), Vol. 4, part 3, pp. 150–185, Berlin–Heidelberg–New York: Springer (1962).

Trible, W. M., Morse, A. E.: Transpalatal hypophysectomy. Trans. Amer. Laryngol. Rhinol. Otol. Soc. 188–195 (1965).

Vourc'h, G.: L'anesthésie dans les hypophysectomies. In: Adénomes hypophysaires (Guiot, G., ed.), pp. 181–190. Paris: Masson (1958).

West, J. M.: Die Chirurgie der Hypophysis vom Standpunkt des Rhinologen. Arch. Laryngol. Rhinol. **23,** 288–295 (1910).

West, J. M.: The surgery of the hypophysis from the standpoint of the rhinologist. J.A.M.A. **54,** 1132–1134 (1910).

Wilson, C. B., Dempsey, L. C.: Transsphenoidal microsurgical removal of 250 pituitary adenomas. J. Neurosurg. **48,** 13–22 (1978).

Yamamoto, I., Rhoton, Al., Jr., Peace, D. A.: Microsurgery of the third ventricle: Part I. Microsurgical anatomy. Neurosurgery **8,** 334–356 (1981).

Zervas, N. T.: Stereotaxic thermal hypophysectomy. Progr. Neurol. Surg. **6,** 217–251 (1975).

Chapter 2

Abbie, A. A.: The clinical significance of the anterior choroidal artery. Brain **56,** 233–246 (1933).

Agati, D.: Ipertrofie etmoido-sfenoidali a protundenza endocranica. Radiol. Med. **32,** 151–154 (1946).

Arnold, F.: Handbuch der Anatomie des Menschen. Vol. **2,** pt. 1, p. 465. Freiburg i. Br.: Herder'sche Verlagshandlung (1847) (Cited by Meyer, 1887).

Bacon, T., Duchesneau, P. M., Weinstein, M. A.: Demonstration of the superior ophthalmic vein by high resolution computed tomography. Radiology **124,** 129 (1977).

Balèiaux-Wada, D., Mortelmans, L. L., Dupont, M. G., et al.: The use of coronal scans for computed tomography of the orbits. Neuroradiology **14,** 89 (1977).

Bedford, M. A.: The "cavernous sinus". Brit. J. Ophthal. **50,** 41–46 (1966).

Bendescu, T.: Beiderseitige Optikusatrophie verursacht durch Pneumosinus dilatans der rechten Keilbeinhöhle. Z. Augenheilk. **79,** 41–50 (1932).

Bergland, R., Ray, S.: The arterial supply of the human optic chiasm. J. Neurosurg. **31,** 327–334 (1969).

Bonnal, J., Thibaut, A., Brotchi, J., et al.: Invading meningiomas of the sphenoid ridge. J. Neurosurg. **53,** 587–599 (1980).

Bonnet, P.: La loge caverneuse et les syndromes de la loge caverneuse. Arch. Ophtalmol. (Paris) **15,** 357–372 (1955).

Brismar, J., Brismar, G., Davis, K. R.: Superior ophthalmic vein at computed tomography. Acta Radiol. (Stock.) **18,** 273 (1977).

Butler, H.: The development of certain human dural venous sinuses. J. Anat. **91,** 510–526 (1957).

Cabanis, E. A., Iba-Zizen, M. T., et al.: Tomodensiometric anatomy of the orbital blood vessels. Bull. Soc. Ophthalmol. Fr. **6–7,** 511 (1979).

Christensen, J. B., Telford, I. R.: Synopsis of Gross Anatomy with Clinical Correlations, ed. **3,** p. 275, New York: Harper and Row (1978).

Clay, C., Vignaut, J., Aubin, M. L., et al.: Phlébographie orbitaire et du sinus caverneux. Gaz. Med. France **80,** 2073–2086 (1973).

Crafts, R. D.: A Textbook of Human Anatomy, ed. **2,** pp. 503–505. New York: J. Wiley and Sons (1979).

Craig, W. M., Gogela, L. J.: Meningioma of the optic foramen as a cause of slowly progressive blindness. Report of three cases. J. Neurosurg. **7,** 44–48 (1950).

van Damme, W., Kosman, P., Wackenheim, A.: A standardized method for computed tomography of the orbits. Neuroradiology **13,** 139 (1977).

Dandy, W. E.: Prechiasmal intracranial tumors of the optic nerves. Am. J. Ophthalmol. **5,** 169–188 (1922).

Dawson, B. H.: The blood vessels of the human optic chiasm and their relation to those of the hypophysis and hypothalamus. Brain **81,** 207–217 (1958).

DiDio, L. J. A.: Synopsis of Anatomy, p. 394. St. Louis: Mosby (1970).

Duke-Elder, S.: Textbook of Ophthalmology, Vol. 1, pp. 102, 182, 184, 188, 401. London: Kimpton (1932).

Dunker, R. O., Harris, A. B.: Surgical anatomy of the proximal anterior cerebral artery. J. Neurosurg. **44,** 359–367 (1976).

Gardner, E., Gray, D. J., O'Rahilly, R.: Anatomy. A Regional Study of Human Structure, ed. **4,** p. 609. Philadelphia: W. B. Saunders (1975).

Glenn, W. V., Johnson, R. J., et al.: Further investigation and clinical use of advanced CT display capability. Invest. Radiol. **10,** 479 (1975).

Goddé-Jolly, D., Cabanis, E. A., et al.: Tomodensiometric anatomy and physiology of the muscle cone. Bull. Soc. Ophthalmol. Fr. **3,** 215 (1980).

Grant, J. C. B.: A Method of Anatomy, **6**th ed., p. 660. Baltimore: Williams and Wilkins (1958).

Hacker, H.: Venenabflüsse des Gehirns. Deutscher Röntgenkongreß (1967), Part A. Stuttgart: G. Thieme (1968b).

Harris, F. S., Rhoton, A. L., Jr.: Anatomy of the cavernous sinus. A microsurgical study. J. Neurosurg. **45,** 169–180 (1976).

Haverling, M., Johanson, H.: Computed sagittal tomography of the orbit. A. J. R. **131,** 346 (1978).

Hayreh, S. S., Dass, R.: The ophthalmic artery. Brit. J. Ophthal. **46,** 65–97 (1962).

Hollenhorst, R. W., Jr., Hollenhorst, R. W., et al.: Visual prognosis of optic nerve sheath meningiomas producing shunt vessels on the optic disk. Mayo. Clin. Proc. **53,** 84–92 (1978).

Hollinshead, W. H.: Anatomy for Surgeons, Vol. **1,** p. 156. New York: Hoeber (1954).

Hughes, B.: Blood supply of the optic nerves and chiasma and its clinical significance. Brit. J. Ophthal. **42,** 106–125 (1958).

James, B. P., Lawton Smith, J.: Bilateral optic nerve sheath meningiomas presenting as the chiasmal syndrome. Neuro-Ophthalmology Update, pp. 177–183. New York: Masson Publishing USA (1977).

Johnston, T. B., Davies, D. V., Davies, F.: Gray's Anatomy, **32**nd ed., p. 757. London: Longmans Green (1958).

Lang, J.: Klinische Anatomie des Kopfes. Berlin–Heidelberg–New York: Springer (1981).

Lanz, T. von, Wachsmuth, W.: Praktische Anatomie, Vol. 1/1B. Berlin–Heidelberg–New York: Springer (1979).

Lawrence, W., Hirst, M. D., et al.: Sphenoidal pneumosinus dilatans with bilateral optic nerve meningiomas. Case report. J. Neurosurg. **51,** 402–407 (1979).

Leonardi, M., Barbina, V., et al.: Sagittal computed tomography of the orbit. J. Comput. Assist. Tomogr. **1,** 511 (1977).

LeRebellar, M. J., Caillé, J. M., et al.: Tomodensiometric aspects of the normal and pathologic eyeball. Bull. Soc. Ophthalmol. Fr. **80,** 307 (1980).

Liliequist, B.: The subarachnoid cisterns. Anatomic and roentgenologic study. Acta radiol. (Stockh.) Suppl. 185 (1959).

Little, H. L., Chambers, J. W., Walsh, F. B.: Unilateral intracranial optic nerve involvement. Neurosurgical significance. Arch. Ophthalmol. **73,** 331–337 (1965).

Lombardi, G., Passerini, A., Cecchini, A.: Pneumosinus dilatans. Acta Radiol. (Diagn). **7,** 535–542 (1968).

Macialowicz, T.: A case of dilating pneumosinus of the sphenoid sinus and the posterior ethmoid cells. Pol. Rev. Radiolog. Nucl. Med. **33,** 324–330 (1969).

Manelfe, C. L., Pasquini, U., Bank, W. O.: Metrizamide demonstration of the subarachnoid space surrounding the optic nerves. J. Comput. Assist. Tomogr. **2,** 545 (1978).

Manelfe, C., Tremoulet, M., Roulleau, J.: Étude artériographique des branches intracaverneuses de la carotide interne. Neurochirurgie **18,** 581–598 (1972).

Mayer, E. G.: Über Lageanomalien des Planum sphenoidale und ihre diagnostische Bedeutung. Roentgenpraxis **6,** 427–431 (1934).

McGrath, P.: The cavernous sinus; an anatomical survey. Aust. NZ J. Surg. **47,** 601–613 (1977).

Nathan, H., Goldhammer, Y.: The rootlets of the trochlear nerve. Anatomical observations in human brains. Acta Anat. **84,** 590–596 (1973).

Nathan, H., Quaknine, G., Kosary, I. Z.: The abducens nerve. Anatomical variations in its course. J. Neurosurg. **41,** 561–566 (1974).

Palacios, E., Fine, M., Haughton, V. M.: Multiplanar Anatomy of the Head and Neck for Computed Tomography. New York: John Wiley & Sons (1980).

Parkinson, D.: A surgical approach to the cavernous portion of the carotid artery. Anatomical studies and case report. J. Neurosurg. **23,** 474–483 (1965).

Patouillard, P., Vanneuville, G.: Les parois du sinus caverneux. Neurochirurgie **18,** 551–560 (1972).

Paturet, G.: Traité d'Anatomie Humaine, Vol. **IV,** pp. 721–722. Système Nerveux. Paris: Masson (1964).

Perlmutter, D., Rhoton, A. L., Jr.: Microsurgical anatomy of the anterior cerebral-anterior communicating-recurrent artery complex. J. Neurosurg. **45,** 259–271 (1976).

Potter, G. D., Trokel, S. L.: The Optic Canal. In: Radiology of the Skull and Brain: Technical Aspects of Computed Tomography (Newton, T. H., Potts, D. G., eds.), Vol. **5.** St. Louis: Mosby (1981).

Prives, M. G., Lisenkov, N. K., Bushkovich, V. I.: Human Anatomy, ed. **7,** 815 pp. Leningrad: Izdatelstvo "Medisina" (1969).

Quiroz-Gutiérrez, F.: Tratado de Anatomia Humana, Vol. **II,** pp. 146–389. Mexico City: Editorial Porrua (1965).

Rabischong, P., Clay, C., Vignaud, J., et al.: Approche hémodynamique de la signification fonctionnelle du sinus caverneux. Neurochirurgie **18,** 613–622 (1972).

Rhoton, A. L., Jr., Hardy, D. G., Chambers, S. M.: Microsurgical anatomy and dissection of the sphenoid bone, cavernous sinus and sellar region. Surg. Neurol. **12,** 63–104 (1979).

Ridley, H.: The Anatomy of the Brain, p. 39. London: Smith and Walford (1695).

Romanes, G. J.: Cunningham's Textbook of Anatomy, ed. **12,** p. 953. London: Oxford University Press (1981).

Rouvière, H.: Anatomie Humaine. Descriptive et Topographique, ed. **10,** Vol. III, p. 678. Paris: Masson (1970).

Salvolini, U., Cabanis, E. A., et al.: Computed tomography of the optic nerve: Part 1. Normal results. J. Comput. Assist. Tomogr. **2,** 141 (1978).

Samii, M., Draf, W.: Course on Surgery of the Skull Base. Hannover, West Germany (1979).

Samii, M., Draf, W.: Course in the Surgery of the Anterior Skull Base. Hannover, West-Germany (1980).

Samii, M., Draf, W.: Course on the Surgery of the Middle Skull Base. Hannover, West-Germany (1981).

Samii, M., Jannetta, P. J.: Symposium on Cranial Nerves. Hannover, West-Germany (1980).

Schaeffer, J. P.: Morris's Human Anatomy, **11**th ed., p. 658. New York: McGray-Hill (1953).

Schott: On some affections of the optic nerve. Arch. Ophthalmol. **6,** 262–283 (1877).

Seeger, W.: Atlas of Topographical Anatomy of the Brain and Surrounding Structures. Wien–New York: Springer (1978).

Seeger, W.: Microsurgery of the Brain. Anatomical and Technical Principles, Vol. 1 + 2. Wien–New York: Springer (1980).

Sinelnikov, P. D.: Atlas of Human Anatomy, Vol. **2,** p. 154. Moscow: Izdatelstvo "Medisina" (1958).

Snell, R. S.: Clinical Anatomy for Students, ed. **2,** Fig. 43. Boston: Little, Brown and Co. (1981).

Sundt, T. M., Jr., Murphey, F.: Clipcrafts for aneurysm and small vessel surgery. Part 3: Clinical experience in intracranial carotid artery aneurysms. J. Neurosurg. **31,** 59–71 (1969).

Sugita, K., Hirota, T., Iguchi, I., et al.: Transient amaurosis under decreased atmospheric pressure with sphenoidal sinus dysplasia. Case report. J. Neurosurg. **46,** 111–114 (1977).

Tadmor, R., New, F. J.: Computed tomography of the orbit with special emphasis on coronal sections: Part 1. Normal anatomy. J. Comput. Assist. Tomogr. **2,** 24 (1978).

Testut, L., Latarjet, A.: Tratado de Anatomia Humana, Vol. **II,** p. 441. Angiologia-Sistema Nervioso Central. Barcelona: Salvat Editores (1974).

Theron, J.: Les affluents du plexus caverneux. Neurochirurgie **18,** 623–638 (1972).

Thompson, J. S.: Core Textbook of Anatomy, pp. 204–206. Philadelphia: J. B. Lippincott (1977).

Thorek, P.: Anatomy in Surgery, p. 58. Philadelphia: J. B. Lippincott (1951).

Trobe, J. D., Glaser, J. S., Post, J. D., et al.: Bilateral optic canal meningiomas: a case report. Neurosurgery **3,** 68–74 (1978).

Umansky, F., Nathan, H.: The lateral wall of the cavernous sinus. J. Neurosurg. **56,** 228–234 (1982).

Unsöld, R.: Computed Tomography in Ophthalmology, Vol. **22,** No. 4, pp. 45–80. Boston, Massachusetts: Little, Brown and Company (1982).

Unsöld, R.: On the CT diagnosis of optic nerve lesions. Differential diagnostic criteria. Albrecht von Graefes Arch. Klin. Exp. Ophthalmol. **281,** 124 (1982).

Unsöld, R., DeGroot, J., Newton, T. H.: Images of the optic nerve: Anatomic-CT correlation. Am. J. Neuroradiol. **1,** 317 (1980).

Unsöld, R., Newton, T. H., Berninger, W.: The Value and Clinical Application of Multiplanar Computer Reformations in Orbital Diagnosis. In: Diagnostic Radiology 1980. Proceedings of the Annual Postgraduate Course in Diagnostic Radiology, San Francisco, Mar. 3–7, 1980 (Margulis, A. R., Gooding, C. A., eds.). San Francisco: University of California, Department of Radiology (1980).

Unsöld, R., Newton, T. H., DeGroot, J.: CT evaluation of extraocular muscles: Anatomic-CT correlations. Albrecht von Graefes Arch. Klin. Exp. Ophthalmol. **214,** 155 (180).

Unsöld, R., Newton, T. H., Hoyt, W. F.: CT examination technique of the optic nerve. J. Comput. Assist. Tomogr. **4** (4), 560 (1980).

Unsöld, R., Norman, D., Berninger, W.: Multiplanar evaluation of the optic canal from axial transverse CT sections. J. Comput. Assist. Tomogr. **4** (3), 418 (1980).

Vignaud, J., Aubin, M.-L.: Coronal (frontal) sections in computerized tomography of the orbit. J. Neuroradiol. **5,** 161 (1978).

Vignaud, J., Clay, C., Aubin, M. L., et al.: Opacification du sinus caverneux. Intérèt de la tomographie simultanée. J. Radiol. Electrol. Med. Nucl. **53,** 51–53 (1972).

Vignaud, J., Clay, C., Kujas, A., et al.: Phlebo-tomographies simultanées du sinus caverneux. Neurochirurgie **18,** 665–675 (1972).

Vignaud, J., Doyon, D., Aubin, M. L., et al.: Opacification du sinus caverneux par voix postérieure. Neurochirurgie **18,** 649–664 (1972).

Walsh, F. B.: Meningiomas primary within the orbit and the optic canal in Lawton Smith J. (ed.): Neuro-Ophthalmology, Symposium of the University of Miami and the Bascom Palmer Eye Institute, Vol. **V,** pp. 240–266. Hallandale, Florida: Huffman Publishing (1970).

Warwick, R., Williams, P. L. (eds.): Gray's Anatomy, ed. **35,** p. 695. Edinburgh: Longman (1973).

Warwick, R.: In: Anatomy of the Eye and Orbit (Wolff, E., Last, R. J., eds.), 7th ed. London: H. K. Lewis (1976).

Watanabe, T. J., LaMasters, D., et al.: Contrast Enhancement of the Normal Orbit. In International Workshop on Contrast Media in Computed Tomography, Berlin 1981. International Congress Series No. **561.** Amsterdam: Excerpta Medica (1981).

Weinberger, L. M., Adler, F. H., Grant, F. C.: Primary pituitary adenoma and the syndrome of the cavernous sinus. A clinical and anatomic study. Arch. Ophthalmol. **24,** (NS), 1196–1236 (1940).

Weinstein, M. A., Modic, M. T., Risius, B., et al.: Visualization of arteries, veins and nerves of the orbit by sector computed tomography. Radiology **138,** 83 (1981).

Weizenhoffer, A.: Contralateral cavernous sinus thrombosis. NY State J. Med. **32,** 139–142 (1932).

Williams, F. P., Shawker, T. H., Lora, J.: Pneumosinus dilatans of the sphenoid sinus. Bull. Los Angeles Neurol. Soc. **40,** 45–48 (1975).

Winslow, J. B.: Exposition anatomique de la structure du corps humain, Vol. **2,** p. 31. London: Prevost (1732).

Wolff, E.: The Anatomy of the Eye and Orbit, 4th ed., pp. 14, 287, 288, 370. London: Lewis (1954).

Wood Jones, F.: Buchanan's Manual of Anatomy, 8th ed., p. 1175. London: Baillière, Tindall and Cox (1949).

Zozulia, Y. A., Romodanov, S. A., Patsko, Y. V.: Diagnosis and surgical treatment of benign craniobasal tumours involving the cavernous sinus. Acta Neurochir. (Wien) Suppl. **28,** 387–390 (1979).

Chapter 3

Bostroem, A., Spatz, H.: Über die von der Olfactoriusrinne ausgehenden Meningeome und über die Meningeome im allgemeinen. Nervenarzt **2,** 505–521 (1929).

Bradac, G. B.: Some aspects of the venous drainage dynamics with tumors at the bone of the skull in the anterior and middle fossae. Neuroradiology **12,** 115–120 (1976).

Dandy, W. E.: Prechiasmal intracranial tumors of the optic nerve. Amer. J. Ophthal. **5,** 169–188 (1922).

Dietz, H.: Die frontobasale Schädelhirnverletzung. Berlin–Heidelberg–New York: Springer (1970). See there further literature before 1970.

Ehlers, N., Malmros, R.: The suprasellar meningioma. Acta Ophthalmol. (Copenhagen) Suppl. 121 (1973).

Hacker, H.: Venenabflüsse des Gehirns. Deutscher Röntgenkongreß (1967), Part A. Stuttgart: G. Thieme (1968b).

Haensel, G., Seeger, W.: Die mikrochirurgische Behandlung der sogenannten Tuberculum sellae-Meningeome. Acta Neurochir. (Wien) **37,** 111–123 (1977).

Hughes, B.: Blood supply of the optic nerves and chiasma and its clinical significance. Brit. J. Ophthal. **42,** 106–125 (1958).

Kaplan, H. A.: The lateral perforating branches of the anterior and middle cerebral arteries. J. Neurosurg. **23,** 305–310 (1965).

Kaplan, H. A., Browder, J.: Benign tumors of the cerebral dural sinuses. J. Neurosurg. **37,** 576–579 (1972).

Kaplan, H. A., Browder, J.: Atresia of the rostral superior sagittal sinus: substitute parasagittal venous channels. J. Neurosurg. **38,** 602–607 (1973).

Kaplan, H. A., Browder, A., Browder, J.: Nasal venous drainage and the Foramen caecum. Laryngoscope **83,** 327–329 (1973).

Krause, F.: Die spezielle Chirurgie der Gehirnkrankheiten. Bd. 2b u. 3. In: Neue Deutsche Chirurgie, Bd. 49b u. 50. Stuttgart: F. Enke (1941, 1932).

Lang, J.: Klinische Anatomie des Kopfes. Berlin–Heidelberg–New York: Springer (1981).

Lanz, T. von, Wachsmuth, W.: Praktische Anatomie, Vol. 1/1B. Berlin–Heidelberg–New York: Springer (1979).

Liliequist, B.: The subarachnoid cisterns. Anatomic and roentgenologic study. Acta radiol. (Stockh.) Suppl. 185 (1959).

Logue, V.: Surgery of Meningiomas. In: Operative Surgery Fundamental International Techniques Neurosurgery (Symon, L., ed.), pp. 128–173. London–Boston–Sydney–Wellington–Durban–Toronto: Butterworths (1979).

Love, J. G., Gay, J. R.: Resection of the superior longitudinal sinus. J. Neurosurg. **4,** 182–188 (1947).

McCord, G. M., Goree, J. A., Jimenez, J. P.: Venous drainage to the inferior sagittal sinus. Radiology **105,** 583–589 (1972).

Maltby, G. L.: Resection of longitudinal sinus posterior to the rolandic area for complete removal of a meningioma. Arch. Neurol. Psychiat. **42,** 1135–1139 (1939).

Marc, J. A., Schechter, M. M.: Cortical venous rerouting in parasagittal meningiomas. Radiology **112,** 85–92 (1974).

Okonek, G.: Beitrag zur Erkennung und Behandlung basaler Meningeome. Zbl. Chir. **22,** 1912–1025 (1941).

Olivecrona, H.: The Surgical Treatment of Intracranial Tumors. In: Handbuch der Neurochirurgie 4/IV (Olivecrona, H., Tönnis, W., eds.), pp. 181–184. Berlin–Heidelberg–New York: Springer (1967).

Palacios, E., Fine, M., Haughton, V. M.: Multiplanar Anatomy of the Head and Neck for Computed Tomography. New York: John Wiley & Sons (1980).

Perlmutter, D., Rhoton, A. L., Jr.: Microsurgical anatomy of the anterior cerebral-anterior communicating-recurrent artery complex. J. Neurosurg. **45,** 259–271 (1976).

Poppen, J. L.: An Atlas of Neurosurgical Techniques. Philadelphia–London: W. B. Saunders Company (1960).

Probst, Ch.: Frontobasale Verletzungen. Pathogenetische, diagnostische und therapeutische Probleme aus neurochirurgischer Sicht. Bern–Stuttgart–Wien: Hans Huber (1971). See there further literature up till 1971.

Samii, M., Draf, W.: Course on Surgery of the Skull Base. Hannover, West Germany (1979).

Samii, M., Draf, W.: Course on the Surgery of the Anterior Skull Base. Hannover, West-Germany (1980).

Samii, M., Jannetta, P. J.: Symposium on Cranial Nerves. Hannover, West-Germany (1980).

Seeger, W.: Atlas of Topographical Anatomy of the Brain and Surrounding Structures. Wien–New York: Springer (1978).

Seeger, W.: Microsurgery of the Brain. Anatomical and Technical Principles, Vol. 1+2. Wien–New York: Springer (1980).

Stephens, R. B., Stilwell, D. L.: Arteries and Veins of the Human Brain. Springfield, Ill.: Ch. C Thomas (1969).

Symon, L.: Olfactory groove and suprasellar meningiomas. In: Advances and Technical Standards in Neurosurgery (Krayenbühl, H., et al., eds.), Vol. **4,** pp. 67–91. Wien–New York: Springer (1977).

Towne, E. B.: Invasion of intracranial venous sinuses by meningioma (dural endothelioma). Ann. Surg. **83,** 321–327 (1926).

Wilson, McClure: The Anatomical Foundation of Neurology of the Brain Subarachnoid Spaces, Chapter 4, pp. 93–103. Boston: Little, Brown (1963 and 1972).

Chapter 4

Ausman, J. I., Diaz, F. G., et al.: Superficial temporal to proximal superior cerebellar artery anastomosis for basilar artery stenosis. Neurosurgery **9,** 56–59 (1981).

Ausman, J. I., Lee, M. C., et al.: Stroke: what's new? Cerebral revascularization. Minn. Med. **59,** 223–227 (1976).

Ausman, J. I., Lindsay, W., et al.: Ipsilateral subclavian to external carotid and STA-MCA bypasses for retinal ischemia. Surg. Neurol. **9,** 5–8 (1978).

Ausman, J. I., Nocoloff, D. M., Chou, S. N.: Posterior fossa revascularization: anastomosis of vertebral artery to PICA with interposed radial artery graft. Surg. Neurol. **9,** 281–286 (1978).

Barner, H. B., Judd, D. R., et al.: Late failure of arterialized in situ saphenous vein. Arch. Surg. **99,** 781–786 (1969).

Barnes, W. T., Jacoby, G. E.: Aneurysm of the common carotid artery due to cystic medial necosis treated by excision and graft. Ann. Surg. **155,** 82–85 (1962).

Baxter, Th. J., O'Brien, B., et al.: The histopathology of small vessels following microvascular repair. Brit. J. Surg. **59,** 617 (1972).

Beall, A. C., Jr., Crawford, E. S., et al.: Extracranial aneurysms of the carotid artery. Report of seven cases. Postgrad. Med. **32,** 93–102 (1962).

Brambilla, G., Paoletti, P., Rodriguez y Baena, R.: Extracranial-intracranial arterial bypass in the treatment of inoperable giant aneurysms of the internal carotid artery. Report of a Case. Acta Neurochir. (Wien) **60,** 63–69 (1982).

Chater, N. L., Popp, J.: Microsurgical vascular bypass for occlusive cerebrovascular disease: Review of 100 cases. Surg. Neurol. **6,** 115–118 (1976).

Chater, N. L., Reichmann, O. H., Tew, J.: Cerebral Revascularization – Scientific Exhibit. American Association of Neurological Surgeons. Los Angeles (1972).

Chater, N. L., Reichmann, O. H., Tew, J.: Cerebral Revascularization for Occlusive Cerebrovascular Disease. Presented at the meeting of the American Association of Neurological Surgeons. Los Angeles, April 8–11 (1973).

Chater, N. L., Spetzler, R.: Anatomical Studies of the Cerebral Cortical Vasculature of Microvascular Surgical Significance. Presented at the international Symposium on Neurosurgery Through the Microscope. Mount Sinai School of Medicine, City University of New York. New York City, June 11–14 (1973).

Chater, N. L., Spetzler, R., Tonnenmacher, K., et al.: Microvascular bypass surgery. Part I: Anatomical studies. J. Neurosurg. **44,** 712–714 (1976).

Chater, N. L., Yaşargil, M. G.: Results of Temporal Artery Bypass Procedures in Treatment of Cerebrovascular Disease. Presented at Congress of Neurological Surgeons. Miami, Florida, October 1971.

DeBakey, M. E.: Concepts underlying surgical treatment of cerebrovascular insufficiency. Clin. Neurosurg. **10,** 310–340 (1964).

De Weese, J. A., Robb, C. G.: Autogenous venous bypass grafts five years later. Ann. Surg. **174,** 346–356 (1971).

Donaghy, R. M. P., Yaşargil, M. G. (eds.): Microvascular Surgery, pp. 75–86. Report of First Conference 1966. St. Louis: Mosby (1967).

Drake, C.: The Intracranial Use of the 'Hunterian' Proximal Ligation in the Treatment of Giant Aneurysm. Presented at American Association of Neurological Surgeons, Toronto, Canada (1977).

Drake, C. G.: Giant intracranial aneurysms: experience with surgical treatment in 174 patients. Clin. Neurosurg. **26,** 12–95 (1979).

Ferguson, G. G., Drake, C. G., Peerless, S. J.: Extracranial-intracranial arterial bypass in the treatment of "giant" intracranial aneurysms. Stroke **8,** 11, 1977 (Abstract).

Fields, W. S.: Selection of stroke patient for arterial reconstructive surgery. Am. J. Surg. **125,** 527–529 (1973).

Galbraith, J. G., McDowell, H. A.: Stroke and occlusive cerebrovascular disease: review and surgical results in 265 cases. J. Med. Assoc. Alabama **38,** 1107–1111 (1969).

Garmella, J. J., Lynch, M. F., et al.: Endarterectomy and thrombectomy for the totally occluded extracranial internal carotid artery: use of Fogarty balloon catheters. Ann. Surg. **164,** 325–333 (1966).

Gelber, B. J., Sundt, T. M., Jr.: Treatment of intracavernous and giant carotid aneurysms by combined internal carotid ligation and extra- to intracranial bypass. J. Neurosurg. **52,** 1–10 (1980).

Gilsbach, J. M.: Intraoperative Doppler Sonography in Neurosurgery. Wien–New York: Springer (1983).

Gratzl, O., Schmiedek, P., Oeteanu-Nube, V.: Long-term clinical results following extra-intracranial arterial bypass surgery. In: Microsurgery for Stroke (Schmiedek, P., Gratzl, O., Spetzler, R., eds.), pp. 271–275. Berlin–Heidelberg–New York: Springer (1977).

Henschen, C.: XXXVIII. Operative Revaskularisation des zirkulatorisch geschädigten Gehirns durch Auflage gestielter Muskellappen (Encephalo-Myo-Synangiose). Basel, pp. 392–401.

Holbach, K. H., Wassmann, H., Bonatelli, A. P.: A method to identify and treat reversible ischemialterations of brain tissue. In: Microsurgery for Stroke (Schmiedek, P., Gratzl, O., Spetzler, R., eds.), pp. 169–176. Berlin–Heidelberg–New York: Springer (1977).

Hopkins, L. N., Grand, W.: Extracranial-intracranial arterial bypass in the treatment of aneurysms of the carotid and middle cerebral arteries. Neurosurgery **5,** 21–31 (1979).

Horváth, M., Pásztor, E., Vajda, J., Nyáry, I.: Posterior fossa revascularization by superficial temporal artery (STA) – superior cerebellar artery (SCA) anastomosis. Acta Neurochir. (Wien) **66,** 43–53 (1982).

International Symposium on Microneurosurgical Anastomosis for Cerebral Ischemia. Loma Linda University School of Medicine Loma Linda Calif. June 14–15 (1973).

Jacobson, J. H., Suarez, E.: Microsurgery in anastomosis of small vessels. Surgical Forum **11,** 243 (1960).

Khodadad, G.: Occipital artery-posterior inferior cerebellar artery anastomosis. Surg. Neurol. **5,** 225–227 (1976).

Khodadad, G.: Short- and long-term results of microvascular anastomosis in the vertebrobasilar system: A critical analysis. Neurol. Res. **3,** 33–65 (1981).

Khodadad, G., Singh, R. S., Olinger, C. P.: Possible prevention of brain stem stroke by microvascular anastomosis in the vertebrobasilar system. Stroke **8,** 316–321 (1977).

Kletter, G., Koos, W. Th.: Zur Technik der arteriellen experimentellen extra-intra-kraniellen Anastomose. Acta Chir. Austriaca **8,** 83 (1975).

Kletter, G., Matras, H., Dinges, H. P.: Zur partiellen Klebung von Mikrogefäßanastomosen im intrakraniellen Bereich. Wien. klin. Wschr. **90,** 415–419 (1978).

Kletter, G., Meyermann, R.: Histological Case Control of Microanastomosis. Clinical Microneurosurgery 234. Stuttgart: G. Thieme (1976).

Kletter, G., Meyermann, R.: Histologische Veränderungen nach Mikrogefäßanastomosen. Acta Chirurg. Austriaca **2,** 35 (1977).

Kletter, G., Meyermann, R., Koos, W. Th., Schuster, H.: L'importance de la structure histologique de l'artère temporale superficielle pour la fonction de l'anastomose arterielle extra-intracrânienne. Neurochirurgie (Paris) **21,** 551 (1975).

Kopaniky, D., Spetzler, R. F.: Severe otorrhagia resulting from a ruptured aneurysm of the extracranial internal carotid artery (in preparation).

Krayenbühl, H.: Comments on the history of external-internal anastomosis for cerebral ischemia. In: Microsurgery for Stroke (Schmiedek, P., Gratzl, O., Spetzler, R., eds.), pp. 3–7. Berlin–Heidelberg–NewYork: Springer (1977).

Lang, J.: Klinische Anatomie des Kopfes. Berlin–Heidelberg–New York: Springer (1981).

Lanz, T. von, Wachsmuth, W.: Praktische Anatomie, Vol. 1/1B. Berlin–Heidelberg–New York: Springer (1979).

Lazar, M. L., Clark, K.: Microsurgical cerebral revascularization: concept and practice. Surg. Neurol. **1,** 355–359 (1973).

Lougheed, W. M., Marshall, B. M., et al.: Common carotid to intracranial internal carotid bypass venous graft. J. Neurosurg. **34,** 114–118 (1971).

Matras, H., Chiari, F., et al.: Zur Klebung von Mikrogefäßanastomosen. Bericht d. 13. Jtgg. d. Dtsch. Ges. f. plast. und Wiederherstellungschir., 1975, S. 357. Stuttgart: G. Thieme (1977).

Matras, H., Chiari, F., et al.: Neue Wege in der Mikrogefäßchirurgie (eine experimentelle Studie). Bericht d. 17. Tagung der Österr. Ges. f. Chir., Salzburg, 1976. Acta Chir. Austr. Sonder-Supplement S. 458 (1976/77).

Matras, H., Chiari, F., et al.: Zur Klebung kleinster Gefäße im Tierversuch. Dtsch. Z. Mund-Kiefer-Gesichts-Chir. **1,** 19 (1977).

Meyermann, R., Kletter, G.: Causes of Stenosis and Embolic Occlusions in Microsurgical Anastomosis. Advances in Neurosurgery **2,** 322 (1975).

Miller, C. F. II, Spetzler, R. F., Kopaniky, D. J.: Middle meningeal to middle cerebral arterial bypass for cerebral revascularization. Case report. J. Neurosurg. **50,** 802–804 (1979).

Nunn, D. B., Chun, B., et al.: Autogeneous veins as arterial substitutes: A study of their histologic fate with special attention to endothelium. Ann. Surg. **160,** 14–22 (1964).

Ohara, I., Utsumi, N., Ouchi, H.: Resection of extracranial internal carotid artery aneurysms with arterial reconstruction. J. Cardiovasc. Surg. **9,** 365–373 (1968).

Palacios, E., Fine, M., Haughton, V. M.: Multiplanar Anatomy of the Head and Neck for Computed Tomography. New York: John Wiley & Sons (1980).

Peerless, S. J., Chater, N. L., Ferguson, G. G.: Multiple-vessel occlusions in cerebro-vascular disease – A further follow up of the effects of microvascular bypass on the quality of life and the incidence of stroke. In: Microsurgery for Stroke (Schmiedek, P., Gratzl, O., Spetzler, R., eds.), pp. 251–259. Berlin–Heidelberg–New York: Springer (1977).

Raphael, H. A., Bernatz, P. E., Spittell, J. A., Jr., et al.: Cervical carotid aneurysms: treatment by excision and restoration of arterial continuity. Am. J. Surg. **105,** 771–778 (1963).

Reichmann, O. H.: Experimental lingual-basilar arterial microanastomosis. J. Neurosurg. **34,** 500–505 (1971).

Reichmann, O. H.: Extracranial-intracranial arterial anastomosis. In: Cerebral Vascular Diseases: Ninth Conference (Whisnant, J. P., Sandok, B. A., eds.), pp. 175–185. New York: Grune and Stratton (1975).

Roski, R., Spetzler, R. F., et al.: Reversal of documented seven-year old visual field defect with extracranial-intracranial arteriel anastomosis. Surg. Neurol. **10,** 267–268 (1978).

Roski, R. A., Spetzler, R. F., et al.: Occipital artery to posterior inferior cerebellar artery bypass for vertebrobasilar ischemia. Neurosurgery **10,** No. 1, 44–49 (1982).

Samii, M., Draf, W.: Course on Surgery of the Skull Base. Hannover, West Germany (1979).

Samii, M., Jannetta, P. J.: Symposium on Cranial Nerves. Hannover, West-Germany (1980).

Samson, S., Neuwelt, E. A., et al.: Failure of extracranial-intracranial arterial bypass in acute middle cerebral artery occlusion. Case report. Neurosurgery **6,** 185–188 (1980).

Schmiedek, P., Gratzl, O., et al.: Selection of patients for extracranial arterial bypass surgery based on rCBF measurements. J. Neurosurg. **44,** 303–312 (1976).

Seeger, W.: Atlas of Topographical Anatomy of the Brain and Surrounding Structures. Wien–New York: Springer (1978).

Seeger, W.: Microsurgery of the Brain. Anatomical and Technical Principles, Vol. 1 + 2. Wien–New York: Springer (1980).

Spetzler, R. F.: Extracranial-intracranial arterial anastomosis for cerebrovascular disease. Surg. Neurol. **11,** 157–161 (1979).

Spetzler, R. F., Chater, N. L.: Occipital artery-middle cerebral anastomosis for cerebral artery occlusive disease. Surg. Neurol. **2,** 235–238 (1974).

Spetzler, R., Chater, N.: Microvascular bypass surgery. Part 2: Physiological studies. J. Neurosurg. **45,** 508–513 (1976).

Spetzler, R. F., Chater, N. L.: Microvascular arterial bypass in cerebrovascular occlusive disease. In: Clinical Microneurosurgery (Koos, W. Th., Bock, F. W., Spetzler, R. F., eds.), pp. 242–246. Stuttgart: G. Thieme (1976).

Spetzler, R., Chater, N. L., Mani, J.: The spectrum of intracranial occlusive disease suitable for microvascular bypass. J. Radiol. (submitted).

Spetzler, R. F., Iversen, A. A.: Alleable microsurgical suction device: Technical note. J. Neurosurg. **54,** 704–705 (1981).

Spetzler, R. F., Owen, M. P.: Extracranial-intracranial arterial bypass to a single branch of the middle cerebral artery in the management of a traumatic aneurysm. Neurosurgery **4,** 334–337 (1979).

Spetzler, R. F., Rhodes, R. S., et al.: Subclavian to middle cerebral artery saphenous vein bypass graft. J. Neurosurg. **53,** 465–469 (1980).

Spetzler, R. F., Roski, R. A., et al.: The 'bonnet bypass'. J. Neurosurg. **53,** 707–709 (1980).

Spetzler, R. F., Schuster, H., Roski, R. A.: Elective extracranial-intracranial arterial bypass in the treatment of inoperable giant aneurysms of the internal carotid artery. J. Neurosurg. **53,** 22–27 (1980).

Story, J. L., Brown, W. E., Jr., et al.: Cerebral revascularization: common carotid to distal middle cerebral artery bypass. Neurosurgery **2,** 131–134 (1978).

Story, J. L., Brown, W. E., Jr., et al.: Cerebral revascularization: proximal external carotid to distal middle cerebral artery bypass with a synthetic tube graft. Neurosurgery **3,** 61–65 (1978).

Story, J. L., Brown, W. E., Jr., et al.: Cerebral revascularization: cervical carotid-intracranial arterial long graft bypass. In: Advances in Neurosurgery, Vol. 7 (Marguth, F., Brock M., Kazner, E., et al., eds.), pp. 15–23. Berlin–Heidelberg–New York: Springer (1979).

Sundt, T. M., Piepgras, D. G.: Occipital to posterior inferior cerebellar artery bypass surgery. J. Neurosurg. **48,** 916–928 (1978).

Sundt, T. M., Siekert, R. G., et al.: Bypass surgery for vascular disease of the carotid system. Mayo Clinic Rochester Minn. **51,** 677–692 (1976).

Sundt, T. M., Whisnat, J. P., Piepgras, D. G., et al.: Intracranial bypass grafts for vertebral-basilar ischemia. Mayo Clin. Proc. **53,** 12–18 (1978).

Sundt, T. M., Jr.: Editorial comment to Reference 1. Neurosurgery **9,** 59–60 (1981).

Sundt, T. M., Jr., Campbell, J. K., Houser, O. W.: Transpositions and anastomoses between the posterior cerebral and superior cerebellar arteries. J. Neurosurg. **55,** 967–970 (1981).

Sundt, T. M., Jr., Houser, O. W., et al.: Interposition saphenous vein grafts between the external carotid artery and the proximal posterior cerebral artery for advanced occlusive disease and large aneurysms in the posterior circulation. J. Neurosurg. **56,** 1982 (in press).

Sundt, T. M., Jr., Piepgras, D. G.: Surgical approach to giant intracranial aneurysms. Operative experience with 80 cases. J. Neurosurg. **51,** 731–742 (1979).

Sundt, T. M., Jr., Smith, H. C., et al.: Transluminal angioplasty for basilar artery stenosis. Mayo Clin. Proc. **55,** 673–680 (1980).

Tew, J. M., Jr.: Reconstructive intracranial vascular surgery for prevention of stroke. Clin. Neurosurg. **22,** 264–280 (1975).

Thompson, J. E., Austin, D. J.: Endarterectomy of the totally occluded carotid artery for stroke: Results in 100 operations. Arch. Surg. **95,** 791–801 (1967).

Weinstein, P. R., Chater, N. L., et al.: Extra- to intracranial arterial bypass for occlusive vertebro-basilar cerebrovascular disease. Presented at the meeting of American Association of Neurological Surgeons. Miami, April 1975.

Wilson, J. R., Jordan, P. H., Jr.: Excision of an internal carotid artery aneurysm: restitution of continuity by substitution of external for internal carotid artery. Ann. Surg. **154,** 45–47 (1961).

Yaşargil, M. G., Krayenbühl, H. A., Jacobson, J. H.: Microsurgery Applied to Neurosurgery, 230 pp. Stuttgart: G. Thieme (1969).

Yaşargil, M. G., Krayenbühl, H. A., Jacobson, J. H. II: Microneurosurgical arterial reconstruction. Surgery **67,** 221–233 (1970).

Yaşargil, M. G., Yonekawa, Y.: Results of microsurgical extra-intracranial arterial bypass in the treatment of cerebral ischemia. Neurosurgery **1,** 22–24 (1977).

Chapter 5

Apfelbaum, R. I.: A comparison of percutaneous radiofrequency trigeminal neurolysis and microvascular decompression of the trigeminal nerve for the treatment of tic douloureux. Neurosurgery **1,** 16–21 (1977).

Apfelbaum, R. I.: Surgical management of disorders of lower cranial nerves. In: Current Techniques in Operative Neurosurgery, 2nd ed. (Schmidek, H. H., ed.). New York: Grune/Stratton (1982).

Atkinson, W. J.: The anterior inferior cerebellar artery: Its variations, pontine distributions, and significance in the surgery of cerebello-pontine angle tumors. J. Neurol. Neurosurg. Psychiat. **12,** 137–151 (1949).

Burchiel, K. J., Steege, T. D., Howe, J. F., Loeser, J. D.: Comparison of percutaneous radiofrequency gangliolysis and microvascular decompression for the surgical management of tic douloureux. Neurosurgery **9,** 111–119, (1981).

Campbell, E., Keedy, C.: Hemifacial spasm: A note of the etiology in two cases. J. Neurosurg. **4,** 342–347 (1944).

Cushing, H.: The major trigeminal neuralgias and their surgical treatment based on experiences with 332 gasserian operations; the varieties of facial neuralgia. Am. J. Med. Sci. **160,** 157–184 (1920).

Dandy, W. E.: An operation for the cure of tic douloureux. Partial section of the sensory root at the pons. Arch. Surg. **18,** 687–734 (1929).

Dandy, W. E.: The treatment of trigeminal neuralgia by the cerebellar route. Ann. Surg. **96,** 787–795 (1932).

Dandy, W. E.: Concerning the cause of trigeminal neuralgia. Am. J. Surg. **24,** 447–455 (1934).

Dandy, W. E.: Trigeminal neuralgia and trigeminal tic douloureux. In: Lewis' Practice of Surgery, Vol. 12, pp. 167–187. Hagerstown, Md.: W. F. Prior (1946).

Fisch, U.: The surgical anatomy of the so-called internal auditory artery. In: Disorders of the Skull Base Region; Proceedings: Nobel Symposium, 10th, Stockholm, 1968 (Hamberger, C.-A., Wersäll, J., eds.), pp. 121–130. Stockholm: Almqvist and Wiksell, New York: Wiley (1968).

Gardner, W. J.: The mechanism of tic douloureux. Trans. Am. Neurol. Assoc. **78,** 168–173 (1953).

Gardner, W. J.: Concerning the mechanism of trigeminal neuralgia and hemifacial spasm. J. Neurosurg. **19,** 947–957 (1962).

Gardner, W. J., Miklos, W. V.: Response of trigeminal neuralgia to 'decompression' of sensory route: Discussion of cause of trigeminal neuralgia. JAMA **170,** 1773–1776 (1959).

Gardner, W. J., Sava, G. A.: Hemifacial spasm – A reversible pathophysiologic state. J. Neurosurg. **20,** 240–247 (1962).

German, W. J.: Surgical treatment of spasmodic facial tic. Surgery **11,** 912–914 (1942).

Granit, R., Skoglund, C. R., Leksell, L.: Fibre interaction in injured or compressed region of nerve. Brain **67,** 125–140 (1944).

Haines, S. J., Jannetta, P. J., Zorub, D. S.: Microvascular relations of the trigeminal nerve: An anatomical study with clinical correlation. J. Neurosurg. **52,** 381–386 (1980).

Haines, S. J., Martinez, A. J., Jannetta, P. J.: Arterial cross compression of the trigeminal nerve at the pons in trigeminal neuralgia: Case report with autopsy findings. J. Neurosurg. **50,** 257–259 (1979).

Hanraets, P. R.: Surgical treatment of trigeminal neuralgia following the method of Dandy. Psychiatr. Neurol. Neurochir. **73,** 441–446 (1970).

Hardy, D. G., Rhoton, A. L.: Microsurgical relationships of the superior cerebellar artery and the trigeminal nerve. J. Neurosurg. **49,** 669–678 (1978).

Jannetta, P. J.: Arterial compression of the trigeminal nerve at the pons in patients with trigeminal neuralgia. J. Neurosurg. (Suppl.) **26,** 159–162 (1967).

Jannetta, P. J.: Microsurgical exploration and decompression of the facial nerve in hemifacial spasm. Curr. Topics Surg. Res. **2,** 217–220 (1970).

Jannetta, P. J.: Trigeminal and glossopharyngeal neuralgia. Curr. Diagnosis **3,** 849–850 (1971).

Jannetta, P. J.: Neurovascular compression of the facial nerve in hemifacial spasm. Relief by microsurgical technique. In: Reconstructive Surgery of Brain Arteries (Merei, R. T., ed.), pp. 193–199. Budapest, Hungary: Akademiai Kiado (1974).

Jannetta, P. J.: Neurovascular cross-compression in patients with hyperactive dysfunction symptoms of the eighth cranial nerve. Surg. Forum **26,** 467–469 (1975).

Jannetta, P. J.: Microsurgical approach to the trigeminal nerve for tic douloureux. In: Progress in Neurological Surgery, Vol. 7: Pain – Its Neurosurgical Management (Krayenbühl, H., Maspes, P. S., Sweet, W. H., eds.), pp. 180–200. Basel: S. Karger (1976).

Jannetta, P. J.: Observations on the etiology of trigeminal neuralgia, hemifacial spasm, acoustic nerve dysfunction and glossopharyngeal neuralgia: Definitive microsurgical treatment and results in 117 patients. Neurochirurgia (Stuttg.) **20,** 145–154 (1977).

Jannetta, P. J.: Treatment of trigeminal neuralgia by suboccipital and transtentorial cranial operations. Clin. Neurosurg. **24,** 538–549 (1977).

Jannetta, P. J.: Microsurgery of cranial nerve cross-compression. Clin. Neurosurg. **26,** 607–615, (1979).

Jannetta, P. J.: Treatment of trigeminal neuralgia. Neurosurgery **4,** 93–94 (1979).

Jannetta, P. J., Abbasy, M., Maroon, J. C., Ramos, F. M., Albin, M. S.: Hemifacial spasm: Etiology and definitive microsurgical treatment of hemifacial spasm. Operative techniques and results in 47 patients. J. Neurosurg. **47,** 321–328 (1977).

Jannetta, P. J., Hackett, E., Ruby, J. R.: Electromyographic and electron microscopic correlates in hemifacial spasm treated by microsurgical relief of neurovascular compression. Surg. Forum **21,** 449–451 (1970).

Jannetta, P. J., Rand, R. W.: Microanatomy of the trigeminal nerve. Anat. Rec. 154–362 (1966).

Jannetta, P. J., Rand, R. W.: Transtentorial retro-gasserian rhizotomy in trigeminal neuralgia by microneurosurgical technique. Bull., L. A. Neurol. Soc. **31,** 93–99 (1966).

Lang, J.: Klinische Anatomie des Kopfes. Berlin–Heidelberg–New York: Springer (1981).

Lanz, T. von, Wachsmuth, W.: Praktische Anatomie, Vol. 1/1B. Berlin–Heidelberg–New York: Springer (1979).

Lee, F. C.: Trigeminal neuralgia. J. Med. Assoc. Georgia **26,** 431 (1937).

Lewy, F. H., Grant, F. C.: Physiopathologic and pathoanatomic aspects of major trigeminal neuralgia. Arch. Neurol. Psychiat. **40,** 1126–1134 (1938).

Liliequist, B.: The subarachnoid cisterns. Anatomic and roentgenologic study. Acta radiol. (Stockh.) Suppl. 185, 1959.

Martin, R. G., Grant, J. L., Peace, D., Theiss, C., Rhoton, A. L.: Microsurgical relationships of the anterior inferior cerebellar artery and the facial-vestibulocochlear nerve complex. Neurosurgery **6,** 483–507 (1980).

Matsushima, Y., et al.: A new surgical treatment of moyamoya disease in children: a preliminary report. Surg. Neurol. **15,** 313–320 (1981).

Mazzoni, A.: Internal auditory canal: Arterial relations at the porus acusticus. Ann. Otol. Rhinol. Laryngol. **78,** 797–814 (1969).

Nager, G. T.: Origins and relations of the internal auditory artery and the subarcuate artery. Ann. Otol. Rhinol. Laryngol. **63,** 51–61 (1954).

Naidich, T. P., Kricheff, I. I., George, A. E., Lin, J. P.: The anterior inferior cerebellar artery in mass lesions: Preliminary findings with emphasis on the lateral projection. Radiology **119,** 375–383 (1976).

Nieuwenhuys, R., Voogd, J., van Juijzen, Chr.: The Human Central Nervous System. A Synopsis and Atlas. Berlin–Heidelberg–New York: Springer (1978).

Palacios, E., Fine, M., Haughton, V. M.: Multiplanar Anatomy of the Head and Neck for Computed Tomography. New York: John Wiley & Sons (1980).

Rand, R. W.: Microneurosurgery. 2nd ed. St. Louis: Mosby (1978).

Rand, R. W.: Functional and Anatomic Localization in the Trigeminal Root: in Support of Dandy. In: Current Controversies in Neurosurgery (Morley, T. P., ed.), pp. 533–538. Philadelphia: Saunders (1976).

Rand, R. W.: Microsurgical operations in the treatment of trigeminal neuralgia. J. Microsurg. **1,** 101–107 (1979).

Rand, R. W.: Gardner neurovascular decompression of the trigeminal and facial nerves for tic douloureux and hemifacial spasm. Surg. Neurol. **16,** 329–332 (1981).

Rand, R. W., Jannetta, P. J.: Microneurosurgery: application of the binocular surgical microscope in brain tumors, intracranial aneurysms, spinal cord disease and nerve reconstruction. Clin. Neurosurg. **15,** 319–342 (1967).

Rhoton, A. L.: Microsurgical removal of acoustic neuromas. Surg. Neurol. **6,** 211–219 (1976).

Rhoton, A. L.: Microsurgical neurovascular decompression for trigeminal neuralgia and hemifacial spasm. J. Fla. Med. Assoc. **65,** 425–428 (1978).

Samii, M., Draf, W.: Course on Surgery of the Skull Base. Hannover, West Germany (1979).

Samii, M., Draf, W.: Course on the Surgery of the Posterior Skull Base. Hannover, West-Germany (1982).

Samii, M., Jannetta, P. J.: Symposium on Cranial Nerves. Hannover, West-Germany (1980).

Scoville, W. B.: Partial extracranial section of seventh nerve for hemifacial spasm. J. Neurosurg. **31,** 106–108 (1969).

Seeger, W.: Atlas of Topographical Anatomy of the Brain and Surrounding Structures. Wien–New York: Springer (1978).

Seeger, W.: Microsurgery of the Brain. Anatomical and Technical Principles, Vol. 1 + 2. Wien–New York: Springer (1980).

Spiller, W. G., Frazier, C. H.: Tic douloureux; anatomic and clinical basis for subtotal section of sensory root of trigeminal nerve. Arch. Neurol. Psychiat. **29,** 50–55 (1933).

Sunderland, S.: The arterial relations of the internal auditory meatus. Brain **68,** 23–27 (1945).

Taarnhøj, P.: Decompression of the trigeminal root and the posterior part of the ganglion as treatment in trigeminal neuralgia. Preliminary communication. J. Neurosurg. **9,** 288–290 (1952).

Taarnhøj, P.: Ny operation ved trigeminus neuralgi. Decompression af trigeminusroden og gangliets bageste del. Nord. Med. **47,** 360–361 (1952).

Taarnhøj, P.: Decompression of the trigeminal root. J. Neurosurg. **11,** 299–305 (1954).

Taarnhøj, P.: Trigeminal neuralgia and decompression of the trigeminal root. Surg. Clin. North. Am. **36 (4),** 1145–1157 (1956).

Waga, S., Marikawa, A., Kojima, T.: Trigeminal neuralgia: Compression of the trigeminal nerve by an elongated and dilated basilar artery. Surg. Neurol. **11,** 13–16 (1979).

Watt, J. C., McKillip, A. N.: Relation of arteries to roots of nerves in posterior cranial fossa in man. Arch. Surg. **30,** 336–345 (1935).

Willis, T.: The Anatomy of the Brain and Nerves. Tercentenary ed. 1664, Feindel, W. Montreal: McGill University Press. 1965.

Wilson, McClure: The Anatomical Foundation of Neurology of the Brain Subarachnoid Spaces. Chapter 4, pp. 93–103. Boston: Little, Brown. 1963 and 1972.

Wilson, C. B., Torke, C., Prioleiau, G.: Microsurgical vascular decompression for trigeminal neuralgia and hemifacial spasm. West. J. Med. **132,** 481–484 (1980).

Wolf, B. S., Huang, Y. P., Newman, C. M.: Lateral anastomotic mesencephalic vein and other variations in drainage of basal cerebral vein. Amer. J. Roentgenol. **89,** 411–422 (1963).

Yaşargil, M. G., Fox, J. L.: The microsurgical approach to acoustic neuromas. Surg. Neurol. **2,** 393–398 (1974).

Chapter 6

Krause, F.: Die spezielle Chirurgie der Gehirnkrankheiten, Bd. 2b u. 3. In: Neue Deutsche Chirurgie, Bd. 49b u. 50. Stuttgart: F. Enke (1941, 1932).

Lang, J.: Klinische Anatomie des Kopfes. Berlin–Heidelberg–New York: Springer (1981).

Lanz, T. von, Wachsmuth, W.: Praktische Anatomie, Vol. 1/1B. Berlin–Heidelberg–New York: Springer (1979).

Liliequist, B.: The subarachnoid cisterns. Anatomic and roentgenologic study. Acta radiol. (Stockh.) Suppl. 185 (1959).

Logue, V.: Surgery of Meningiomas. In: Operative Surgery Fundamental International Techniques Neurosurgery (Symon, L., ed.), pp. 128–173. London, Boston, Sydney, Wellington, Burban, Toronto: Butterworths (1979).

Nieuwenhuys, R., Voogd, J., van Juijzen, Chr.: The Human Central Nervous System. A Synopsis and Atlas. Berlin–Heidelberg–New York: Springer (1978).

Okonek, G.: Beitrag zur Erkennung und Behandlung basaler Meningeome. Zbl. Chir. **22,** 1912–1925 (1941).

Olivecrona, H.: The Surgical Treatment of Intracranial Tumors. In: Handbuch der Neurochirurgie 4/IV (Olivecrona, H., Tönnis, W., eds.), pp. 181–184. Berlin–Heidelberg–New York: Springer (1967).

Palacios, E., Fine, M., Haughton, V. M.: Multiplanar Anatomy of the Head and Neck for Computed Tomography. New York: John Wiley & Sons (1980).

Poppen, J. L.: An Atlas of Neurosurgical Techniques. Philadelphia–London: W. B. Saunders Company (1960).

Samii, M., Draf, W.: Course on Surgery of the Skull Base. Hannover, West-Germany (1979).

Samii, M., Draf, W.: Course on the Surgery of the Posterior Skull Base. Hannover, West-Germany (1982).

Samii, M., Jannetta, P. J.: Symposium on Cranial Nerves. Hannover, West-Germany (1980).

Seeger, W.: Atlas of Topographical Anatomy of the Brain and Surrounding Structures. Wien–New York: Springer (1978).

Seeger, W.: Microsurgery of the Brain. Anatomical and Technical Principles, Vol. 1+2. Wien–New York: Springer (1980).

Seeger, W.: Microsurgery of the Spinal Cord and Surrounding Structures. Anatomical and Technical Principles. Wien–New York: Springer (1982).

Stephens, R. B., Stilwell, D. L.: Arteries and Veins of the Human Brain. Springfield, Ill.: Ch. C Thomas (1969).

Willis, T.: The Anatomy of the Brain and Nerves. Tercentenary ed. 1664, Feindel, W. Montreal: McGill University Press (1965).

Wilson, McClure: The Anatomical Foundation of Neurology of the Brain Subarachnoid Spaces, Chapter 4, pp. 93–103. Boston: Little, Brown (1963 and 1972).

Wolf, B. S., Huang, Y. P., Newman, C. M.: Lateral anastomotic mesencephalic vein and other variations in drainage of basal cerebral vein. Amer. J. Roentgenol. **89,** 411–422 (1963).

Subject Index

Abocat plastic cannula 292, 325
Adhesions 252
Ala vomeris 12, 14
Anastomosis from A. occipitalis to A. cerebelli inf. post. 314
Anastomosis techniques, variants 310
Aneurysmatic bone cyst 390
Aneurysms of A. basilaris 1
Anosmia 200, 234
Aortography 314
Apertura mediana (MAGENDI) 327
Apertura piriformis 2, 4
Apertura piriformis, narrow 36, 38
Apertura sphenoidalis 12, 14
Aponeurosis temporalis, incision 244
Arachnoidea cover of tumor 206
Arachnoidea, outer layer 206
Arcus atlantis post. 320
A. basilaris loop 360
A. carotis int. 22, 24
A. carotis int. in Can. caroticus 198
A. carotis int., penetration point 108
A. carotis int., relation structures, variants 140
A. cerebelli inf. post. 314
A. cerebelli sup. loop 358
A. cubitalis angiography 314
A. occipitalis 314, 322, 330
A. occipitalis and A. cerebelli inf. post., suture 332
A. ophthalmica 186
A. ophthalmica aneurysm 110
A. ophthalmica aneurysms, various types 118, 120
A. ophthalmica, variants 106
A. temp. superfic. 272
A. vertebralis 320

Ballon sella, N.II + N.V2 28
Blood flow/min. 324
Bone resection over Sinus sigmoideus 348
Brachium pontis 354
Brain edema 246
Bulb-headed probe 232, 254

Cartilago septi nasi 4
Cavum Meckeli 194
Cavum Meckeli-meningioma 192
Cerebral vein to Sinus sagittalis sup. 248
Chiasma 190, 218
Cistern chamber 376
Cisterna ambiens 382
Cisterna interpeduncularis 382
Cisterna optica (arachnoidea) 218, 220
Clivus 370
Compression by veins 344
Compression of N. facialis by arteries 340
Compression of N. trigeminus by arteries 340
Compressions of other basal cranial nerves 340
Concha sup. 16
Corpora quadrigemina 372, 382, 386
Crista galli 208
Crus cerebri 384
Curvatura ant. of A. carotis int. 52
Curvatura post. of A. carotis int. 52

Decompression of N. V and N. VII 336
Dental mirror 232, 254
Diabetes insipidus 254
Donor vessel 296, 298, 330
Doppler sonogram 270
Doppler sonographic check of anastomosis 334
Doppler sonographic marking 274
Doppler sonography, defining of A. occipitalis 320
Doppler ultrasonic localization of artery 276
Doppler ultrasonographic check of A. cerebri media 286
Ductus fronto-nasalis 224
Dura defect 218

Edge of Tentorium 336
Encephalomalacia 246
Enostosis 208, 218, 220
Epidermoid, pre- and paramedullary, pre- and parapontine, pre- and paramesencephalic 370
External type of blood flow 274

Facial tic 360
Falx 208, 214, 236, 246
Fascia and Aponeurosis temporalis, sutured 244
Fascia temporalis, incision 244
Fibrinogen concentrate 224, 268, 358, 368, 398
Fibrinogen glue 266
Fissura horizontalis cerebelli 350, 382
Fissura lateralis Sylvii 272
Fissura lateralis Sylvii with temporal branch of A. cerebri media 286
Flatly enlarged sella, N.II + N.V2 28
Flocculus 354
Foramen coecum 230
Foramen lacerum 194
Foramen occipitale 320
Foramen ovale 194
Fronto-basal fracture 234

Galea aponeurotica 202
Galea strip containing artery 282
Ganglion semilunare (Gasseri) 194
Gelfoam 398
Gilsbach, J. M., 1983 310
Gingiva 2
Gingiva incision 30
Glomus tumors of Foramen jugulare 1
Graft closure of dura 222

Hypophyseal stalk 218
Hypophysis operation, disc flap 86
Hypophysis operation, grossly enlarged sella 50
Hypophysis operation, incision and preparation of mucosa 64
Hypophysis operation, liquorrhea 94
Hypophysis operation, local anesthesia 62
Hypophysis operation, locating Corpus sphenoidale 74
Hypophysis operation, opening up of sella space 80
Hypophysis operation, positioning of patient 60
Hypophysis operation, resection of Septum nasi 70
Hypophysis operation, tamponage 88
Hypophysis operation, tumor extirpation 82
Hyposmia 200

Immuno 266, 268, 358, 368, 398
Impressio trigemini 194, 336
Impression fracture 236
Incisura mastoidea 318
Infundibulum 254
Instruments for oronasal hypophysis operation (HARDY) 54
Internal type of blood flow 274
Intrasellar processus 22

Knee of Sinus transversus/sigmoideus 336

Labium sup. 2
Lacuna 248
Lacuna near sinus 350

Lamina cribrosa 212, 232
Lamina cribrosa, gaps, bone bulging, excavations 230
Lamina mediana 4, 12, 14
Leptomeningeal adhesions 250, 252
Liquor fistula 200, 230, 232, 234
Liquor fistula, periosteum flaps 258
Lobulus biventer 327, 350
Lobulus quadrangularis 336, 350, 354
Lobulus semilunaris inf. 350
Lobulus semilunaris sup. 350
Looping of A. cerebelli sup. 344

Meatus nasalis inf. 6
Medulla oblongata 327
Membrana atlanto-occipitalis post. 320
Microvascular Doppler MF 20 270
Midline, determination 44
Midline on the sitting patient 320
M. digastricus 318
M. epicranius 202
M. epicranius, Pars frontalis 238
Musculus frontalis 202

Nails (Riechert's method) 226, 228
Nasal cavity, floor 6
Nasal mucosa 32
Nasal sinuses 232
Nasion 204
Neck musculature 320
N. maxillaris 22, 26
N. occ. maj. 323
N. oculomotorius 372
N. II 23, 26
N. III 197
N. IV 197
N. V 336
N. VII/VIII 336
N. VII, frontal branch 238

Occlusion of A. carotis int. 270
Olfactorius meningioma 200
Olfactorius meningioma, skin incision to trepanation 202
Operative approach to N. V 362
Operative approach to N. VII 362
Os petrosum 400
Os sphenoidale preparation 46

Palatum durum 6
Parahippocampus region 382
Parasellar area 102
Periosteum frontal 240
"PICA" 314
Planum nuchae 320
Planum sphenoidale 16, 18, 232
Planum sphenoidale, defect 220
Plexus chorioideus 364
Pneumatization 232
Pneumosinus dilatans 128
Pneumosinus dilatans, anatomy 122, 124
Pneumosinus dilatans, clinical example 126
Pneumosinus dilatans, microsurgical site 132
Porus acusticus int. 336
Prepontine cistern 382
Processus alveolaris sup. 2
Processus clinoideus ant., drilling 114
Processus clinoideus ant., radix 156
Processus clinoideus ant., resection 176
Processus mastoideus 318
Processus spinosus axis 320
Protub. occipitalis ext. 320

Ramus angularis 274
Ramus front. of A. temp. superfic. 272
Ramus pariet. of A. temp. superfic. 272
Ramus zygomaticus of A. temp. superfic. 272
Receiver vessel 298, 330
Reclination of A. basilaris 364
Reclination of cerebellum 352
Reclination of Sinus sagittalis sup. and cerebral veins 246
Reclination of Tonsilla cerebelli 376
Rubber foil 288, 304, 328, 332

Sella wall 218, 232
Septum nasi 10
Septum nasi, asymmetrical 46
Septum nasi, resection 34
Septum nasi, tear of mucosa 40
Septum sphenoidale 18, 20
Sinus cavernosus 144
Sinus cavernosus, anatomy 100
Sinus cavernosus area, bone preparation 142
Sinus cavernosus, area, bone resection 152
Sinus cavernosus area, dura area tumor-infiltrated, excision 170
Sinus cavernosus area, four tumor types 160
Sinus cavernosus area, site after tumor removal 178
Sinus cavernosus, area, tumor located between Canalis opticus and Fissura orbitalis sup. 172
Sinus cavernosus area, tumors 138
Sinus cavernosus, bone reaction 148, 158
Sinus cavernosus, frontal sections 146
Sinus cavernosus, inoperable tumor 188
Sinus cavernosus tumor, superficial 162
Sinus frontalis 204, 232
Sinus frontalis, mucosa 204, 242
Sinus petrosus sup. 336
Sinus sagitt. sup. 206, 236, 246, 260
Sinus sigmoideus displacement 390, 392, 394
Sinus sigmoideus gaps 398
Sinus sphenoidalis 12, 218
Sinus sphenoidalis floor, resection 44
Sinus sphenoidalis, mucosa 48
Sinus sphenoidalis, opening up 48
Sinus sphenoidalis, ridges in the floor 16, 18
Spina nasalis ant. 6
Spina nasalis ant., variants 8
Squama frontalis, fragments 240
"STAMCA" (Robertson, J. H., Robertson, J. T., 1978, Rosenbaum und Sundt, 1977) 312
"STAMCA", suture 300
"STAMCA" (Yaşargil, Spetzler and others) 310
Sucker instead of spatula 252
Sulcus a. occip. 318
Sulcus a. vertebralis 320
Sulcus caroticus 20
Sulcus sagittalis 230

Temporary clip to A. occipitalis 324
Temporary clipping 290, 292, 298, 302
Tentorium 194, 198
Thrombin-calcium-solution 358
TIA's 270
Tissue glue 224
Tonsilla cerebelli 327
Trigeminal neuralgia 342, 360
Trigonum lemnisci 382, 338
Truncus brachiocephalicus 270
Tuberculum jugulare 376
Tumor hollowing 208

Vascular anastomosis 294
V. petrosa sup. 338, 352, 354
Vertebral steal syndrome 270
Vestibulum oris 2

Wall of Canalis opticus 20

Printed by Ferdinand Berger & Söhne Gesellschaft m.b.H., A-3580 Horn

By the same author:

Microsurgery of the Spinal Cord and Surrounding Structures

Anatomical and Technical Principles

1982. 201 figures. VII, 410 pages.
Format: 24,2 cm × 31,2 cm.
ISBN 3-211-81648-8

Distribution rights for Japan: Nankodo Co. Ltd., Tokyo

This book is primarily concerned with operative interventions of extra and intradural tumors, angiomas, and malformations of the spinal canal (and some typical lesions occurring there). Since Dr. Seeger believes that a thorough familiarity with topographical anatomy is a prerequisite to successful microsurgery, precise anatomical models of each procedure are provided.

These help to elucidate the principles of the operation as well as depict neighboring structures generally not visible from the surgeon's perspective, but which nevertheless can play an important role in a particular maneuver.

Special emphasis is placed on preoperative localization techniques, designed to avoid the failures often contingent upon conventional modes. Various procedures are described which will assist surgeons in avoiding unnecessary laminectomies and hemilaminectomies, and thus prevent subsequent disturbances of static function leading to further complications. The book concludes with some typical computer tomography sections showing possible sources of error in diagnosis.

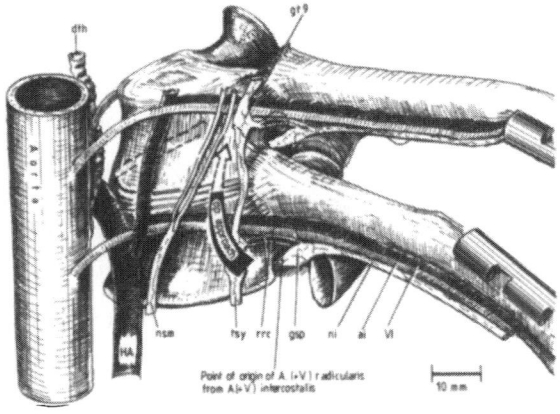

Ventral (transpleural) approach to thoracic spine. Topographical relationships between bony structures and surrounding vessels and nerves.

Microsurgery of the Brain

Anatomical and Technical Principles

1980. 351 figures. XI, IV, 727 pages.
In two volumes, not sold separately.
Format: 24,2 cm × 31,2 cm.
ISBN 3-211-81573-2

Distribution rights for Japan: Nankodo Co. Ltd., Tokyo

Thoralf M. Sundt Jr. in *Journal of Neurosurgery:*

"Seldom does one have the opportunity to review a book of this quality. It is indeed a solid contribution to the neurosurgical literature and one that should be in all department libraries and readily available for the resident staff. Experienced neurosurgeons will also find it most interesting and probably would find it useful for their own personal library as well.
The book is prepared by a master anatomist and artist. The drawings are oriented according to surgical exposures and if the term 'practical or surgical anatomy' really deserves a separate category, this book would certainly qualify as a classic in that field ... It is well worth the asking price."

Atlas of Topographical Anatomy of the Brain and Surrounding Structures

for Neurosurgeons, Neuroradiologists, and Neuropathologists

1978. 258 figures. IX, 544 pages.
Format: 24,2 cm × 31,2 cm.
ISBN 3-211-81447-7

Distribution rights for Japan: Nankodo Co. Ltd., Tokyo
Distribution rights for Socialist Countries: J. A. Barth, Leipzig

John M. Van Buren in *Journal of Neurosurgery:*

"... This book is particularly recommended for the neurosurgeon in training since it provides a comprehensive visual review of the difficult spatial relationships of the brain and cranium. It should also find an appreciative audience among neuroradiologists and surgeons in the ear, nose, and throat, and maxillofacial fields who work about the base of the skull."

JAMA:

"This book does an excellent job of presenting the anatomy as it is seen by neurosurgeons at the operating table today."

Springer-Verlag Wien New York